OXFORD READERS

Ethics

Peter Singer was born in Melbourne, Australia in 1946, and educated at the University of Melbourne and the University of Oxford. He has taught at the University of Oxford, New York University, the University of Colorado at Boulder, the University of California at Irvine, and La Trobe University. He is now Professor of Philosophy, Co-Director of the Institute of Ethics and Public Affairs, and Deputy Director of the Centre for Human Bioethics at Monash University, Melbourne. He is best known for his book *Animal Liberation*, sometimes described as 'the Bible of the Animal Liberation movement'. His other books include: *Democracy and Disobedience; Practical Ethics; The Expanding Circle; Marx; Hegel; Animal Factories* (with Jim Mason); *The Reproduction Revolution* (with Deane Wells); *Should the Baby Live?* (with Helga Kuhse); and *How Are We to Live?* Books he has edited or co-edited include *Test-Tube Babies; In Defence of Animals; Applied Ethics; Animal Rights and Human Obligations; Embryo Experimentation; A Companion to Ethics;* and *The Great Ape Project: Equality Beyond Humanity*. He is the author of the major article on Ethics in the current edition of the *Encylopaedia Britannica*, and, with Helga Kuhse, co-editor of the journal *Bioethics*.

OXFORD **READERS**

Ethics

Edited by Peter Singer

Oxford · New York

OXFORD UNIVERSITY PRESS

1994

Oxford University Press, Walton Street, Oxford OX2 6DP

Oxford New York Toronto
Delhi Bombay Calcutta Madras Karachi
Kuala Lumpur Singapore Hong Kong Tokyo
Nairobi Dar es Salaam Cape Town
Melbourne Auckland Madrid
and associated companies in
Berlin Ibadan

Oxford is a trade mark of Oxford University Press

British Library Cataloguing in Publication Data
Data available

Library of Congress Cataloging in Publication Data

Ethics / edited by Peter Singer.
    p.   cm. — (Oxford readers)
Includes bibliographical references and index.
1. Ethics.   I. Singer, Peter   II. Series.
BJ1012.E8865   1994   170—dc20   93–2949
ISBN 0–19–289245–2

1 3 5 7 9 10 8 6 4 2

Typeset by Pure Tech Corporation, Pondicherry, India
Printed in Great Britain
on acid-free paper by
Bookcraft (Bath) Ltd
Midsomer Norton, Avon

Acknowledgements

Some sections of this anthology are a by-product of research I have been carrying out on the origins and nature of ethics. This research has been supported by a grant from the Australian Research Council, for which I am most grateful.

At every stage in the selection and production of the anthology, I have been ably assisted by Margaret Parnaby. Without her help it would have been a much inferior volume, if indeed I had been able to complete it at all.

Contents

iii Sexual Morality

C. The Role of Reason

PART II: THE CONTENT OF ETHICS: JUDGING GOOD OUTCOMES AND RIGHT ACTS

A. Ultimate Good

B. Deciding What Is Right

Ethics

Introduction

Ethics is about how we ought to live. What makes an action the right, rather than the wrong, thing to do? What should our goals be? These questions are so fundamental that they lead us on to further questions. What is ethics anyway? Where does it come from? Can we really hope to find a rational way of deciding how we ought to live? If we can, what would it be like, and how are we going to know when we have found it?

This book draws together some of the high points of (roughly) the first two and half millennia of thinking about these questions. It is not a conventional reader in moral philosophy. I have tried to capture the essentials of what we know about the origins and nature of ethics, whether this knowledge comes from philosophy, anthropology, history, ethology, the theory of evolution, or game theory. I have taken most of my selections from the Western tradition, since writings in that tradition are understood more easily by the majority of readers of English; but there are selections from other traditions, too, in part to show the universal nature of the problems of ethics—and, in some cases, to show the common elements of the solutions offered to these problems as well.

In addition to including the most important of the answers offered to the questions mentioned above, I have tried to construct a book that will convey something of the intellectual excitement of the search for answers to these basic questions about how we ought to live. This book invites its readers to join in an ancient quest for something that—if it can really be found—would be more valuable than any sacred relic. The goal is wisdom about how to live our lives, and the search has already engaged an extraordinary list of thinkers: Plato, Aristotle, Mencius, Buddha, Confucius, Jesus, Aquinas, Hume, Kant, Bentham, Mill . . . and many others, right down to the present day.

Though the quest is the most serious one possible, that does not preclude good reading and some lighter moments. Within the constraints of space and the need for adequate coverage of the major issues, I have tried to provide a treasury of some of the finest pieces of writing, old and new, in and about ethics. I also wanted to include passages that have been influential in ethical thought and are often referred to, but not so often read. That is why this anthology includes several pieces not usually found in collections of this kind, among them Pascal's attack on the natural law casuistry of the Jesuits, Voltaire's tale of the wise Brahmin and the old woman, Bentham's assessment of the relative merits of push-pin and poetry, W. E. H. Lecky's compilation of the extraordinary practices of the Christian ascetics, Dostoevsky's challenge to utilitarianism in *The Karamazov*

Brothers, the debate between the Controller and the Savage from Huxley's *Brave New World*, and Camus's portrayal of Sisyphus as an existential hero.

Our apparent failure to make progress in ethics is sometimes contrasted unfavourably with the situation in the natural sciences. How is it that those studying moral philosophy still go to Aristotle's *Ethics* as a source of insight and illumination, whereas no scientist would consider his *Physics* as anything but a historical curiosity? The point has some substance, but modern writings in ethics often do give a clearer understanding of the problems with which they deal than Aristotle did in his *Ethics*, and they reach more enlightened conclusions. We can see through Aristotle's facile defence of slavery, for example, and even those who believe in our right to exploit animals for our own ends are hardly likely to accept Aristotle's comfortable idea that this, like slavery, is justified because the less rational beings exist 'for the sake of' the more rational. Similarly, Aristotle's claim that it is wrong and unnatural to earn interest on financial loans is now as laughable as anything he wrote about physics. Not everything that Aristotle wrote about ethics is as obsolete as these doctrines. On the whole, though, I am convinced that progress in ethics is not only possible, but has actually been made. That is why recent work is well-represented in this selection. I have, however, avoided including those academic philosophers who write only for their colleagues, and so lose sight of the large issues of general interest; also omitted are those who approach their topics in ways likely to be inaccessible to readers unfamiliar with the technical terms of the writer's discipline.

What is ethics? The word itself is sometimes used to refer to the set of rules, principles, or ways of thinking that guide, or claim authority to guide, the actions of a particular group; and sometimes it stands for the systematic study of reasoning about how we ought to act. In the first of these senses, we may ask about the sexual ethics of the people of the Trobriand Islands, or speak about the way in which medical ethics in The Netherlands has come to accept voluntary euthanasia. In the second sense, 'ethics' is the name of a field of study, and often of a subject taught in university departments of philosophy. The context usually makes clear which sense is intended: for example, the readings in the first section of this book are about the origins of the rules, principles, or ways of thinking that guide actions, not about the development of systematic thinking on these matters.

Some writers use the term 'morality' for the first, descriptive, sense in which I am using 'ethics'. They would talk of the morality of the Trobriand islanders when they want to describe what the islanders take to be right or wrong. They would reserve 'ethics' (or sometimes, 'moral philosophy') for the field of study or the subject taught in departments of philosophy. I have not adopted this usage. Both 'ethics' and 'morality' have their roots in a word for 'customs', the former being a derivative of the Greek term from which we get 'ethos', and the latter from the Latin root that gives us 'mores', a word still used sometimes to describe the customs of a people. 'Morality' brings with it a particular, and sometimes inappropriate, resonance today. It suggests a stern set of duties that require us to subordinate our natural desires—and our sexual desires get particular emphasis here—in order to obey the moral law. A failure to fulfil our duty brings with it a heavy sense of guilt. Very often, morality is assumed to have a religious basis. These connotations of 'morality' are features of a particular conception of ethics, one linked to the Jewish and Christian traditions, rather than an inherent feature of any ethical system.

Ethics has no necessary connection with any particular religion, nor with religion in general. Some religious leaders and writers are included in this anthology because they have spoken or written in a significant way about central questions in ethics, but as the selections in this book show, ethics exists in all human societies, and perhaps even among our closest non-human relatives as well. We have no need to postulate gods who hand down commandments to us, because we can understand ethics as a natural phenomenon that arises in the course of the evolution of social, intelligent, long-lived mammals who possess the capacity to recognize each other and to remember the past behaviour of others.

This understanding of ethics as a natural phenomenon is presented in Part I of this book, which covers the origins of ethics, the varied forms it takes, and its rational basis. For much of the past century, philosophers have regarded the question of the origin of ethics as something outside their terrain. Since Darwin, there has been a widely supported scientific theory that offers an explanation of the origin of ethics. This led to a flurry of interest in the evolutionary theory among some philosophers. The attempt to draw ethical implications from evolution led to 'Social Darwinism', which in turn was seen as justifying the free-market competition of nineteenth-century capitalism, and was used as an ideological weapon against government regulation of the market. Once Social Darwinism ceased to be fashionable, however, philosophers tended to leave the question of the origin of ethics to scientists. But since ethics leaves no fossils, scientists for several decades after Darwin did not have a lot to say about the origin of ethics. Then, in the 1970s, the rise of sociobiology—evolutionary theory applied to social behaviour—turned our attention to the question of how altruism and, more generally, ethical behaviour can be fitted into evolutionary theory. Some sociobiologists sought to draw ethical premises out of the new discoveries in evolutionary theory. In doing so, they moved effortlessly from factual statements to judgements of value. In a famous passage, David Hume had pointed out the need to explain how any such transition could be possible; by the twentieth century, this had hardened into a conviction, in the minds of most philosophers, that no statements of fact could ever entail any ethical judgement. Philosophers therefore returned to the topic of evolution and ethics, but—at first—only to rebut the philosophical howlers of the sociobiologists-turned-ethicists. A genuine interest in what we can learn about ethics from evolutionary theory was slow to emerge.

Once we admit that Darwin was right when he argued that human ethics evolved from the social instincts that we inherited from our non-human ancestors, we can put aside the hypothesis of a divine origin for ethics. Further questions then arise. If we see ethics as part of our common human heritage, we may expect that there will be ethical universals, principles that hold, in some form, among all human societies. That expectation is in sharp contrast to the prevailing opinion of the nineteenth and early twentieth centuries, when a flood of anthropological reports from all over the world conveyed an overwhelming impression of endless diversity in ethics. While distinct societies obviously do hold different ethical views on many subjects, it is now clear that on some important points, almost all societies are in agreement. That does not mean, of course, that we have to accept as right the ethical views on which societies agree. Until very recently, one of the points on which virtually every society agreed was that a married woman should obey her husband; and if we were to go back further into the past, we could find many equally objectionable 'ethical universals'. The fact that a practice is universal does not determine whether that practice is right or whether it ought to be discouraged to the maximum possible extent, perhaps even prohibited. But just as understanding the origin of ethics helps us to grasp the nature of the phenomenon with which we are dealing, so, too, our understanding is increased by knowledge of the degree of diversity and uniformity in ethical systems between different societies— and even between human societies and those of other social animals, especially our closest relatives, the chimpanzees. Hence the inclusion in this book of the section 'Common Themes in Primate Ethics', which comprises readings on kinship, reciprocity, and sexual ethics.

In bringing together, as forms of 'primate ethics', observations of the social behaviour of human beings and non-human animals, I am suggesting that we abandon the assumption that ethics is uniquely human. Some will resist this suggestion. We have always been reluctant to recognize similarities between our own behaviour and that of non-human animals. We claimed that we were the only tool-using animal, until we discovered that other animals use tools, too. Then we made a similar claim about language, only to find that the great apes can learn to communicate with us in sign language. Surely, it will be said, ethics at least remains a purely human phenomenon. Recall Immanuel Kant's conception of duty, based on our capacity as a rational being to grasp the moral law. What can the interactions of a group of chimpanzees possibly have to do with this? To compare the instinctive or habitual behaviour of chimpanzees with the consciously chosen ethical standards of humans is, it will be said, to degrade and insult our own species.

That there is an immense gulf between the kind of ethic described by Kant and that revealed by the behaviour of the most intellectually gifted chimpanzee is undeniable; but, from the existence of this gulf, it does not follow that we have nothing to learn about our own behaviour from observations of chimpanzees. Kant's ideas are foreign not only to chimpanzee communities, but to most human communities as well. Philosophical systems of ethics are highly sophisticated elaborations of more widespread concepts which have themselves evolved from prehuman social behaviour. To know more about the prehuman basis of ethics will surely help in understanding and assessing the systems of ethics that have grown from it; and the best clues as to what prehuman ethics may have been like will come from observations of those animals with whom we share relatively close common ancestors.

To this, Kant and his followers might reply that since the moral law is based on reason, any apparent parallels between our ethics and that of non-human animals is a mere superficial coincidence. We should no more consider the behaviour of animals to have something to do with ethics than we should think of the web of the spider as a work of art. But on this point the philosophical tradition begins to diverge. Kant represents only one side of a debate over the role that reason can play in our practical life and our ethical decisions. If, for example, we take David Hume's view that the basis of ethics is to be found in our emotions or, as he calls them, passions, then reason becomes much less significant in ethics, and the parallels between our own ethics and that of non-human animals become correspondingly closer. Hence to deny the possibility of 'primate ethics' because of the role that reason plays in ethics is to assume that Kant, and not Hume, was correct on this issue. That may well be the wrong assumption.

The debate between Hume and Kant on the role of reason in ethics sets the theme for the section of this book that takes us to the heart of the most fundamental of all the questions that can be raised about the nature of ethics: whether ethics is objective or subjective. Different terms have been used to frame this question, but behind it always lies the division between, on the one hand, those who hold that there is somehow a true, correct, or best-justified answer to the question 'What ought I to do?', no matter who asks the question; and, on the other hand, those who hold that when different individuals or different societies disagree on ethical issues, then there is no standard by which one could possibly judge one answer to be better than another.

Philosophers have not always seen that this debate between ethical objectivists and ethical subjectivists is, in the end, a question about the role that reason plays in ethics. Kant's assertion that the moral law is a law of reason was based on his own peculiar metaphysics. He saw human nature as eternally divided. On one side is our natural or physical self, trapped in the world of desires. On the other is our intellectual or spiritual self, which partakes of the world of reason from which the moral law derives. Those philosophers who wanted to defend the objectivity of ethics, but did not accept Kant's overall philosophical system, needed to show that there could be another way of knowing what is objectively right. For a long time, defenders of ethical objectivity argued that our ethical judgements were derived from an immediate intellectual grasp of a self-evident truth. Thus, they thought, we can know intuitively that an act is right, in much the same way that we know, without having to think about it, that one and one make two. One the other side, those arguing that ethics is subjective asserted—as Hume does—that ethics is based on feeling or emotion, and not on anything objective or 'out there' in the universe.

But can we really know anything through intuition? The defenders of ethical intuitionism argued that there was a parallel in the way we know, or could immediately grasp, the basic truths of mathematics: that one plus one equals two, for instance. This argument suffered a blow when it was shown that the self-evidence of the basic truths of mathematics could be explained in a different and more parsimonious way, by seeing mathematics as a system of tautologies, the basic elements of which are true by virtue of the meanings of the terms used. On this view, now widely, if not universally, accepted, no special intuition is required to establish that one plus one equals two—this is a logical truth, true by virtue of the meanings we give to the integers 'one' and 'two', as well as 'plus' and 'equals'. So the idea that intuition provides some substantive kind of knowledge of right and wrong lost its only analogue.

It might still be the case that ethical intuition, uniquely among forms of intuition, is a source of genuine knowledge. Yet there is another, even more serious problem with defending the objectivity of ethics in this way. This problem lies in the fact that ethical judgements are supposed to lead to action. For if *knowing* what is right did not carry with it a tendency to motivate us to *do* what is right, ethics would seem to have lost its point. Ethics would then be a system of conduct, rather like etiquette is for most people today. I may know that it is not considered good manners to begin eating before all the other guests have been served, but if I don't happen to care about what others take to be good manners, and I prefer my food piping hot, then I have no reason for waiting. Those who hold that ethical judgements are a special kind of intuition do not intend to relegate ethics to the status of etiquette. They want to say that if I know that something is wrong, I have a reason for not doing it, whether I happen to care about ethics or not. So they must show how the knowledge that we gain through intuition provides us with a reason that can motivate us to do what we see to be right.

There is something obscure, however, about how any kind of knowledge can, by itself, *necessarily* motivate us to act. Of course, if someone tells me that there is a nest of large, stinging ants where I am about to sit, that does usually give me a reason to choose another spot for my picnic. We can presuppose that any normal person prefers not to be stung by ants, and so this information will provide any normal person with a reason for acting; but it operates as a reason because it is relevant to a preference that we have. If, after carefully considering all the consequences, I decide that I do, after all, prefer being stung to sitting anywhere else, the knowledge of the location of the ants ceases to be a reason for me to change my plans.

Kant referred to those imperatives that depend on whether the individual has a given desire as 'hypothetical imperatives'. 'If you don't want to be stung, sit elsewhere' is an example of a hypothetical imperative. The issue between Hume and Kant could then be posed by asking whether all imperatives are hypothetical. Are there any imperatives that are, as Kant put it, 'categorical'—that is, imperatives that apply to every rational being, irrespective of what desires he or she has? Kant thought that if ethics is to be anything more than a delusion, there must be categorical imperatives— for does not morality tell us that we ought to do what is right, irrespective of our desires? If the intuitionists are to succeed in showing that we gain knowledge of objective ethical truth through intuition, they must show that this knowledge gives rise to a categorical imperative. That is why the crucial issue between intuitionists and their subjectivist opponents turns out, in the end, to be the same as the issue between Hume and Kant: are there objective reasons for action, not dependent on our desires?

On this issue, the passing of two centuries since the time of Hume and Kant has not resolved the dispute between the two basic positions that they put forward. The selections in this book show the varying ways in which, over this period, some have maintained that reason is, as Hume put it, 'the slave of the passions', while others have insisted that reason has a significant role to play in ethics, independently of whatever desires one may happen to have. Yet although the debate has not been resolved, we understand the issues better than we did before, and there are even some signs of a convergence. Objectivists no longer seek strange moral facts known only by intuition, but try to sort out the reasons for action that we would accept if we were reasoning under certain idealized conditions—for example, if we were fully informed, not swayed by our own interests, and could vividly imagine what it would be like to be in the position of all others affected by our action. Subjectivists today rarely maintain that ethics is entirely a matter of feelings or desires; they recognize the need to allow scope for disagreement and reasoned argument about ethics. Hence, while they continue to take the view that ethical judgements are based on our desires, they will not allow just any desire to form this basis. Rather, they acknowledge that to count as ethical, desires must be passed through a screen that filters out those that do not meet certain conditions of impartiality and reasonableness. The current debate therefore has a much tighter focus: namely, on the kind of limits that we can put on desires if they are to count as ethical, and whether these limits are sufficient to allow us to reach—in principle, if not in practice—agreement on what we ought to do.

The field of ethics is commonly divided into two parts, meta-ethics and normative ethics. In terms of that division, Part I of this reader, which we have just been discussing, is meta-ethics, and Part II is normative ethics. The term 'meta-ethics' implies that we are not taking part in the practice of ethics itself, but are reflecting on that practice, as if from a different level from which we can view it as a whole, and see what is going on when people are, say, arguing about the rights and wrongs of eating meat, or considering how to respond to a former friend who has acted badly but is now in need of help. In arguing about the nature or basis of ethics, we are asking questions *about* ethics, not arguing *within* ethics. For example, at the level of meta-ethics, we might ask whether there could possibly be a true or correct answer to these questions within ethics. On the other hand, to take part in discussions about substantive issues like vegetarianism or how we ought to treat a former friend is to engage in normative ethical argument— 'normative' refers to 'norms': in other words, values, rules, standards, or principles that should guide our decisions about what we ought to do.

Normative ethics seeks to influence our actions. There are many ways in which one could divide up the immense amount that has been written in this area, but perhaps the most fundamental division consists of answers to two different questions. The first question is: what kinds of thing are ultimately good? The second question is: how do we decide what actions are right?

At first glance, one might think that the answer to the second question will follow immediately from the answer to the first question. For example, suppose that we were to decide that happiness is the only thing that is good in itself. Everything else, we might believe, is not good in itself, but good because it is a means of obtaining happiness (like money, for example). Would it follow immediately that we could decide whether an action is right by asking if it does more to increase happiness than any other action that the agent could do?

That is what the classical utilitarians, like Jeremy Bentham, John Stuart Mill, and Henry Sidgwick, would have wanted to say: but others might agree that happiness, and nothing but happiness, is ultimately valuable, without thereby committing themselves to the classical utilitarian approach to ethics. For it is at least possible that there are rules of ethics that we ought never to break, even when breaking them is the way to maximize whatever is of ultimate value. These rules may not actually be values, but constraints on what we may do to obtain what is of ultimate value. Imagine that you are a surgeon who thinks that human life, at least when it is of reasonable quality, is an ultimate value. One day you walk into the hospital and find that you have a patient who will die shortly because she needs a heart transplant and there are no hearts available. In the next ward is another patient who has an equally pressing need for a liver transplant, but, again, you cannot do the operation because there is no prospect of finding a suitable liver donor in time. In a third ward is a patient on whom you are about to operate to remove a brain tumour. You have done many of these operations, and have no doubt that you can perform the operation successfully on this patient, but you also know that you could contrive a little slip, for which no one could really blame you, that would result in the death of your patient's brain. Then the patient would become a suitable donor of both heart and liver. Thus you would take one life, but save two. All three lives in question could be expected to be of similar quality and length, and all three have much the same kind of family connections. If human life is the only thing of ultimate value, you would have maximized ultimate value. But does it follow that you would be right to do this? Many would say that it does not; for a surgeon deliberately to kill a patient who wants to go on living would be wrong, even if, on balance, it would lead to more lives being saved.

The difference between a value and a rule is that it makes sense to maximize a value—to increase it as much as possible—whereas we can only comply with a rule. So if I value happiness, I can choose between acts that will lead to there being more or less happiness in the world, but if I accept the rule that one should never kill an innocent human being, I can only comply with this rule, or break it. (There is one complication: I might try to reduce the amount of killing of innocent human beings. Is my goal then to maximize a value, or to comply with a rule? Consider this question: should I be ready to kill an innocent human being if, by doing so, I can somehow prevent the killing of several other innocent human beings? An affirmative answer suggests that you regard the reduction of killing of innocent human beings as a value; only a negative answer is consistent with treating the non-killing of innocent human beings as a rule.)

The distinction between values and rules or constraints means that we need to discuss not only what is of ultimate value, but also how we can decide what actions are right. Radically different answers have been given to both of these questions. The nature of the ultimate good for human beings has been discussed by teachers, both religious and secular, for as long as human beings have been able to reflect and speculate on their goals. Precisely because it is *ultimate* values that are in question here, assertion often takes the place of argument, and differences between alternative views are not easy to resolve. Is it happiness that gives everything value, or living a life of rational contemplation? Is the best life one of spiritual purity and self-denial, or a life dedicated to the appreciation of beauty or the enjoyment of friendship, or simply a life in which we get whatever we happen to want? More recent philosophical discussion has sharpened the issues between distinct views, but it has done little to resolve them.

Once we have formed a view about what things are good, we still need to settle the issue to which I have just referred: whether to judge actions as right or wrong on the basis of their compliance with some rules or principles, irrespective of their consequences; or to judge them solely in terms of whether they produce the best consequences. On the side of the first of these alternatives, we find proponents of a natural law ethic, like Thomas Aquinas and the many (mainly Roman Catholic) twentieth-century advocates of this approach to ethics. Also taking this view are defenders of inviolable rights—for example, John Locke (in some of his writings) and contemporary philosophers like Robert Nozick—and those who follow Kant in insisting on the absolute nature of duty. On the other side are consequentialists in general and utilitarians in particular; the tradition of the classical utilitarians has been further developed, and in some respects altered, by modern utilitarians such as J. J. C. Smart and R. M. Hare.

There have been attempts to bridge the gap between those who judge right and wrong on the basis of rules, and those who pay attention only to the consequences of actions. Thus some defenders of an ethics based on rules have acknowledged the need for exceptions, when following the rules would lead to catastrophic consequences; others are prepared to go further still, and regard rules or principles as carrying some weight, but not necessarily an overriding weight, so that consideration of the consequences of our acts is always part of the process of forming an ethical judgement. At the same time, utilitarians have insisted that they can recognize the longer-term good consequences of treating some basic rights and moral rules as if they were, for all practical purposes, inviolable. Yet these explanations often seem a little stretched, and in at least some cases a consequentialist ethic and a more conventional, rule-based ethic give distinct and irreconcilable answers to the question of what we ought to do. The readings included in Part IIB show the different positions taken by, on the one hand, defenders of an ethic of rules—whether based on the theory of natural law, on the idea of natural rights, on Kant's categorical imperative, or on W. D. Ross's idea of prima facie duties—and, on the other hand, consequentialists, and especially utilitarians. Also included among the readings are some of the more important objections to each of these positions, as well as a short section on the twentieth-century revival of social contract ethics, inspired largely by the work of the American philosopher John Rawls, who attempts to stake out a distinct ethical vision based on what rational individuals would sanction if, starting from a position of fundamental equality, they had to reach agreement on basic ethical principles.

One important part of normative ethics is missing from this book. That is the area of applied ethics, which deals with quite practical questions, like abortion, euthanasia, whether we are justified in rearing and killing animals for food, and our obligations to share our wealth with those who live in extreme poverty in other countries. The marked revival of interest in applied ethics that has taken place in Western philosophical thought over the past two decades is one of the more important philosophical developments in twentieth-century ethics. If it finds no place in this book, that is only because I have already edited a collection of essays in this field.[1] To try to cover the same ground in this volume would have made it even more difficult to find the space for all the other writings in ethics that I wanted to include in this anthology. To obtain an overview of the major themes of ethics, the two books should be taken together.

P. S.

[1] Peter Singer (ed.), *Applied Ethics* (Oxford University Press, Oxford, 1986).

PART I

The Nature of Ethics: Its Origins, Variations, and Basis

The Long Search for the Origins of Ethics

INTRODUCTION

Where does ethics come from? is a question that has been asked for thousands of years by thinkers from many different traditions. In Athens, two and a half thousand years ago, the sophist Thrasymachus argued that ethics is something imposed on the weaker by the stronger. In the dialogue between Thrasymachus and Socrates that opens this section, Socrates soon manages to tie the unfortunate Thrasymachus in knots—at least, that is how Plato, Socrates' disciple, describes the scene. But for all Socrates' skill in argument, his victory may be an empty one. Socrates argues that the ruler, *qua* ruler, is not concerned with his own interest, but with that of his subject. If, however, that is what a ruler does, *qua* ruler, then maybe there simply are no rulers, so defined. Thrasymachus' sceptical view of the nature of ethics remains a possibility.

More than two thousand years later, in the shadow of the English Civil War, Thomas Hobbes took an equally sceptical approach to the whole question of the origin of ethics, but reached a different answer. Ethics does, in Hobbes's view, give the ruler a right to command and to be obeyed, but it is in the interests of us all, not only in the interests of the ruler, that this should be so. For if we understand that life without a ruler is 'solitary, poor, nasty, brutish and short', we will see that ethics as we know it can only exist if we all agree on a kind of social contract, which requires a ruler to enforce it.

Hobbes's view of human nature is harsh. The debate over whether humans are good by nature or by training is an old one. Aristotle, writing just after Plato, thought that virtue has to be taught and then practised, so that it becomes a habit. The Chinese philosopher Mencius, who lived at about the same time as Aristotle, debated this question with Chinese sages of his time. Like Aristotle, they argued that human nature must be trained to be good, as a willow tree must be carved to make it into a bowl. Mencius, however, saw human beings as naturally compassionate and with an innate sense of right and wrong. When they do evil, it is because adverse conditions have corrupted their nature. Here Mencius anticipates the eighteenth-century vision of the French philosopher Rousseau, who presents us with the classic portrait of the 'noble savage', a human being whose simple needs are satisfied by the bounty of nature and who has no cause to quarrel with the other inhabitants of his forest. Indeed, these 'savages' are, for Rousseau, anything but savage; their innate feelings of compassion make them naturally ethical beings. It is civilization, and particularly the introduction of property, that introduces evil into the world.

Rousseau, Hume, and Kant form a kind of eighteenth-century triad: each one among the greatest of his country's thinkers, and each with a distinctive view of the origins of ethics. Hume shared with Rousseau the conviction that the origins of ethics are to be found in certain natural feelings or sentiments; but he saw a less pleasant side to human nature as well. We are torn, he thought, between our sentiments of humanity and our avarice and ambition; so the function of ethics is to reinforce those sentiments that meet with the general approval of all, and ensure that our selfish desires are kept under control.

Kant rejected utterly the link between ethics and feelings, on which Rousseau and Hume were in agreement. For Kant, the origin of ethics does not lie in feelings or sentiments at all. Instead, the 'pure moral law' is something quite independent of all inclinations or feelings, something we can recognize only because, in so far as we are rational beings, we can free ourselves from the causal necessity of the ordinary world of feelings and inclinations, and can follow the pure moral law, given by reason alone. The extracts from Hume and Kant in this opening section are, however, only appetizers for a main course that comes later in this book: the debate between them over the role of reason in ethics, presented in Part IC.

The next four extracts present the views on the origin of ethics of the most influential thinkers of the nineteenth and early twentieth centuries: Karl Marx, Charles Darwin, Friedrich Nietzsche, and Sigmund Freud. For Marx and his co-author Friedrich Engels, the answer to the question about the origins of ethics is provided by the materialist conception of history, which is probably their greatest contribution to human thought. They reject the idea, embraced most clearly by Kant but assumed by many other moral philosophers as well, that morality is in some way independent of the material circumstances of human life. Instead, they see morality, as they see religion and every other achievement of the human intellect, as caused and conditioned by the economic arrangements under which human beings live: the way in which they produce their food, whether they use simple hand-tools or large-scale machines, and—corresponding to these means of production—whether they live in a feudal or a capitalist economy. Though it is an oversimplification to compare Marx's views with those put by Thrasymachus so much earlier, if we interpret Thrasymachus as saying that our standard concepts of justice and injustice are moulded to serve the interests of the ruling class, it is easy to see him as a precursor of Marx.

References to ethics or morality in the works of Marx tend to be fleeting; he focused on economics instead, and obviously thought that the origins and nature of morality were not worth his detailed investigation. Darwin, on the other hand, devoted an entire chapter of *The Descent of Man* to the origin of the moral sense. For him, it was important to show not only that our anatomy gives ample evidence of our descent from other animals, but also that our mental powers, including our moral sense, are compatible with this hypothesis. If they were not, then his opponents would have been able to argue that we must, after all, suppose a separate—and presumably divine—act of creation for human beings. Darwin's approach, if not his style, is remarkably modern. He assembles data from observers of non-human animals to show that these animals have social instincts which lead them to behave in ways that—if they were human beings—would certainly be praised as ethical. So he traces the gradual evolution of ethics from these instincts in our non-human ancestors to the most advanced philosophical conceptions of ethics, as advocated by philosophers such as Kant. As the next section shows, more recent data give strong support to Darwin's suggestions.

Nietzsche is no more favourably inclined towards our standard conception of morality than Marx, but he wants to go 'beyond good and evil' for precisely the opposite reasons. For Nietzsche, morality is the creation of 'the herd'—the great mass of ordinary people, led more by fear than by hope, afraid to stand out from the crowd. Morality is the means by which the herd restricts the superior and independent human spirits, from whom alone (Nietzsche thinks) greatness can come, and drags them down to its own level.

As befits the father of psychoanalysis, Sigmund Freud writes mostly of conflicts within the minds of individual human beings; in *Civilization and its Discontents*, however, he takes human society as a whole, and diagnoses an illness within it. The discontents of civilization arise from the conflict between the aggression which he thinks is innate within us all and the 'cultural super-ego', or the collective authority of the community. In this situation, Freud writes, ethics emerges as 'a therapeutic attempt' to resolve the conflict. Given that Freud postulates a natural aggressiveness in human nature, his analysis can perhaps be seen—if stripped of his medical metaphor—as a modern variant on the position laid out by Thomas Hobbes.

Is the search for the origins of ethics over? Is it now just a matter of refining and developing the Darwinian view? In one sense, the answer is 'yes'. The modern scientific approach to the origin of ethics that began with *The Descent of Man* has become much more sophisticated in the past two decades. We are beginning to understand the extent to which humans are ethical by nature. We know that we were neither purely good by nature nor purely evil, but ambivalent. No social contract was ever required, because we were social primates before we were human beings. Nevertheless, we tend to compete with each other for food, sexual partners, and status. Though Darwin did not clear up all the mysteries of the origins of ethics (the interplay between reason and desire raises issues that he did not explore sufficiently), he did provide the general outline of what is surely the right answer to the question with which I began this introduction.

Now other, more specific, questions unfold. The final reading in this section indicates one fruitful area for further investigation. In seeking the origin of ethics, the writers included in this section have all assumed that ethics has a single source, for all human beings. The last writer challenges this assumption. Could there be not human ethics, but man's ethics and woman's ethics? Carol Gilligan—who is, not coincidentally, the only woman included in this section—argues that much of what men have written about ethics has presented only a partial picture, because it has taken the masculine view of ethics as the only possible one. Gilligan holds that the moral sense of women is generally different from that of men. Whether she is right, remains to be seen; if her suggestions stand up to further scrutiny, they will provide a fresh perspective from which we can re-examine the origins and nature of ethics.

1 Morality as the Advantage of the Stronger: A Debate between Socrates and Thrasymachus

'All right, then, listen to this,' [Thrasymachus] said. 'My claim is that morality is nothing other than the advantage of the stronger party . . . Well, why aren't you applauding? No, you won't let yourself do that.'

'First I need to understand your meaning,' I told him. 'I don't yet. You say that right is the advantage of the stronger party, but what on earth do you mean by this, Thrasymachus? Surely you're not claiming, in effect, that if Poulydamas the pancratiast is stronger than us and it's to his advantage, for the sake of his physique, to eat beef, then this food is advantageous, and therefore right, for us too, who are weaker than him?'

'Foul tactics, Socrates,' he said, 'to interpret what I say in the way which allows you unscrupulously to distort it most.'

'No, you've got me wrong, Thrasymachus,' I said. 'I just want you to explain yourself better.'

'Don't you know, then,' he said, 'that some countries are dictatorships, some are democracies, and some are aristocracies?'

'Of course I do.'

'And that what has power in any given country is the government?'

'Yes.'

'Now, each government passes laws with a view to its own advantage: a democracy makes democratic laws, a dictatorship makes dictatorial laws, and so on and so forth. In so doing, each government makes it clear that what is right and moral for its subjects is what is to its own advantage; and each government punishes anyone who deviates from what is advantageous to itself as if he were a criminal and a wrongdoer. So, Socrates, this is what I claim morality is: it is the same in every country, and it is what is to the advantage of the current government. Now, of course, it's the current government which has power, and the consequence of this, as anyone who thinks about the matter correctly can work out, is that morality is everywhere the same—the advantage of the stronger party.'

'Now I see what you mean,' I said. 'And I'll try to see whether or not your claim is true. Your position too, Thrasymachus, is that morality is advantage—despite the fact that you ruled this answer out for me—except that you immediately add "of the stronger party".'

'Hardly a trivial addition,' he said.

'Whether or not it is important isn't yet clear. What *is* clear is that we must try to find out whether your claim is true. The point is that I agree that morality is some kind of advantage, but you are qualifying this and claiming that it is the advantage of the stronger party; since I haven't made up my mind about this qualified version, we must look into the matter.'

'Go ahead,' he said.

'All right,' I said. 'Here's a question for you: you're also claiming, I assume, that obedience to the government is right?'

'Yes, I am.'

'And is the government in every country infallible, or are they also capable of error?'

'They are certainly capable of error,' he said.

'So when they turn to legislation, they sometimes get it right, and sometimes wrong?'

'Yes, I suppose so.'

'When they get it right, the laws they make will be to their advantage, but when they get it wrong, the laws will be to their disadvantage. Is that what you're saying?'

'Yes.'

'And you're also saying that their subjects must act in accordance with any law that is passed, and that this constitutes doing right?'

'Of course.'

'Then it follows from your line of argument that it is no more right to act to the advantage of the stronger party than it is to do the opposite, to act to their disadvantage.'

'What are you saying?' he asked.

'Exactly the same as you, I think; but let's have a closer look. We're agreed that sometimes, when a government orders its subjects to do things, it is utterly mistaken about its own best interest, but that it's right for the subjects to act in accordance with any order issued by the government. Isn't that what we agreed?'

'Yes, I suppose so.'

'Then you must also suppose', I continued, 'that you have agreed that it is right to do things which are not to the advantage of the government and the stronger party. When the rulers mistakenly issue orders which are bad for themselves, and since you claim that it is right for people to act in conformity with all the government's orders, then, my dear Thrasymachus, doesn't it necessarily follow that it is right to do the opposite of what your position affirmed? I mean, the weaker party is being ordered to do what is disadvantageous to the stronger party, obviously.'

'Yes, Socrates,' said Polemarchus, 'that's perfectly clear.'

'Of course,' Cleitophon interrupted, 'if you're going to act as a witness for Socrates.'

'There's no need for a witness,' Polemarchus replied. 'Thrasymachus himself admits that rulers sometimes issue orders which are bad for themselves, and that it's right for people to carry out these orders.'

'That's because Thrasymachus maintained that it was right to carry out the rulers' instructions, Polemarchus.'

'Yes, Cleitophon, and he also maintained that right is the advantage of the stronger party. And once he'd affirmed both of these propositions, he also agreed that sometimes the stronger party tells the weaker party, which is subject to it, to do things which are disadvantageous to it. And from these premisses it follows that morality is no more what is advantageous to the stronger party than it is what is disadvantageous to the stronger party.'

'But,' Cleitophon said, 'what he meant by the advantage of the stronger party was what the stronger party *thinks* is to its advantage. This is what he was maintaining the weaker party ought to do, and this is what he was maintaining morality is.'

'But that's not what he said,' Polemarchus remarked.

'Never mind, Polemarchus,' I said. 'If this is what Thrasymachus is saying now, then let's accept it as his view. But do please tell me, Thrasymachus: *did* you mean to define morality as what appears to the stronger party to be to its advantage, whether or not it really is to its advantage? Is that how we are to understand your meaning?'

'Absolutely not!' he protested. 'Do you suppose I would describe someone who makes mistakes as the stronger party when he is making a mistake?'

'Yes,' I replied, 'I did think you were saying this, when you agreed that rulers are not infallible, but also make mistakes.'

'That's because you're a bully in discussions, Socrates,' he said. 'I mean, to take the first example that comes to mind, do you describe someone who makes mistakes about his patients as a doctor in virtue of the fact that he makes mistakes? Or do you describe someone who makes mistakes in his calculations as a mathematician, at precisely the time when he is making a mistake, and in virtue of the mistake that he is making? It's true that the expression is in our language: we say that a doctor or a mathematician or a teacher makes mistakes; but in fact, in my opinion, to the extent that each of them is what we call him, he never makes mistakes. And the consequence of this is that, strictly speaking—and you're the stickler for verbal precision—no professional makes mistakes: a mistake is due to a failure of knowledge, and for as long as that lasts he is not a professional. Professional, expert, ruler—no ruler makes a mistake at precisely the time when he is ruling, despite the universal usage of expressions like "The doctor made a mistake" or "The ruler made a mistake". So, when I stated my position to you recently, you should appreciate that I too was speaking like that; but the most precise formulation is in fact that a ruler, to the extent that he is a ruler, does not make mistakes; and in not making mistakes he passes laws which are in his best interest; and any subject of his should act in conformity with these laws. Consequently, as I said in the first place, my position is that morality is acting to the advantage of the stronger party.'

'Well, Thrasymachus,' I said, 'so you think I'm a bully, do you?'

'Yes, I do,' he said.

'And that's because you think my questions were premeditated attempts to wrong you?'

'I'm certain of it,' he said. 'And you won't gain any advantage from it, firstly because I'm aware of your unscrupulous tactics, and secondly because as long as I am aware of them, you won't be able to use the argument to batter me down.'

'My dear Thrasymachus,' I protested, 'the idea would never even occur to me! But we must make sure that this situation doesn't arise again, so please would you make something perfectly clear? Is it, according to you, the ruler and the stronger person in the loose sense, or in what you were just calling the precise sense, whose interest, since he is the stronger party, it is right for the weaker party to act in?'

'I'm talking about the ruler in the most precise sense possible,' he replied. 'You can do anything you like, as far as I'm concerned, so try your unscrupulous and bullying tactics on that, if you can! But you don't stand a chance.'

'Do you think I'm crazy enough to try to shave a lion and bully Thrasymachus?' I asked.

'Well, you tried just now,' he said, 'even though you're a nonentity at that too.'

'That's enough of that sort of remark,' I said. 'But let's take this doctor you were talking about a short while ago—the one who's a doctor in the strict sense of the term. Is he a businessman, or someone who attends to sick people? Think about the genuine doctor, please.'

'He attends to sick people,' he replied.

'What about a ship's captain? Is the true captain in charge of sailors or a sailor?'

'In charge of sailors.'

'In other words, we shouldn't take any account of the fact that he is on board a ship and describe him as a sailor. I mean, it isn't because he's on a ship that he's called a captain, but because of his expertise and because he has authority over the sailors.'

'True,' he said.

'Now, does each of the various parties in these situations have a particular advantage to gain?'

'Yes.'

'And isn't it the case,' I went on, 'that the *raison d'être* of a branch of expertise is to consider the welfare and interest of each party and then procure it?'

'Yes, that is what expertise is for,' he answered.

'Is there anything which is in the interest of any branch of expertise except being as perfect as possible?'

'I don't understand the question.'

'For instance,' I said, 'suppose you were to ask me whether it's enough for the body just to be the body, or whether it needs anything else. I'd reply, "There's no doubt at all that it needs something else. That's why the art of medicine has been invented, because the body is flawed and it isn't enough for it to be like that. The branch of expertise has been developed precisely for the purpose of procuring the body's welfare." Would this reply of mine be correct, do you think, or not?' I asked.

'Yes, it would,' he said.

'Well now, is medicine itself flawed? Are all branches of expertise imperfect? For instance, eyes need sight and ears need hearing, and that's why they need a branch of expertise to consider their welfare in precisely these respects and to procure it. Is expertise itself somehow inherently flawed as well, so that each branch of expertise needs a further branch to consider its welfare, and this supervisory branch needs yet another one, and so on *ad infinitum*? Or does every art consider its own interest and welfare? Or is the whole question of it, or another art, being needed to consider its welfare in view of its flaws irrelevant, in the sense that no branch of expertise is flawed or faulty in the slightest, and it's inappropriate for any branch of expertise to investigate the welfare of anything other than its own area of expertise? In other words, any branch of expertise is flawless and perfect, provided it's a genuine branch of expertise—that is, as long as it wholly is what it is, nothing more and nothing less. Please consider this issue with the same strict use of language we were using before, and tell me: am I right or not?'

'I think you're right,' he said.

'It follows, then,' I said, 'that medicine does not consider the welfare of medicine, but the welfare of the body.'

'Yes,' he said.

'And horsemanship considers the welfare of horses, not of horsemanship. In short, no branch of expertise considers its own advantage, since it isn't deficient in any respect: it considers the welfare of its area of expertise.'

'So it seems,' he said.

'But surely, Thrasymachus, the branches of expertise have authority and power over their particular areas of expertise.'

He gave his assent to this with extreme reluctance.

'So no branch of knowledge considers or enjoins the advantage of the stronger party, but the advantage of the weaker party, which is subject to it.'

Eventually, he agreed to this too, although he tried to argue against it. Once he'd agreed, however, I said, 'Surely, then, no doctor, in his capacity as doctor, considers or enjoins what is advantageous to the doctor, but what is advantageous to the patient? I mean, we've agreed that a doctor, in the strict sense of the term, is in charge of bodies, not a businessman. Isn't that what we agreed?'

He concurred.

'And a ship's captain too is, strictly speaking, in charge of sailors, not a sailor?'

He agreed.

'So since captains are like this and wield authority in this way, they won't consider and enjoin the interest of the captain, but what is advantageous to the sailor, the subject.'

He reluctantly agreed.

'Therefore, Thrasymachus,' I said, 'no one in any other kind of authority either, in his capacity as ruler, considers or enjoins his own advantage, but the advantage of his subject, the person for whom he practises his expertise. Everything he says and everything he does is said and done with this aim in mind and with regard to what is advantageous to and appropriate for this person.'

[*Republic*, trans. Robin Waterfield (Oxford University Press: Oxford, 1993), 18–25. Written *c*.390 BC.]

ARISTOTLE

2 Moral Virtue, How Produced

Virtue, then, being of two kinds, intellectual and moral, intellectual virtue in the main owes both its birth and its growth to teaching (for which reason it requires experience and time), while moral virtue comes about as a result of habit, whence also its name (ἠθική) is one that is formed by a slight variation from the word ἔθος (habit). From this it is also plain that none of the moral virtues arises in us by nature; for nothing that exists by nature can form a habit contrary to its nature. For instance the stone which by nature moves downwards cannot be habituated to move upwards, not even if one tries to train it by throwing it up ten thousand times; nor can fire be habituated to move downwards, nor can anything else that by nature be-haves in one way be trained to behave in another. Neither by nature, then, nor contrary to nature do the virtues arise in us; rather we are adapted by nature to receive them, and are made perfect by habit.

Again, of all the things that come to us by nature we first acquire the potentiality and later exhibit the activity (this is plain in the case of the sen-ses; for it was not by often seeing or often hearing that we got these senses, but on the contrary we had them before we used them, and did not come to have them by using them); but the virtues we get by first exercising them, as also happens in the case of the arts as well. For the things we have to learn before we can do them, we learn by doing them, e.g. men become builders by building and lyre-players by playing the lyre; so too we become just by doing just acts, temperate by doing temperate acts, brave by doing brave acts.

This is confirmed by what happens in states; for legislators make the citizens good by forming habits in them, and this is the wish of every legislator, and those who do not effect it miss their mark, and it is in this that a good constitution differs from a bad one.

Again, it is from the same causes and by the same means that every virtue is both produced and destroyed, and similarly every art; for it is from playing the lyre that both good and bad lyre-players are produced. And the corresponding statement is true of builders and of all the rest; men will be good or bad builders as a result of building well or badly. For if this were not so, there would have been no need of a teacher, but all men would have been born good or bad at their craft. This, then, is the case with the virtues also; by doing the acts that we do in our transactions with other men we become just or unjust, and by doing the acts that we do in the presence of danger, and by being habituated to feel fear or confidence, we become brave or cowardly. The same is true of appetites and feelings of anger; some men become temperate and good-tempered, others self-indulgent and irascible, by behaving in one way or the other in the appropriate circumstances. Thus, in one word, states of character arise out of like activities. This is why the activities we exhibit must be of a certain kind; it is because the states of character correspond to the differences between these. It makes no small difference, then, whether we form habits of one kind or of another from our very youth; it makes a very great difference, or rather *all* the difference.

[*The Nicomachean Ethics of Aristotle*, trans. and introd. W. D. Ross (Oxford University Press: London, 1959), 28–9. Written *c*.340 BC.]

MENCIUS

3 Are Humans Good by Nature? A Debate between Chinese Sages

Kao Tzu said, 'Human nature is like the willow tree, and righteousness is like a cup or a bowl. To turn human nature into humanity and righteousness is like turning the willow into cups and bowls.' Mencius said, 'Sir, can you follow the nature of the willow tree and make the cups and bowls, or must you violate the nature of the willow tree before you can make the cups and bowls? If you are going to violate the nature of the willow tree in order to make cups and bowls, then must you also violate human nature in order to make it into humanity and righteousness? Your words, alas!

would lead all people in the world to consider humanity and righteousness as calamity [because they required the violation of human nature]!'

Kao Tzu said, 'Man's nature is like whirling water. If a breach in the pool is made to the east it will flow to the east. If a breach is made to the west it will flow to the west. Man's nature is indifferent to good and evil, just as water is indifferent to east and west.' Mencius said, 'Water, indeed, is indifferent to the east and west, but is it indifferent to high and low? Man's nature is naturally good just as water naturally flows downward. There is no man without this good nature; neither is there water that does not flow downward. Now you can strike water and cause it to splash upward over your forehead, and by damming and leading it, you can force it uphill. Is this the nature of water? It is the forced circumstance that makes it do so. Man can be made to do evil, for his nature can be treated in the same way.' [. . .]

Kung-tu Tzu said, 'Kao Tzu said that man's nature is neither good nor evil. Some say that man's nature may be made good or evil, therefore when King Wen and King Wu were in power the people loved virtue, and when Kings Yu and Li were in power people loved violence. Some say that some men's nature is good and some men's nature is evil. Therefore even under (sage-emperor) Yao there was Hsiang [who daily plotted to kill his brother], and even with a bad father Ku-sou, there was [a most filial] Shun (Hsiang's brother who succeeded Yao), and even with (wicked king) Chou as nephew and ruler, there were Viscount Ch'i of Wei and Prince Pi-kan. Now you say that human nature is good. Then are those people wrong?'

Mencius said, "If you let people follow their feelings (original nature), they will be able to do good. This is what is meant by saying that human nature is good. If man does evil, it is not the fault of his natural endowment. The feeling of commiseration is found in all men; the feeling of shame and dislike is found in all men; the feeling of respect and reverence is found in all men; and the feeling of right and wrong is found in all men. The feeling of commiseration is what we call humanity; the feeling of shame and dislike is what we call righteousness; the feeling of respect and reverence is what we call propriety (li); and the feeling of right and wrong is what we call wisdom. Humanity, righteousness, propriety, and wisdom are not drilled into us from outside. We originally have them with us. [. . .]

Mencius said, 'The trees of the Niu Mountain were once beautiful. But can the mountain be regarded any longer as beautiful since, being in the borders of a big state, the trees have been hewed down with axes and hatchets? Still with the rest given them by the days and nights and the nourishment provided them by the rains and the dew, they were not without buds and sprouts springing forth. But then the cattle and the sheep pastured upon them once and again. That is why the mountain looks so bald. When people see that it is so bald, they think that there was never any timber on the mountain. Is this the true nature of the mountain? Is there not [also] a heart of humanity and righteousness originally existing in man? The way in which he loses his originally good mind is like the way in which the trees are hewed down with axes and hatchets. As trees are cut down day after day, can a mountain retain its beauty? To be sure, the days and nights do the healing, and there is the nourishing air of the calm morning which keeps him normal in his likes and dislikes. But the effect is slight, and is disturbed and destroyed by what he does during the day. When there is repeated disturbance, the restorative influence of the night will not be sufficient to preserve (the proper goodness of the mind). When the in-fluence of the night is not sufficient to preserve it, man becomes not much different from the beast. People see that he acts like an animal, and think that he never had the original endowment (for goodness). But is that his true character? Therefore with proper nourishment and care, everything grows, whereas without proper nourishment and care, everything decays. Confucius said, "Hold it fast and you preserve it. Let it go and you lose it. It comes in and goes out at no definite time and without anyone's knowing its direction." He was talking about the human mind.' [. . .]

[Mencius said] 'I like life and I also like righteousness. If I cannot have both of them, I shall give up life and choose righteousness. I love life, but there is something I love more than life, and therefore I will not do anything improper to have it. I also hate death, but there is something I hate more than death, and therefore there are occasions when I will not avoid danger. If there is nothing that man loves more than life, then why should he not employ every means to preserve it? And if there is nothing that man hates more than death, then why does he not do anything to avoid danger? There are cases when a man does not take the course even if by taking it he can preserve his life, and he does not do anything even if by doing it he can avoid danger. Therefore there is something men love more than life and there is something men hate more than death. It is not only the worthies alone who have this moral sense. All men have it, but only the worthies have been able to preserve it.

[*The Book of Mencius*, from *A Source Book in Chinese Philosophy*, trans. and comp. Wing-Tsit Chan (Princeton University Press: Princeton, NJ, 1963), 51–7. Written c.350 BC.]

THOMAS HOBBES

4 **Of the Natural Condition of Mankind and the Laws of Nature**

Nature hath made men so equal, in the faculties of the body and mind; as that though there be found one man sometimes manifestly stronger in body, or of quicker mind than another, yet when all is reckoned together, the difference between man and man, is not so considerable, as that one man can thereupon claim to himself any benefit, to which another may not pretend, as well as he. For as to the strength of body, the weakest has strength enough to kill the strongest, either by secret machination, or by confederacy with others, that are in the same danger with himself.

And as to the faculties of the mind, setting aside the arts grounded upon words, and especially that skill of proceeding upon general and infallible rules, called science; which very few have, and but in few things; as being not a native faculty, born with us; nor attained, as prudence, while we look after somewhat else, I find yet a greater equality amongst men than that of strength. For prudence is but experience; which equal time, equally bestows on all men, in those things they equally apply themselves unto. That which may perhaps make such equality incredible, is but a vain conceit of one's own wisdom, which almost all men think they have in a greater degree than the vulgar; that is, than all men but themselves, and a few others, whom by fame or for concurring with themselves, they approve. For such is the nature of men, that howsoever they may acknowledge many others to be more witty, or more eloquent, or more learned; yet they will hardly believe there be many so wise as themselves; for they see their own wit at hand, and other men's at a distance. But this proveth rather that men are in that point equal, than unequal. For there is not ordinarily a greater sign of the equal distribution of anything, than that every man is contented with his share.

From this equality of ability, ariseth equality of hope in the attaining of our ends. And therefore if any two men desire the same thing, which nevertheless they cannot both enjoy, they become enemies; and in the way to their end, which is principally their own conservation, and sometimes their delectation only, endeavour to destroy or subdue one another. And from hence it comes to pass, that where an invader hath no more to fear than another man's single power; if one plant, sow, build, or possess a convenient seat, others may probably be expected to come prepared with forces united, to dispossess and deprive him, not only of the fruit of his labour, but also of his life or liberty. And the invader again is in the like danger of another.

And from this diffidence of one another, there is no way for any man to secure himself, so reasonable, as anticipation; that is, by force, or wiles, to master the persons of all men he can, so long, till he see no other power great enough to endanger him: and this is no more than his own conservation requireth, and is generally allowed. Also because there be some, that taking pleasure in contemplating their own power in the acts of conquest, which they pursue farther than their security requires; if others, that otherwise would be glad to be at ease within modest bounds, should not by invasion increase their power, they would not be able, long time, by standing only on their defence, to subsist. And by consequence, such augmentation of dominion over men being necessary to a man's conservation, it ought to be allowed him.

Again, men have no pleasure, but on the contrary a great deal of grief, in keeping company, where there is no power able to overawe them all. For every man looketh that his companion should value him, at the same rate he sets upon himself: and upon all signs of contempt, or undervaluing, naturally endeavours, as far as he dares, (which amongst them that have no common power to keep them in quiet, is far enough to make them destroy each other,) to extort a greater value from his contemners, by damage; and from others, by the example.

So that in the nature of man, we find three principal causes of quarrel. First, competition; secondly, diffidence; thirdly, glory.

The first, maketh men invade for gain; the second, for safety; and the third, for reputation. The first use violence, to make themselves masters of other men's persons, wives, children, and cattle; the second, to defend them; the third, for trifles, as a word, a smile, a different opinion, and any other sign of undervalue, either direct in their persons, or by reflection in their kindred, their friends, their nation, their profession, or their name.

Hereby it is manifest, that during the time men live without a common power to keep them all in awe, they are in that condition which is called war; and such a war, as is of every man, against every man. For 'war' consisteth not in battle only, or the act of fighting; but in a tract of time, wherein the will to contend by battle is sufficiently known: and therefore the notion of 'time' is to be considered in the nature of war, as it is in the nature of weather. For as the nature of foul weather lieth not in a shower or two of rain, but in an inclination thereto of many days together; so the nature of war consisteth not in actual fighting, but in the known disposition thereto during all the time there is no assurance to the contrary. All other time is 'peace.'

Whatsoever therefore is consequent to a time of war, where every man is enemy to every man, the same is consequent to the time wherein men live without other security than what their own strength and their own invention shall furnish them withal. In such condition there is no place for industry, because the fruit thereof is uncertain, and consequently no culture of the earth; no navigation, nor use of the commodities that may be imported by sea; no commodious building; no instruments of moving and removing such things as require much force; no knowledge of the face of the earth; no account of time; no arts; no letters; no society; and, which is worst of all, continual fear and danger of violent death; and the life of man, solitary, poor, nasty, brutish, and short.

It may seem strange to some man, that has not well weighed these things, that Nature should thus dissociate, and render men apt to invade and destroy one another; and he may therefore, not trusting to this inference, made from the passions, desire perhaps to have the same confirmed by experience. Let him therefore consider with himself, when taking a journey, he arms himself, and seeks to go well accompanied; when going to sleep, he locks his doors; when even in his house, he locks his chests; and this when he knows there be laws, and public officers, armed, to revenge all injuries shall be done him; what opinion he has of his fellow-subjects, when he rides armed; of his fellow-citizens, when he locks his doors; and of his children and servants, when he locks his chests. Does he not there as much accuse mankind by his actions as I do by my words? But neither of us accuse man's nature in it. The desires and other passions of man are in themselves no sin. No more are the actions that proceed from those passions, till they know a law that forbids them; which till laws be made they cannot know, nor can any law be made till they have agreed upon the person that shall make it.

It may peradventure be thought there was never such a time nor condition of war as this; and I believe it was never generally so, over all the world, but there are many places where they live so now. For the savage people in many places of America, except the government of small families, the concord whereof dependeth on natural lust, have no government at all, and live at this day in that brutish manner, as I said before. Howsoever, it may be perceived what manner of life there would be, where there were no common power to fear, by the manner of life which men that have formerly lived under a peaceful government, use to degenerate into in a civil war.

But though there had never been any time, wherein particular men were in a condition of war one against another; yet in all times, kings, and persons of sovereign authority, because of their independency, are in continual jealousies, and in the state and posture of gladiators; having their weapons pointing, and their eyes fixed on one another; that is, their forts, garrisons, and guns upon the frontiers of their kingdoms; and continual spies upon their neighbours; which is a posture of war. But because they uphold thereby the industry of their subjects; there does not follow from it that misery which accompanies the liberty of particular men.

To this war of every man, against every man, this also is consequent; that nothing can be unjust. The notions of right and wrong, justice and injustice, have there no place. Where there is no common power, there is no law: where no law, no injustice. Force and fraud, are in war the two cardinal virtues. Justice and injustice are none of the faculties neither of the body nor mind. If they were, they might be in a man that were alone in the world, as well as his senses, and passions. They are qualities that relate to men in society, not in solitude. It is consequent also to the same condition, that there be no propriety, no dominion, no 'mine' and 'thine' distinct; but only that to be every man's, that he can get; and for so long, as he can keep it. And thus much for the ill condition, which man by mere nature is actually placed in; though with a possibility to come out of it, consisting partly in the passions, partly in his reason.

The passions that incline men to peace, are fear of death; desire of such things as are necessary to commodious living; and a hope by their industry to obtain them. And reason suggesteth convenient articles of peace, upon which men may be drawn to agreement. These articles are they which otherwise are called the Laws of Nature: whereof I shall speak more particularly [. . .]

'The right of Nature,' which writers commonly call *jus naturale*, is the liberty each man hath, to use his own power, as he will himself, for the preservation of his own nature; that is to say, of his own life; and consequently, of doing anything, which in his own judgment and reason he shall conceive to be the aptest means thereunto.

By 'liberty,' is understood, according to the proper signification of the word, the absence of external impediments: which impediments may oft take away part of a man's power to do what he would; but cannot hinder him from using the power left him, according as his judgment and reason shall dictate to him.

A 'law of Nature,' *lex naturalis*, is a precept or general rule, found out by reason, by which a man is forbidden to do that which is destructive of his life, or taketh away the means of preserving the same; and to omit that, by which he thinketh it may be best preserved. For though they that speak of this subject, use to confound *jus* and *lex*, 'right' and 'law:' yet they ought to be distinguished; because 'right,' consisteth in liberty to do, or to forbear; whereas 'law,' determineth and bindeth to one of them; so that law and right differ as much as obligation and liberty; which in one and the same matter are inconsistent.

And because the condition of man, as hath been declared in the precedent chapter, is a condition of war of every one against every one; in which case every one is governed by his own reason; and there is nothing he can make use of, that may not be a help unto him, in preserving his life against his enemies; it followeth, that in such a condition, every man has a right to everything; even to one another's body. And therefore, as long as this natural right of every man to everything endureth, there can be no security to any man, how strong or wise soever he be, of living out the time, which Nature ordinarily alloweth men to live. And consequently it is a precept, or general rule of reason, 'that every man ought to endeavour peace, as far as he has hope of obtaining it; and when he cannot obtain it, that he may seek, and use, all helps, and advantages of war.' The first branch of which rule, containeth the first, and fundamental law of Nature; which is, 'to seek peace, and follow it.' The second, the sum of the right of Nature: which is, 'by all means we can, to defend ourselves.'

From this fundamental law of Nature, by which men are commanded to endeavour peace, is derived this second law; 'that a man be willing, when others are so too, as far-forth, as for peace, and defence of himself he shall think it necessary, to lay down this right to all things; and be contented with so much liberty against other men, as he would allow other men against himself.' For as long as every man holdeth this right, of doing anything he liketh; so long are all men in the condition of war. But if other men will not lay down their right, as well as he; then there is no reason for any one to divest himself of his: for that were to expose himself to prey, which no man is bound to, rather than to dispose himself to peace. This is that law of the Gospel; 'whatsoever you require that others should do to you, that do ye to them.' [. . .]

From that law of Nature, by which we are obliged to transfer to another, such rights, as being retained, hinder the peace of mankind, there followeth a third; which is this, 'that men perform their covenants made;' without which, covenants are in vain, and but empty words; and the right of all men to all things remaining, we are still in the condition of war.

And in this law of Nature consisteth the fountain and original of 'justice.' For where no covenant hath preceded, there hath no right been transferred, and every man has right to everything; and consequently, no action can be unjust. But when a covenant is made, then to break it is 'unjust': and the definition of 'injustice,' is no other than 'the not performance of covenant.' And whatsoever is not unjust, is 'just.'

But because covenants of mutual trust, where there is a fear of not performance on either part, as hath been said in the former chapter, are invalid; though the original of justice be the making of covenants; yet injustice actually there can be none, till the cause of such fear be taken away; which while men are in the natural condition of war, cannot be done. Therefore before the names of just and unjust can have place, there must be some coercive power, to compel men equally to the performance of their covenants, by the terror of some punishment, greater than the benefit they expect by the breach of their covenant; and to make good that propriety, which by mutual contract men acquire, in recompense of the universal right they abandon: and such power there is none before the erection of a commonwealth. And this is also to be gathered out of the ordinary definition of justice in the schools: for they say, that 'justice is the constant will of giving to every man his own.' And therefore where there is no 'own,' that is no propriety, there is no injustice; and where there is no coercive power erected, that is, where there is no commonwealth, there is no propriety; all men having right to all things: therefore where there is no commonwealth, there nothing is unjust. So that the nature of justice, consisteth in keeping of valid covenants: but the validity of covenants begins not but with the constitution of a civil power, sufficient to compel men to keep them; and then it is also that propriety begins.

[*Leviathan*, Thomas Hobbes (Dent: London, 1914), 289–97. First published in 1651.]

JEAN-JACQUES ROUSSEAU

5 The Natural State of Man

As important as it is, in making a true judgement of man's natural state, to consider him from his origins and examine him, so to speak, in the embryo of his species, I do not propose to trace his organic system through all its successive developments. I shall not pause to search the animal system for what he might have been at the beginning in order to become what he is at the end [. . .] I shall suppose him to have been at all times formed as I see him today, walking on two feet, using his hands in the same way we do, casting his gaze over all nature, and measuring with his eyes the vast expanse of the heavens.

In stripping the creature thus constituted of all the supernatural endowments he may have received and all the artificial faculties that he could have acquired only through a long process, and considering him, in short, as he must have emerged from the hands of nature, I see an animal less strong than some, less agile than others, but on the whole the most advantageously constituted of all. I see him eating his fill under an oak tree, quenching his thirst at the first stream, making his bed at the base of the same tree that supplied his meal, and, behold, his needs are met.

The earth, left to its natural fertility and bespread with immense forests never hewn by an axe, everywhere offers storehouses and shelter for animals of every species. Scattered among the beasts, man observes and imitates their activities and so raises himself to the level of their instincts, with the added advantage that though every other species has only its own instinct, man, who perhaps has none peculiar to himself, arrogates them all and nourishes himself equally well on most of the various foods that the other animals divide among themselves, and he thus finds his sustenance more easily than do any of the rest [. . .]

At first glance, it would seem that because in the state of nature men have no kind of moral relationships to each other, nor any recognized duties, they would be neither good nor evil, and could have neither vices nor virtues; unless we took those words in a physical sense and could call an individual's 'vices' those attributes that might be deleterious to his own survival and 'virtues' those that might be propitious for it, in which case we should have to call most virtuous the person who least resisted the simple impulses of nature. But without diverging from ordinary usage, we would do well to suspend judgement on this situation and guard against our own biases until we have observed, with the scales of impartiality in our hands, more virtues than vices among civilized men, whether those men's virtues are more beneficial than their vices are pernicious; or whether the advancement of their knowledge adequately compensates for the harm they do each other, as they learn of the good they should do each other; or whether, all things considered, they would not be in a happier situation, having neither harm to fear from anyone nor good to hope from anyone, rather than subjecting themselves to a universal dependence and obligating themselves to accept everything from those who do not obligate themselves to give them anything.

Above all, let us not conclude with Hobbes that man is naturally wicked because he has no idea of goodness or vice-ridden because he has no knowledge of virtue, that he always withholds from his fellow men services that he does not believe he owes them, or on the strength of his properly claimed right to the things he needs, he madly imagines himself to be the sole owner of the universe. [. . .] I believe I need have no fear of contradiction when I credit man with the one natural virtue that the most intemperate detractor of human virtues has been forced to recognize. I speak of pity, a fitting predisposition for creatures as weak and subject to as many ills as we, a virtue all the more universal and useful to man because it precedes any kind of reflection in him, and so natural that even the beasts themselves sometimes show discernible signs of it. [. . .]

Hence, it is certain that pity is a natural sentiment moderating the action of self-love in each individual and so contributing to the mutual preservation of the whole species. It is pity that sends us unreflecting to the aid of those we see suffering; it is pity that in the state of nature takes the place of laws, moral habits, and virtues, with the added benefit that there no one is tempted to disobey its gentle voice; it will deter a robust savage from robbing a weak child or infirm old person of his hard-won sustenance if the savage himself can hope to find his own elsewhere; it is pity that, in place of that sublime maxim of rational justice, 'Do unto others as you would have them do unto you,' inspires in all men that other maxim of natural goodness, much less perfect but perhaps more useful: 'Do what is good to yourself with as little possible harm to others.' In short, it is to this natural feeling, rather than to any subtle arguments, that we must look for the cause of the aversion that every man feels to doing evil, quite independently of the maxims of education. Although it may be the business of Socrates and others of that stamp to acquire virtue through reason, the human race would long ago have ceased to exist if its preservation had depended strictly on the reasoning power of the individuals who make it up.

[A Discourse on the Origin of Inequality, trans. Franklin Philip (Oxford University Press: Oxford, 1994), 26–7, 43–8. First published in 1755.]

6 Affection of Humanity: The Foundation of Morals

When a man denominates another his *enemy*, his *rival*, his *antagonist*, his *adversary*, he is understood to speak the language of self-love, and to express sentiments, peculiar to himself, and arising from his particular circumstances and situation. But when he bestows on any man the epithets of *vicious* or *odious* or *depraved*, he then speaks another language, and expresses sentiments, in which he expects all his audience are to concur with him. He must here, therefore, depart from his private and particular situation, and must choose a point of view, common to him with others; he must move some universal principle of the human frame, and touch a string to which all mankind have an accord and symphony. If he mean, therefore, to express that this man possesses qualities, whose tendency is pernicious to society, he has chosen this common point of view, and has touched the principle of humanity, in which every man, in some degree, concurs. While the human heart is compounded of the same elements as at present, it will never be wholly indifferent to public good, nor entirely unaffected with the tendency of characters and manners. And though this affection of humanity may not generally be esteemed so strong as vanity or ambition, yet, being common to all men, it can alone be the foundation of morals, or of any general system of blame or praise. One man's ambition is not another's ambition, nor will the same event or object satisfy both; but the humanity of one man is the humanity of every one, and the same object touches this passion in all human creatures.

But the sentiments, which arise from humanity, are not only the same in all human creatures, and produce the same approbation or censure; but they also comprehend all human creatures; nor is there any one whose conduct or character is not, by their means, an object to every one of censure or approbation. On the contrary, those other passions, commonly denominated selfish, both produce different sentiments in each individual, according to his particular situation; and also contemplate the greater part of mankind with the utmost indifference and unconcern. Whoever has a high regard and esteem for me flatters my vanity; whoever expresses contempt mortifies and displeases me; but as my name is known but to a small part of mankind, there are few who come within the sphere of this passion, or excite, on its account, either my affection or disgust. But if you represent a tyrannical, insolent, or barbarous behaviour, in any country or in any age of the world, I soon carry my eye to the pernicious tendency of such a conduct, and feel the sentiment of repugnance and displeasure towards it. No character can be so remote as to be, in this light, wholly indifferent to me. What is beneficial to society or to the person himself must still be preferred. And every quality or action, of every human being, must, by this means, be ranked under some class or denomination, expressive of general censure or applause.

What more, therefore, can we ask to distinguish the sentiments, dependent on humanity, from those connected with any other passion, or to satisfy us, why the former are the origin of morals, not the latter? Whatever conduct gains my approbation, by touching my humanity, procures also the applause of all mankind, by affecting the same principle in them; but what serves my avarice or ambition pleases these passions in me alone, and affects not the avarice and ambition of the rest of mankind. There is no circumstance of conduct in any man, provided it have a beneficial tendency, that is not agreeable to my humanity, however remote the person; but every man, so far removed as neither to cross nor serve my avarice and ambition, is regarded as wholly indifferent by those passions. The distinction, therefore, between these species of sentiment being so great and evident, language must soon be moulded upon it, and must invent a peculiar set of terms, in order to express those universal sentiments of censure or approbation, which arise from humanity, or from views of general usefulness and its contrary. Virtue and Vice become then known; morals are recognized; certain general ideas are framed of human conduct and behaviour; such measures are expected from men in such situations. This action is determined to be conformable to our abstract rule; that other, contrary. And by such universal principles are the particular sentiments of self-love frequently controlled and limited.[1]

['An Enquiry Concerning the Principles of Morals' in L. A. Selby-Bigge (ed.), *Hume's Enquiries*, 2nd edn. (Clarendon Press: Oxford, 1902), 272–5. First published in 1751.]

[1] It seems certain, both from reason and experience, that a rude, untaught savage regulates chiefly his love and hatred by the ideas of private utility and injury, and has but faint conceptions of a general rule or system of behaviour. The man who stands opposite to him in battle, he hates heartily, not only for the present moment, which is almost unavoidable, but for ever after; nor is he satisfied without the most extreme punishment and vengeance. But we, accustomed to society, and to more enlarged reflections, consider, that this man is serving his own country and community; that any man, in the same situation, would do the same; that we ourselves, in like circumstances, observe a like conduct; that, in general, human society is best supported on such maxims: and by these suppositions and views, we correct, in some measure, our ruder and narrower passions. And though much of our friendship and enmity be still regulated by private considerations of benefit and harm, we pay, at least, this homage to general rules, which we are accustomed to respect, that we commonly pervert our adversary's conduct, by imputing malice or injustice to him, in order to give vent to those passions, which arise from self-love and private interest. When the heart is full of rage, it never wants pretences of this nature; though sometimes as frivolous, as those from which Horace, being almost crushed by the fall of a tree, affects to accuse of parricide the first planter of it.

7 The Noble Descent of Duty

Duty! Thou sublime and mighty name that dost embrace nothing charming or insinuating but requirest submission and yet seekest not to move the will by threatening aught that would arouse natural aversion or terror but only holdest forth a law which of itself finds entrance into the mind and yet gains reluctant reverence (though not always obedience)—a law before which all inclinations are dumb even though they secretly work against it: what origin is there worthy of thee, and where is to be found the root of thy noble descent which proudly rejects all kinship with the inclinations and from which to be descended is the indispensable condition of the only worth which men can give themselves?

It cannot be less than something which elevates man above himself as a part of the world of sense, something which connects him with an order of things which only the understanding can think and which has under it the entire world of sense, including the empirically determinable existence of man in time, and the whole system of all ends which is alone suitable to such unconditional practical laws as the moral. It is nothing else than personality, i.e. the freedom and independence from the mechanism of nature regarded as a capacity of a being which is subject to special laws (pure practical laws given by its own reason), so that the person as belonging to the world of sense is subject to his own personality so far as he belongs to the intelligible world. For it is then not to be wondered at that man, as belonging to two worlds, must regard his own being in relation to his second and higher vocation with reverence and the laws of this vocation with the deepest respect.

Many expressions which indicate the worth of objects according to moral ideas are based on this origin. The moral law is holy (inviolable). Man is certainly unholy enough, but humanity in his person must be holy to him. Everything in creation which he wishes and over which he has power can be used merely as a means; only man, and, with him, every rational creature, is an end in itself. He is the subject of the moral law which is holy, because of the autonomy of his freedom. Because of the latter, every will, even the private will of each person directed to himself, is restricted to the condition of agreement with the autonomy of the rational being, namely, that it be subjected to no purpose which is not possible by a law which could arise from the will of the passive subject itself. This condition thus requires that the person never be used as a means except when it is at the same time an end. We may rightly attribute this condition even to the divine will with respect to the rational beings in the world as its creatures, since the condition rests on the personality of these beings, whereby alone they are ends in themselves.

This idea of personality awakens respect; it places before our eyes the sublimity of our own nature (in its [higher] vocation), while it shows us at the same time the unsuitability of our conduct to it, thus striking down our self-conceit. This is naturally and easily observed by the most common human reason. Has not every even fairly honest man sometimes found that he desists from an otherwise harmless lie which would extricate him from a vexing affair or which would even be useful to a beloved and deserving friend simply in order not to have to contemn himself secretly in his own eyes? In the greatest misfortunes of his life which he could have avoided if he could have disregarded duty, does not a righteous man hold up his head thanks to the consciousness that he has honored and preserved humanity in his own person and in its dignity, so that he does not have to shame himself in his own eyes or have reason to fear the inner scrutiny of self-examination? This comfort is not happiness, not even the smallest part of happiness; for no one would wish to have occasion for it, not even once in his life, or perhaps even would desire life itself in such circumstances. But he lives and cannot tolerate seeing himself as unworthy of life. This inner satisfaction is therefore merely negative with reference to everything which might make life pleasant; it is the defense against the danger of sinking in personal worth after the value of his circumstances has been completely lost. It is the effect of a respect for something entirely different from life, in comparison and contrast to which life and its enjoyment have absolutely no worth. He yet lives only because it is his duty, not because he has the least taste for living.

Such is the nature of the genuine incentive of pure practical reason. It is nothing else than the pure moral law itself, so far as it lets us perceive the sublimity of our own supersensuous existence and subjectively effects respect for their higher vocation in men who are conscious of their sensuous existence and of the accompanying dependence on their pathologically affected nature. Now let there be associated with this incentive so many charms and pleasures of life that even for their sake alone the most skilful choice of a reasonable Epicurean, considering the highest welfare of life, would declare himself for moral conduct (and it may even be advisable to connect this prospect of a merry enjoyment of life with that supreme determining motive which is sufficient of itself); but this is only in order to hold a balance against the attractions which vice on the other side does not fail to offer and not in order to place in these prospects even the smallest part of the real moving force when duty is what we are concerned with. For the latter would be simply to destroy the purity of the moral disposition at its source. The majesty of duty has nothing to do with the enjoyment of life; it has its own law, even its own tribunal, and however much one wishes to mix them together, in order to offer the mixture to the sick as though it were a medicine, they nevertheless soon separate of themselves; but, if they do not separate, the moral ingredient has no effect at all, and even if the physical life gained some strength in this way, the moral life would waste away beyond rescue. [. . .]

Two things fill the mind with ever new and increasing admiration and awe, the oftener and more steadily they are reflected on: the starry heavens above me and the moral law within me. I do not merely conjecture them and seek them as though obscured in darkness or in the transcendent region beyond my horizon: I see them before me, and I associate them directly with the consciousness of my own existence. The former begins from the place I occupy in the external world of sense, and it broadens the connection in which I stand into an unbounded magnitude of worlds beyond worlds and systems of systems and into the limitless times of their periodic motion, their beginning and continuance. The latter begins from my invisible self, my personality, and exhibits me in a world which has true infinity but which is comprehensible only to the understanding—a world with which I recognize myself as existing in a universal and necessary (and not only, as in the first case, contingent) connection, and thereby also in connection with all those visible worlds. The former view of a countless multitude of worlds annihilates, as it were, my importance as an animal creature, which must give back to the planet (a mere speck in the universe) the matter from which it came, the matter which is for a little time provided with vital force, we know not how. The latter, on the contrary, infinitely raises my worth as that of an intelligence by my personality, in which the moral law reveals a life independent of all animality and even of the whole world of sense—at least so far as it may be inferred from the purposive destination assigned to my existence by this law, a destination which is not restricted to the conditions and limits of this life but reaches into the infinite.

[*The Critique of Practical Reason and Other Writings in Moral Philosophy*, trans. L. W. Beck (University of Chicago Press: Chicago, 1949), 193–5, 258–9. First published in 1788.]

KARL MARX AND FRIEDRICH ENGELS

8   The Material Basis of Morality

Men can be distinguished from animals by consciousness, by religion, or anything else you like. They themselves begin to distinguish themselves from animals as soon as they begin to produce their means of subsistence, a step which is conditioned by their physical organization. By producing their means of subsistence men are indirectly producing their actual material life.

The way in which men produce their means of subsistence depends first of all on the nature of the actual means of subsistence they find in existence and have to reproduce. This mode of production must not be considered simply as being the production of the physical existence of the individuals. Rather it is a definite form of activity of these individuals, a definite form of expressing their life, a definite mode of life on their part. As individuals express their life, so they are. What they are, therefore, coincides with their production, both with *what* they produce and with *how* they produce. The nature of individuals thus depends on the material conditions determining their production. [. . .]

The production of ideas, of conceptions, of consciousness, is at first directly interwoven with the material activity and the material intercourse of men, the language of real life. Conceiving, thinking, the mental intercourse of men, appear at this stage as the direct efflux of their material behaviour. The same applies to mental production as expressed in the language of politics, laws, morality, religion, metaphysics, etc. of a people. Men are the producers of their conceptions, ideas, etc.—real, active men, as they are conditioned by a definite development of their productive forces and of the intercourse corresponding to these, up to its furthest forms. Consciousness can never be anything else than conscious existence, and the existence of men is their actual life-process. If in all ideology men and their circumstances appear upside-down as in a *camera obscura*, this phenomenon arises just as much from their historical life-process as the inversion of objects on the retina does from their physical life-process.

In direct contrast to German philosophy which descends from heaven to earth, here we ascend from earth to heaven. That is to say, we do not set out from what men say, imagine, conceive, nor from men as narrated, thought of, imagined, conceived, in order to arrive at men in the flesh. We set out from real, active men, and on the basis of their real life-process we demonstrate the development of the ideological reflexes and echoes of this life-process. The phantoms formed in the human brain are also, necessarily, sublimates of their material life-process, which is empirically verifiable and bound to material premisses. Morality, religion, metaphysics, all the rest of ideology and their corresponding forms of consciousness, thus no longer retain the semblance of independence. They have no history, no development; but men, developing their material production and their material intercourse, alter, along with this their real existence, their thinking and the products of their thinking. Life is not determined by consciousness, but consciousness by life.

* * * * * *

The charges against Communism made from a religious, a philosophical, and, generally, from an ideological standpoint, are not deserving of serious examination.

Does it require deep intuition to comprehend that man's ideas, views and conceptions, in one word, man's consciousness, changes with every change in the conditions of his existence, in his social relations and in his social life?

What else does the history of ideas prove, than that intellectual production changes in character in proportion as material production is changed? The ruling ideas of each age have ever been the ideas of its ruling class.

When people speak of ideas that revolutionize society, they do but express the fact, that within the old society, the elements of a new one have been created, and that the dissolution of the old ideas keeps even pace with the dissolution of the old conditions of existence.

When the ancient world was in its last throes, the ancient religions were overcome by Christianity. When Christian ideas succumbed in the 18th century to the ideas of the Enlightenment, feudal society fought its death battle with the then revolutionary bourgeoisie. The ideas of religious liberty and freedom of conscience, merely gave expression to the sway of free competition within the domain of knowledge.

'Undoubtedly,' it will be said, 'religious, moral, philosophical, political, juridical ideas, etc., have been modified in the course of historical development. But religion, morality, philosophy, political science, and law, constantly survived this change.

'There are, besides, eternal truths, such as Freedom, Justice, etc., that are common to all states of society. But Communism abolishes eternal truths, it abolishes all religion, and all morality, instead of constituting them on a new basis; it therefore acts in contradiction to all past historical experience.'

What does this accusation reduce itself to? The history of all past society has consisted in the development of class antagonisms, antagonisms that assumed different forms at different epochs.

But whatever form they may have taken, one fact is common to all past ages, viz., the exploitation of one part of society by the other. No wonder, then, that the social consciousness of past ages, despite all the multiplicity and variety it displays, moves within certain common forms, in forms of consciousness which cannot completely vanish except with the total disappearance of class antagonisms.

[*Karl Marx and Friedrich Engels: The German Ideology*, ed. R. Pascal (International Publishers: New York, 1963), 8, 13–14; *The Communist Manifesto*, ed. David McLellan (Oxford University Press: Oxford, 1992), 24–5. First written in 1845 and 1848 respectively.]

CHARLES DARWIN

9 The Origin of the Moral Sense

I fully subscribe to the judgment of those writers who maintain that of all the differences between man and the lower animals, the moral sense or conscience is by far the most important. This sense, as Mackintosh remarks, has a rightful supremacy over every other principle of human action; it is summed up in that short but imperious word *ought*, so full of high significance. It is the most noble of all the attributes of man, leading him without a moment's hesitation to risk his life for that of a fellow-creature; or after due deliberation, impelled simply by the deep feeling of right or duty, to sacrifice it in some great cause. Immanuel Kant exclaims, 'Duty! Wondrous thought, that workest neither by fond insinuation, flattery, nor by any threat, but merely by holding up thy naked law in the soul, and so extorting for thyself always reverence, if not always obedience; before whom all appetites are dumb, however secretly they rebel; whence thy original?'

This great question has been discussed by many writers of consummate ability; and my sole excuse for touching on it, is the impossibility of here passing it over; and because, as far as I know, no one has approached it exclusively from the side of natural history. The investigation possesses, also, some independent interest, as an attempt to see how far the study of the lower animals throws light on one of the highest psychical faculties of man.

The following proposition seems to me in a high degree probable—namely, that any animal whatever, endowed with well-marked social instincts, the parental and filial affections being here included, would inevitably acquire a moral sense or conscience, as soon as its intellectual powers had become as well, or nearly as well developed, as in man. For, *firstly*, the social instincts lead an animal to take pleasure in the society of its fellows, to feel a certain amount of sympathy with them, and to perform various services for them. The services may be of a definite and evidently instinctive nature; or there may be only a wish and readiness, as with most of the higher social animals, to aid their fellows in certain general ways. But these feelings and services are by no means extended to all the individuals of the same species, only to those of the same association. *Secondly*, as soon as the mental faculties had become highly developed, images of all past actions and motives would be incessantly passing through the brain of each individual; and that feeling of dissatisfaction, or even misery, which invariably results, as we shall hereafter see, from any unsatisfied instinct, would arise, as often as it was perceived that the enduring and always present social instinct had yielded to some other instinct, at the time stronger, but neither enduring in its nature, nor leaving behind it a very vivid impression. It is clear that many instinctive desires, such as that of hunger, are in their nature of short duration; and after being satisfied, are not readily or vividly recalled. *Thirdly*, after the power of language had been acquired, and the wishes of the community could be expressed, the common opinion how each member ought to act for the public good, would naturally become in a paramount degree the guide to action. But it should be borne in mind that however great weight we may attribute to public opinion, our regard for the approbation and disapprobation of our fellows depends on sympathy, which, as we shall see, forms an essential part of the social instinct, and is indeed its foundation-stone, *Lastly*, habit in the individual would ultimately play a very important part in guiding the conduct of each member; for the social instinct, together with sympathy, is, like any other instinct, greatly strengthened by habit, and so consequently would be obedience to the wishes and judgment of the community. These several subordinate propositions must now be discussed, and some of them at considerable length.

It may be well first to premise that I do not wish to maintain that any strictly social animal, if its intellectual faculties were to become as active and as highly developed as in man, would acquire exactly the same moral sense as ours. In the same manner as various animals have some sense of beauty, though they admire widely different objects, so they might have a sense of right and wrong, though led by it to follow widely different lines of conduct. If, for instance, to take an extreme case, men were reared under precisely the same conditions as hive-bees, there can hardly be a doubt that our unmarried females would, like the worker-bees, think it a sacred duty to kill their brothers, and mothers would strive to kill their fertile daughters; and no one would think of interfering. Nevertheless, the bee, or any other social animal, would gain in our supposed case, as it appears to me, some feeling of right or wrong, or a conscience. For each individual would have an inward sense of possessing certain stronger or more enduring instincts, and others less strong or enduring; so that there would often be a struggle as to which impulse should be followed; and satisfaction, dissatisfaction, or even misery would be felt, as past impressions were compared during their incessant passage through the mind. In this case an inward monitor would tell the animal that it would have been better to have followed the one impulse rather than the other. The one course ought to have been followed, and the other ought not; the one would have been right and the other wrong; but to these terms I shall recur.

Sociability. Animals of many kinds are social; we find even distinct species living together; for example, some American monkeys; and united flocks of rooks, jackdaws, and starlings. Man shews the same feeling in his strong love for the dog, which the dog returns with interest. Every one must have noticed how miserable horses, dogs, sheep, &c., are when separated from their companions, and what strong mutual affection the two former kinds, at least, shew on their reunion. It is curious to speculate on the feelings of a dog, who will rest peacefully for hours in a room with his master or any of the family, without the least notice being taken of him; but if left for a short time by himself, barks or howls dismally. We will confine our attention to the higher social animals; and pass over insects, although some of these are social, and aid one another in many important ways. The most common mutual service in the higher animals is to warn one another of danger by means of the united senses of all. [. . .] Social animals perform many little services for each other: horses nibble, and cows lick each other, on any spot which itches: monkeys search each other for external parasites; and Brehm states that after a troop of the *Cercopithecus griseo-viridis* has rushed through a thorny brake, each monkey stretches itself on a branch, and another monkey sitting by, 'conscientiously' examines its fur, and extracts every thorn or burr.

Animals also render more important services to one another: thus wolves and some other beasts of prey hunt in packs, and aid one another in attacking their victims. Pelicans fish in concert. The Hamadryas baboons turn over stones to find insects, &c.; and when they come to a large one, as many as can stand round, turn it over together and share the booty. Social animals mutually defend each other. [. . .] In Abyssinia, Brehm encountered a great troop of baboons, who were crossing a valley: some had already ascended the opposite mountain, and some were still in the valley: the latter were attacked by the dogs, but the old males immediately hurried down from the rocks, and with mouths widely opened, roared so fearfully, that the dogs quickly drew back. They were again encouraged to the attack; but by this time all the baboons had reascended the heights, excepting a young one, about six months old, who, loudly calling for aid, climbed on a block of rock, and was surrounded. Now one of the largest males, a true hero, came down again from the mountain, slowly went to the young one, coaxed him, and triumphantly led him away—the dogs being too much astonished to make an attack. [. . .]

It is certain that associated animals have a feeling of love for each other, which is not felt by non-social adult animals. How far in most cases they actually sympathise in the pains and pleasures of others, is more doubtful, especially with respect to pleasures. [. . .]

Many animals, however, certainly sympathise with each other's distress or danger. This is the case even with birds. Capt. Stansbury found on a salt lake in Utah an old and completely blind pelican, which was very fat, and must have been well fed for a long time by his companions. Mr Blyth, as he informs me, saw Indian crows feeding two or three of their companions which were blind; and I have heard of an analogous case with the domestic cock. We may, if we choose, call these actions instinctive; but such cases are much too rare for the development of any special instinct. I have myself seen a dog, who never passed a cat who lay sick in a basket, and was a great friend of his, without giving her a few licks with his tongue, the surest sign of kind feeling in a dog. [. . .]

Besides love and sympathy, animals exhibit other qualities connected with the social instincts, which in us would be called moral; and I agree with Agassiz that dogs possess something very like a conscience.

Dogs possess some power of self-command, and this does not appear to be wholly the result of fear. As Braubach remarks, they will refrain from stealing food in the absence of their master. They have long been accepted as the very type of fidelity and obedience. But the elephant is likewise very faithful to his driver or keeper, and probably considers him as the leader of the herd. [. . .]

All animals living in a body, which defend themselves or attack their enemies in concert, must indeed be in some degree faithful to one another; and those that follow a leader must be in some degree obedient. [. . .]

It has often been assumed that animals were in the first place rendered social, and that they feel as a consequence uncomfortable when separated from each other, and comfortable whilst together; but it is a more probable view that these sensations were first developed, in order that those animals which would profit by living in society, should be induced to live together, in the same manner as the sense of hunger and the pleasure of eating were, no doubt, first acquired in order to induce animals to eat. The feeling of pleasure from society is probably an extension of the parental or filial affections, since the social instinct seems to be developed by the young remaining for a long time with their parents; and this extension may be attributed in part to habit, but chiefly to natural selection. With those animals which were benefited by living in close association, the individuals which took the greatest pleasure in society would best escape various dangers; whilst those that cared least for their comrades, and lived solitary, would perish in greater numbers. With respect to the origin of the parental and filial affections, which apparently lie at the base of the social instincts, we know not the steps by which they have been gained; but we may infer that it has been to a large extent through natural selection. [. . .]

Man a social animal. Every one will admit that man is a social being. We see this in his dislike of solitude, and in his wish for society beyond that of his own family. [. . .] As man is a social animal, it is almost certain that he would inherit a tendency to be faithful to his comrades, and obedient to the leader of his tribe; for these qualities are common to most social animals. He would consequently possess some capacity for self-command. He would from an inherited tendency be willing to defend, in concert with others, his fellow-men; and would be ready to aid them in any way, which did not too greatly interfere with his own welfare or his own strong desires.

The social animals which stand at the bottom of the scale are guided almost exclusively, and those which stand higher in the scale are largely guided, by special instincts in the aid which they give to the members of the same community; but they are likewise in part impelled by mutual love and sympathy, assisted apparently by some amount of reason. Although man, as just remarked, has no special instincts to tell him how to aid his fellow-men, he still has the impulse, and with his improved intellectual faculties would naturally be much guided in this respect by reason and experience.

Instinctive sympathy would also cause him to value highly the approbation of his fellows; [. . .] Consequently man would be influenced in the highest degree by the wishes, approbation, and blame of his fellow-men, as expressed by their gestures and language. Thus the social instincts, which must have been acquired by man in a very rude state, and probably even by his early ape-like progenitors, still give the impulse to some of his best actions; but his actions are in a higher degree determined by the expressed wishes and judgment of his fellow-men, and unfortunately very often by his own strong selfish desires. But as love, sympathy and self-command become strengthened by habit, and as the power of reasoning becomes clearer, so that man can value justly the judgments of his fellows, he will feel himself impelled, apart from any transitory pleasure or pain, to certain lines of conduct. He might then declare—not that any barbarian or uncultivated man could thus think—I am the supreme judge of my own conduct, and in the words of Kant, I will not in my own person violate the dignity of humanity.

[*The Descent of Man*, 2nd edn. (John Murray: London, 1875), 97–111. First published in 1871.]

FRIEDRICH NIETZSCHE

10   **The Origins of Herd Morality**

After the social structure as a whole is stabilized and secured against external dangers, it is the fear of one's neighbor that creates new perspectives of moral valuations. Certain strong and dangerous drives, such as love for enterprise, foolhardiness, revenge, cunning, rapacity, and love for domination, all of them traits that had just been not only honored as being socially useful (under other names than these, as seem fair enough), but actually cultivated and fostered (because they were constantly needed to overcome the common danger imposed by the common enemy)—now, with the outlet channels gone, are gradually branded as immoral and given over to defamation. Now the antithetical drives and inclinations come into their own so far as morality is concerned. The herd-instinct draws its conclusions, step by step. How much or how little the common good is endangered, the dangers to the status quo that lie in a given opinion, or state, or passion, in a given will or talent—these now furnish the moral perspective. Here too fear is once again the mother of morality. Communal solidarity is annihilated by the highest and strongest drives that, when they break out passionately, whip the individual far past the average low level of the herd-conscience; society's belief in itself, its backbone as it were, breaks. Hence such drives will best be branded and defamed. A superior, independent intellect, a will to stand alone, even a superior rationality, are felt to be dangers; everything that lifts the individual above the herd and causes fear in his neighbor is from now on called *evil;* the fair-minded, unassuming disposition that adapts and equalizes, all mediocrity of desires comes to be called and honored by the name of morality. Finally, when conditions are very peaceful, all opportunity and necessity for cultivating one's feelings for rigor and hardness disappear; now any rigor, even in the operations of justice, begins to disturb men's conscience. Any superior and rigorous distinction and self-responsibility is felt to be almost insulting; it awakens mistrust; the 'lambs' and even more the 'sheep' gain respect.

> [*Beyond Good and Evil*, trans. Marianne Cowan (Henry Regnery Company: Chicago, 1955), 110–11. First published in 1886.]

SIGMUND FREUD

11 The Cultural Super-Ego

Just as a planet revolves around a central body as well as rotating on its own axis, so the human individual takes part in the course of development of mankind at the same time as he pursues his own path in life. But to our dull eyes the play of forces in the heavens seems fixed in a never-changing order; in the field of organic life we can still see how the forces contend with one another, and how the effects of the conflict are continually changing. So, also, the two urges, the one towards personal happiness and the other towards union with other human beings must struggle with each other in every individual; and so, also, the two processes of individual and of cultural development must stand in hostile opposition to each other and mutually dispute the ground. But this struggle between the individual and society is not a derivative of the contradiction—probably an irreconcilable one—between the primal instincts of Eros and death. It is a dispute within the economics of the libido, comparable to the contest concerning the distribution of libido between ego and objects; and it does admit of an eventual accommodation in the individual, as, it may be hoped, it will also do in the future of civilization, however much that civilization may oppress the life of the individual to-day.

The analogy between the process of civilization and the path of individual development may be extended in an important respect. It can be asserted that the community, too, evolves a super-ego under whose influence cultural development proceeds. It would be a tempting task for anyone who has a knowledge of human civilizations to follow out this analogy in detail. I will confine myself to bringing forward a few striking points. The super-ego of an epoch of civilization has an origin similar to that of an individual. It is based on the impression left behind by the personalities of great leaders—men of overwhelming force of mind or men in whom one of the human impulsions has found its strongest and purest, and therefore often its most one-sided, expression. In many instances the analogy goes still further, in that during their lifetime these figures were—often enough, even if not always—mocked and maltreated by others and even despatched in a cruel fashion. In the same way, indeed, the primal father did not attain divinity until long after he had met his death by violence. The most arresting example of this fateful conjunction is to be seen in the figure of Jesus Christ—if, indeed, that figure is not a part of mythology, which called it into being from an obscure memory of that primal event. Another point of agreement between the cultural and the individual super-ego is that the former, just like the latter, sets up strict ideal demands, disobedience to which is visited with 'fear of conscience'. Here, indeed, we come across the remarkable circumstance that the mental processes concerned are actually more familiar to us and more accessible to consciousness as they are seen in the group than they can be in the individual man. In him, when tension arises, it is only the aggressiveness of the super-ego which, in the form of reproaches, makes itself noisily heard; its actual demands often remain unconscious in the background. If we bring them to conscious knowledge, we find that they coincide with the precepts of the prevailing cultural super-ego. At this point the two processes, that of the cultural development of the group and that of the cultural development of the individual, are, as it were, always interlocked. For that reason some of the manifestations and properties of the super-ego can be more easily detected in its behaviour in the cultural community than in the separate individual.

The cultural super-ego has developed its ideals and set up its demands. Among the latter, those which deal with the relations of human beings to one another are comprised under the heading of ethics. People have at all times set the greatest value on ethics, as though they expected that it in particular would produce especially important results. And it does in fact deal with a subject which can easily be recognized as the sorest spot in every civilization. Ethics is thus to be regarded as a therapeutic attempt—as an endeavour to achieve, by means of a command of the super-ego, something which has so far not been achieved by means of any other cultural activities. As we already know, the problem before us is how to get rid of the greatest hindrance to civilization—namely, the constitutional inclination of human beings to be aggressive towards one another; and for that very reason we are especially interested in what is probably the most recent of the cultural commands of the super-ego, the commandment to love one's neighbour as oneself. In our research into, and therapy of, a neurosis, we are led to make two reproaches against the super-ego of the individual. In the severity of its commands and prohibitions it troubles itself too little about the happiness of the ego, in that it takes insufficient account of the resistances against obeying them—of the instinctual strength of the id [in the first place], and of the difficulties presented by the real external environment [in the second]. Consequently we are very often obliged, for therapeutic purposes, to oppose the super-ego, and we endeavour to lower its demands. Exactly the same objections can be made against the ethical demands of the cultural super-ego. It, too, does not trouble itself enough about the facts of the mental constitution of human beings. It issues a command and does not ask whether it is possible for people to obey it. On the contrary, it assumes that a man's ego is psychologically capable of anything that is required of it, that his ego has unlimited mastery over his id. This is a mistake; and even in what are known as normal people the id cannot be controlled beyond certain limits. If more is demanded of a man, a revolt will be produced in him or a neurosis, or he will be made unhappy. The commandment, 'Love thy neighbour as thyself', is the strongest defence against human aggressiveness and an excellent example of the unpsychological proceedings of the cultural super-ego. The commandment is impossible to fulfil; such an enormous inflation of love can only lower its value, not get rid of the difficulty. Civilization pays no attention to all this; it merely admonishes us that the harder it is to obey the precept the more meritorious it is to do so. But anyone who follows such a precept in present-day civilization only puts himself at a disadvantage *vis-à-vis* the person who disregards it. What a potent obstacle to civilization aggressiveness must be, if the defence against it can cause as much unhappiness as aggressiveness itself!

[*Civilization and its Discontents*, trans. James Strachey (W. W. Norton and Co.: New York, 1962), 88–90. First published in 1930.]

CAROL GILLIGAN

12   In a Different Voice

At a time when efforts are being made to eradicate discrimination between the sexes in the search for social equality and justice, the differences between the sexes are being rediscovered in the social sciences. This discovery occurs when theories formerly considered to be sexually neutral in their scientific objectivity are found instead to reflect a consistent observational and evaluative bias. Then the presumed neutrality of science, like that of language itself, gives way to the recognition that the categories of knowledge are human constructions. The fascination with point of view that has informed the fiction of the twentieth century and the corresponding recognition of the relativity of judgment infuse our scientific understanding as well when we begin to notice how accustomed we have become to seeing life through men's eyes.

A recent discovery of this sort pertains to the apparently innocent classic *The Elements of Style* by William Strunk and E. B. White. A Supreme Court ruling on the subject of sex discrimination led one teacher of English to notice that the elementary rules of English usage were being taught through examples which counterposed the birth of Napoleon, the writings of Coleridge, and statements such as 'He was an interesting talker. A man who had traveled all over the world and lived in half a dozen countries,' with 'Well, Susan, this is a fine mess you are in' or, less drastically, 'He saw a woman, accompanied by two children, walking slowly down the road.'

Psychological theorists have fallen as innocently as Strunk and White into the same observational bias. Implicitly adopting the male life as the norm, they have tried to fashion women out of a masculine cloth. It all goes back, of course, to Adam and Eve—a story which shows, among other things, that if you make a woman out of a man, you are bound to get into trouble. In the life cycle, as in the Garden of Eden, the woman has been the deviant.

The penchant of developmental theorists to project a masculine image, and one that appears frightening to women, goes back at least to Freud, who built his theory of psychosexual development around the experiences of the male child that culminate in the Oedipus complex. In the 1920s, Freud struggled to resolve the contradictions posed for his theory by the differences in female anatomy and the different configuration of the young girl's early family relationships. After trying to fit women into his masculine conception, seeing them as envying that which they missed, he came instead to acknowledge, in the strength and persistence of women's pre-Oedipal attachments to their mothers, a developmental difference. He considered this difference in women's development to be responsible for what he saw as women's developmental failure.

Having tied the formation of the superego or conscience to castration anxiety, Freud considered women to be deprived by nature of the impetus for a clear-cut Oedipal resolution. Consequently, women's superego—the heir to the Oedipus complex—was compromised: it was never 'so inexorable, so impersonal, so independent of its emotional origins as we require it to be in men.' From this observation of difference, that 'for women the level of what is ethically normal is different from what it is in men,' Freud concluded that women 'show less sense of justice than men, that they are less ready to submit to the great exigencies of life, that they are more often influenced in their judgements by feelings of affection or hostility'.[1] [. . .]

---

[1] S. Freud, 'Some Psychical Consequences of the Anatomical Distinction between the Sexes' (1925), in *The Standard Edition of the Complete Psychological Works of Sigmund Freud*, trans. and ed. James Strachey (The Hogarth Press: London, 1961), xix. 257–8.

The criticism that Freud makes of women's sense of justice, seeing it as compromised in its refusal of blind impartiality, reappears not only in the work of Piaget but also in that of Kohlberg. While in Piaget's account of the moral judgment of the child, girls are an aside, a curiosity to whom he devotes four brief entries in an index that omits 'boys' altogether because 'the child' is assumed to be male, in the research from which Kohlberg derives his theory, females simply do not exist.[1] Kohlberg's six stages that describe the development of moral judgment from childhood to adulthood are based empirically on a study of eighty-four boys whose development Kohlberg has followed for a period of over twenty years.[2] Although Kohlberg claims universality for his stage sequence, those groups not included in his original sample rarely reach his higher stages.[3] Prominent among those who thus appear to be deficient in moral development when measured by Kohlberg's scale are women, whose judgments seem to exemplify the third stage of his six-stage sequence. At this stage morality is conceived in interpersonal terms and goodness is equated with helping and pleasing others. This conception of goodness is considered by Kohlberg and Kramer to be functional in the lives of mature women insofar as their lives take place in the home. Kohlberg and Kramer imply that only if women enter the traditional arena of male activity will they recognize the inadequacy of this moral perspective and progress like men toward higher stages where relationships are subordinated to rules (stage four) and rules to universal principles of justice (stages five and six).[4]

Yet herein lies a paradox, for the very traits that traditionally have defined the 'goodness' of women, their care for and sensitivity to the needs of others, are those that mark them as deficient in moral development. In this version of moral development, however, the conception of maturity is derived from the study of men's lives and reflects the importance of individuation in their development. Piaget, challenging the common impression that a developmental theory is built like a pyramid from its base in infancy, points out that a conception of development instead hangs from its vertex of maturity, the point toward which progress is traced. Thus, a change in

[1] Jean Piaget, *The Moral Judgement of the Child* (first published 1932; The Free Press: New York, 1965).

[2] Lawrence Kohlberg, 'The Development of Modes of Thinking and Choices in Years 10 to 16', Ph.D. thesis (University of Chicago, 1958); *The Philosophy of Moral Development* (Harper and Row: San Francisco, 1981).

[3] Carolyn P. Edwards, 'Societal Complexity and Moral Development: A Kenyan Study', *Ethos*, 3 (1975), 505–27; Constance Holstein, 'Development of Moral Judgement: A Longitudinal Study of Males and Females', *Child Development*, 47 (1976): 51–61; Elizabeth L. Simpson, 'Moral Development Research: A Case Study of Scientific Cultural Bias', *Human Development*, 17 (1974), 81–106.

[4] L. Kohlberg and R. Kramer, 'Continuities and Discontinuities in Child and Adult Moral Development,' *Human Development*, 12 (1969), 93–120.

the definition of maturity does not simply alter the description of the highest stage but recasts the understanding of development, changing the entire account.[1]

When one begins with the study of women and derives developmental constructs from their lives, the outline of a moral conception different from that described by Freud, Piaget, or Kohlberg begins to emerge and informs a different description of development. In this conception, the moral problem arises from conflicting responsibilities rather than from competing rights and requires for its resolution a mode of thinking that is contextual and narrative rather than formal and abstract. This conception of morality as concerned with the activity of care centers moral development around the understanding of responsibility and relationships, just as the conception of morality as fairness ties moral development to the understanding of rights and rules.

This different construction of the moral problem by women may be seen as the critical reason for their failure to develop within the constraints of Kohlberg's system. Regarding all constructions of responsibility as evidence of a conventional moral understanding, Kohlberg defines the highest stages of moral development as deriving from a reflective understanding of human rights. That the morality of rights differs from the morality of responsibility in its emphasis on separation rather than connection, in its consideration of the individual rather than the relationship as primary, is illustrated by two responses to interview questions about the nature of morality. The first comes from a twenty-five-year-old man, one of the participants in Kohlberg's study:

[*What does the word morality mean to you?*] Nobody in the world knows the answer. I think it is recognizing the right of the individual, the rights of other individuals, not interfering with those rights. Act as fairly as you would have them treat you. I think it is basically to preserve the human being's right to existence. I think that is the most important. Secondly, the human being's right to do as he pleases, again without interfering with somebody else's rights.

[*How have your views on morality changed since the last interview?*] I think I am more aware of an individual's rights now. I used to be looking at it strictly from my point of view, just for me. Now I think I am more aware of what the individual has a right to.

Kohlberg cites this man's response as illustrative of the principled conception of human rights that exemplifies his fifth and sixth stages. Commenting on the response, Kohlberg says: 'Moving to a perspective outside of that of his society, he identifies morality with justice (fairness, rights, the Golden Rule), with recognition of the rights of others as these are defined naturally

---

[1] Jean Piaget, *Structuralism* (Basic Books: New York, 1970).

or intrinsically. The human being's right to do as he pleases without interfering with somebody else's rights is a formula defining rights prior to social legislation'.

The second response comes from a woman who participated in the rights and responsibilities study. She also was twenty-five and, at the time, a third-year law student:

[*Is there really some correct solution to moral problems, or is everybody's opinion equally right?*] No, I don't think everybody's opinion is equally right. I think that in some situations there may be opinions that are equally valid, and one could conscientiously adopt one of several courses of action. But there are other situations in which I think there are right and wrong answers, that sort of inhere in the nature of existence, of all individuals here who need to live with each other to live. We need to depend on each other, and hopefully it is not only a physical need but a need of fulfillment in ourselves, that a person's life is enriched by cooperating with other people and striving to live in harmony with everybody else, and to that end, there are right and wrong, there are things which promote that end and that move away from it, and in that way it is possible to choose in certain cases among different courses of action that obviously promote or harm that goal.

[*Is there a time in the past when you would have thought about these things differently?*] Oh, yeah, I think that I went through a time when I thought that things were pretty relative, that I can't tell you what to do and you can't tell me what to do, because you've got your conscience and I've got mine.

[*When was that?*] When I was in high school. I guess that it just sort of dawned on me that my own ideas changed, and because my own judgment changed, I felt I couldn't judge another person's judgment. But now I think even when it is only the person himself who is going to be affected, I say it is wrong to the extent it doesn't cohere with what I know about human nature and what I know about you, and just from what I think is true about the operation of the universe, I could say I think you are making a mistake.

[*What led you to change, do you think?*] Just seeing more of life, just recognizing that there are an awful lot of things that are common among people. There are certain things that you come to learn promote a better life and better relationships and more personal fulfillment than other things that in general tend to do the opposite, and the things that promote these things, you would call morally right.[1]

This response also represents a personal reconstruction of morality following a period of questioning and doubt, but the reconstruction of moral understanding is based not on the primacy and universality of individual rights, but rather on what she describes as a 'very strong sense of being responsible to the world.' Within this construction, the moral dilemma changes from how to exercise one's rights without interfering with the

[1] L. Kohlberg, 'Continuities and Discontinuities in Childhood and Adult Moral Development Revisited', in *Collected Papers on Moral Development and Moral Education* (Moral Education Research Foundation: Harvard University, Cambridge, Mass., 1973), 29–30.

rights of others to how 'to lead a moral life which includes obligations to myself and my family and people in general.' The problem then becomes one of limiting responsibilities without abandoning moral concern. When asked to describe herself, this woman says that she values 'having other people that I am tied to, and also having people that I am responsible to. I have a very strong sense of being responsible to the world, that I can't just live for my enjoyment, but just the fact of being in the world gives me an obligation to do what I can to make the world a better place to live in, no matter how small a scale that may be on.' Thus while Kohlberg's subject worries about people interfering with each other's rights, this woman worries about 'the possibility of omission, of your not helping others when you could help them.'

The issue that this woman raises is addressed by Jane Loevinger's fifth 'autonomous' stage of ego development, where autonomy, placed in a context of relationships, is defined as modulating an excessive sense of responsibility through the recognition that other people have responsibility for their own destiny. The autonomous stage in Loevinger's account witnesses a relinquishing of moral dichotomies and their replacement with 'a feeling for the complexity and multifaceted character of real people and real situations'[1] Whereas the rights conception of morality that informs Kohlberg's principled level (stages five and six) is geared to arriving at an objectively fair or just resolution to moral dilemmas upon which all rational persons could agree, the responsibility conception focuses instead on the limitations of any particular resolution and describes the conflicts that remain.

Thus it becomes clear why a morality of rights and noninterference may appear frightening to women in its potential justification of indifference and unconcern. At the same time, it becomes clear why, from a male perspective, a morality of responsibility appears inconclusive and diffuse, given its insistent contextual relativism. Women's moral judgments thus elucidate the pattern observed in the description of the developmental differences between the sexes, but they also provide an alternative conception of maturity by which these differences can be assessed and their implications traced. The psychology of women that has consistently been described as distinctive in its greater orientation toward relationships and interdependence implies a more contextual mode of judgment and a different moral understanding. Given the differences in women's conceptions of self and morality, women bring to the life cycle a different point of view and order human experience in terms of different priorities.

[*In a Different Voice: Psychological Theory and Women's Development* (Harvard University Press: Cambridge, Mass., 1982), 6–22.]

[2] Jane Loevinger and Ruth Wessler, *Measuring Ego Development* (Jossey-Bass: San Francisco, 1970), 6.

Common Themes in Primate Ethics

INTRODUCTION

The ancient Greeks cremated their dead. The Greek historian Herodotus tells how Darius, King of Persia, once asked some Greeks how much he would have to pay them to induce them to eat their fathers' dead bodies. They were shocked by the question, and would not do so for any sum of money. Darius then called in some Indians, whose custom it was to eat the bodies of their parents, and asked them how much they wanted to burn their fathers' bodies. The Indians implored Darius not to mention so dire a deed. The story illustrates the existence of diversity in ethics, but also of the interest that this diversity holds for Darius, for Herodotus, and, down through the centuries, for the modern reader.

Perhaps, however, in being so impressed by diversity, we overlook the more significant common elements in ethics. There seems to be a popular belief that the taboo on incest is the only moral rule that holds everywhere. The reality is that some much more significant ethical principles carry weight in virtually every human community. These include: obligations on members of a family to support their kin; obligations of reciprocity, to return favours done and gifts received; and constraints on sexual relationships. The readings in this section illustrate the widespread acceptance of these obligations and constraints from the time of Hammurabi to our own times, from the China of Confucius to the Melanesian islanders of the Western Pacific, and from the !Kung people of the Kalahari to Martin Luther. (The '!' indicates a kind of clicking noise that precedes the initial letter.) These common elements of human ethics manifest themselves in even the most unpromising circumstances, as Tony Ashworth shows in his study of reciprocity across the opposed trench lines of World War I. The precise form of the obligations or constraints varies from one society to another, but the significance of these universals lies in the fact that obligations of kinship, reciprocity, and sexual relationships form the core of all human ethical systems—and they also guide the behaviour of our close non-human relatives.

The scientific approach to the origin of ethics that began with *The Descent of Man* has become much more sophisticated in the past two decades. So in seeking the origins of the social rules that apply across a wide range of primate societies, we can now turn to evolutionary theory. Our knowledge of genetics makes the existence of obligations between kin totally unsurprising; it also offers a possible explanation for the widespread 'double standard' of sexual morality, which judges female promiscuity more harshly than similar conduct by males. With regard to the evolution of co-operation, biological scientists have been able to draw on findings from another area of thought, known variously as decision theory, rational choice theory, or game theory. The work of Robert Trivers on reciprocal altruism broke new ground here; and Robert Axelrod's ingenious explorations of a situation known as the Prisoner's Dilemma (to be found in the selection from Axelrod that appears below) give us a sharper insight into the logic of reciprocity. This in turn helps to explain why reciprocity is found amongst all social mammals with long memories who live in stable communities and recognize each other as individuals; a description that has applied to human beings for most of their evolutionary history. It also shows that an ethic of 'turn the other cheek' is not only impracticable, but positively harmful.

To pursue questions about the origins and nature of ethics without looking at the full range of possible explanations is to remain wilfully ignorant. Yet, for most of this century, philosophers writing on ethics have focused on what other philosophers writing on ethics have written. The discipline has become ingrown, scrutinizing narrowly framed questions that can be advanced by careful reasoning and argument, while ignoring whole bodies of knowledge about the nature of ethics that have accumulated in other fields of study. Against that background, the readings in this section suggest a case for a change of direction. I write 'suggest' deliberately: the readings are no more than snapshots, taken almost at random, of the ethical practices of different societies. Much more work would need to be done to explore the suggested common themes of primate ethics. Then, when that was done, and we had drawn together all that we know about the nature of primate ethics, we would still have to make a serious attempt to incorporate this knowledge into our philosophical understanding of the subject.

At the same time, we must be careful to establish exactly what it is that the evolutionary explanations show, and what relevance they have to questions about how we ought to live. Attempts to deduce a 'scientific ethics' from the theory of evolution go back to the first reviews of Darwin's *Origin of Species*. Darwin himself rejected the idea that his theory can in any way support the view that 'might makes right', or that 'more evolved' means better. Some of his followers, however, have been so excited by the ability of their discipline to explain some aspects of human behaviour that they have leapt to embrace sweeping claims about the ability of science to eliminate or replace ethics entirely. Such claims are unfounded. We are thinking beings, able to make choices about what we do, choices that are based on our values. No recital of biological facts can dictate to us what our values must be (though we may well want to take such facts into account in our reflections on why we hold the values we do hold, and on the likely consequences of our choices). But the extravagant claims of some over enthusiastic evolutionary theorists should not lead us to ignore the valuable insights that evolutionary theory can provide. As long as we remain on the level of the explanation of ethics, rather than the justification of a particular view about what we ought to do, evolutionary theory has an important role to play in helping us to understand the characteristics common to primate ethics, and why ethics exists at all.

i. Kinship

JANE GOODALL

13 Helping Kin in Chimpanzees

July 1974. Observer Eslom Mpongo followed Madam Bee as she headed slowly for Kahama Stream. Her two daughters, young adult Little Bee and adolescent Honey Bee, were far ahead along the trail that led to a stand of *Saba florida* vines with their large, lemonlike fruits. Madam Bee looked old and sick. Her arm, paralyzed by polio, dragged and several half-healed wounds were visible on her back, head, and one leg. It was very hot that summer, and food was relatively scarce so that the chimpanzees sometimes had to travel considerable distances from one feeding place to the next. Again and again Madam Bee stopped to rest. When soft food calls indicated that the two young females had arrived at the food site, Madam Bee moved a little faster; but when she got there, it seemed that she was too tired or weak to climb. She looked up at her daughters, then lay on the ground and watched as they moved about, searching for ripe fruits. After about ten minutes Little Bee climbed down. She carried one of the fruits by its stem in her mouth and had a second in one hand. As she reached the ground, Madam Bee gave a few soft grunts. Little Bee approached, also grunting, and placed the fruit from her hand on the ground beside her mother. She then sat nearby and the two females ate together.

[L]et me give some examples of helping and altruism in chimpanzee society. An early report is that of Savage and Wyman (1843–44).[1] They describe how a female chimpanzee jumped hastily down from a tree when approached by hunters, but then returned for her infant. She 'took him into her arms, at which moment she was shot.' At Gombe a mother will risk severe punishment by attacking an adult male who is harming her child (during a charging display, for instance). Melissa even leaped at alpha male Mike as he dragged her infant during excitement; he let go of the infant and attacked Melissa. Another time, when the high-ranking and unusually aggressive adult male Humphrey attacked the adolescent Little Bee, her mother and younger sister both hurled themselves at the aggressor—who fled! There are many occasions when an infant or juvenile tries to help his or her mother when she is being attacked. Sometimes this merely involves following at a distance and uttering loud waa-barks, but there are occasions when a child will actually hit or bite the aggressor, even when this is an adult male.

---

[1] T. S. Savage and J. Wyman, 'Observations on the External Character and Habits of the *Troglodytes niger* Geoff., and on its Organization', *Boston Journal of Natural History*, 4 (1843–4), 362–6.

Adults of either sex are likely to go to the aid of their mothers if they happen to be nearby. Goblin once ran some 200 meters when he heard the loud screams of his mother, Melissa, who was being attacked by another female. When he arrived, he displayed toward and attacked his mother's aggressor. Adult males often support their younger siblings, especially brothers, during aggressive incidents: thus Faben and Jomeo frequently hurried to help Figan and Sherry, respectively. Evered was very supportive of his grown sister, Gilka, and almost always intervened on her behalf if he was in the vicinity when she got into social difficulties. Other adult males too occasionally aided their sisters.

[*The Chimpanzees of Gombe* (Harvard University Press: Cambridge, Mass., 1986), 357, 376–7.]

EDWARD WESTERMARCK

14 A Universal Duty

There is one duty so universal and obvious that it is seldom mentioned: the mother's duty to rear her children, provided that they are suffered to live. Another duty—equally primitive, I believe, in the human race—is incumbent on the married man: the protection and support of his family. [. . .]

The parents' duty of taking care of their offspring is, in the first place, based on the sentiment of parental affection. That the maternal sentiment is universal in mankind is a fact too generally admitted to need demonstration; not so the father's love of his children. Savage men are commonly supposed to be very indifferent towards their offspring; but a detailed study of facts leads us to a different conclusion. It appears that, among the lower races, the paternal sentiment is hardly less universal than the maternal, although it is probably never so strong and in many cases distinctly feeble. But more often it displays itself with considerable intensity even among the rudest savages. In the often-quoted case of the Patagonian chief who, in a moment of passion, dashed his little son with the utmost violence against the rocks because he let a basket of eggs which the father handed to him fall down, we have only an instance of savage impetuosity. The same father would, at any other time, have been the most daring, the most enduring, and the most self-devoted in the support and defence of his child. Similarly the Central Australian natives, in fits of sudden passion, when hardly knowing what they do, sometimes treat a child with great severity; but as a rule, to which there are very few exceptions, they are kind and considerate to their children, the men as well as the women carrying them when they get tired on the march, and always seeing that they get a good share of any food. All authorities agree that the Australian Black is affectionate to his children. 'From observation of various tribes in far distant parts of Australia,' says Mr Howitt, 'I can assert confidently that love for their children is a marked feature in the aboriginal character. I cannot recollect having ever seen a parent beat or cruelly use a child; and a short road to the goodwill of the parents is, as amongst us, by noticing and admiring their children. No greater grief could be exhibited, by the fondest parents in the most civilised community at the death of some little child, than that which I have seen exhibited in an Australian native camp, not only by the immediate parents, but by the whole related group.' Other representatives of the lowest savagery, as the Veddahs and Fuegians, are likewise described as tender parents. Though few peoples have acquired a worse reputation for cruelty than the Fijians, even the greatest censurer of their character admits that the exhibition of parental love among them 'is sometimes such as to be worthy of admiration'; whilst, according to another authority, 'it is truly touching to see how parents are attached to their children.' The Bangala of the Upper Congo, 'swayed one moment by a thirst for blood and indulging in the most horrible orgies, . . . may yet the next be found approaching their homes looking forward with the liveliest interest to the caresses of their wives and children.' Carver asserts that he never saw among any other people greater proofs of parental or filial tenderness than among the North American Naudowessies. Among the Point Barrow Eskimo 'the affection of parents for their children is extreme'; and the same seems to be the case among the Eskimo in general. Concerning the Aleuts Veniaminof wrote long ago:—'The children are often well fed and satisfied, while the parents almost perish with hunger. The daintiest morsel, the best dress, is always kept for them.' Mr Hooper, again, found parental love nowhere more strongly exemplified than among the Chukchi; 'the natives absolutely doat upon their children.' Innumerable facts might indeed be quoted to prove that paternal affection is not a late product of civilisation, but a normal feature of the savage mind as it is known to us. [. . .]

We have further to consider the duty of assisting brothers and sisters and more distant relatives. Among the Aleuts, says Veniaminof, a brother 'must always aid his brother in war as well as in the chase, and each protect the other; but if anybody, disregarding this natural law, should go to live apart, caring only for himself, such a one should be discarded by his relatives in case of attack by enemies or animals, or in time of storms; and such dishonourable conduct would lead to general contempt.' Among the Point Barrow Eskimo 'the older children take very good care of the smaller ones'; and of the Sia Indians (Pueblos) we are told that 'a marked trait is their loving kindness and care for younger brothers and sisters.' Dr Schweinfurth writes:—'Notwithstanding . . . that certain instances may be alleged which seem to demonstrate that the character of the Dinka is unfeeling, these cases never refer to such as are bound by the ties of kindred. Parents do not desert their children, nor are brothers faithless to brothers, but are ever prompt to render whatever aid is possible.' I presume that these examples of fraternal relations may, on the whole, be regarded as expressive of universal facts. According to Confucius, the love which brother should bear to brother is second only to that which is due from children to parents.

The duty of assisting more distant relatives is much more variable. It may be said that, as a general rule, among savages and barbarians—with the exception, perhaps, of those who live in small family-groups—as also among the peoples of archaic culture, this duty is more prominent and extends further than amongst ourselves. The blood-tie has much greater strength, related families keep more closely together for mutual protection and aid.

[*The Origin and Development of the Moral Ideas* (Macmillan: London, 1906), i. 526–39.]

DAVID BARASH

15 The Genetic Basis of Kinship

A number of years ago, the great biologist J. B. S. Haldane was asked one day in a pub if he would give up his life for his brother. No, said Haldane, he wouldn't do that, but he would sacrifice himself for *three* brothers or, failing that, nine cousins. His reasoning: humans share one-half their genes with brothers (or sisters), one-quarter with half-siblings, one-eighth their genes with cousins, and so forth. Therefore, any gene that influenced its carrier to risk its body in order to save three brothers (or nine cousins) would result in making more copies of itself than would be lost, even if the individual died in the attempt. Each of us is likely to have more copies of our own genes in the bodies of three siblings or nine cousins than we have within ourselves. In most cases, of course, the choices are not nearly so stark as life and death. But, any time a behavior involves a cost in terms of fitness, we are justified in looking for a benefit in terms of fitness. (Both costs and benefits are measured in the same way, in units of fitness—numbers of genes projected into future generations.)

Actually, relatedness between two individuals is not the only factor determining whether one will be altruistic toward the other. There are two other important considerations: the cost to the altruist in performing the act and the benefit derived by the recipient. Kin selection is a rather complex equation. If we could eavesdrop on a gene's advice to its body, it would go something like this: 'You should be more inclined to help someone the more closely related to him you are. At the same time, you should be more inclined to help him if he really will benefit from it and less inclined if the risk to you is high.' Expressing it quantitatively, we can say that for altruism to evolve via kin selection, the benefit gained by the recipient multiplied by the proportion of genes shared by the would-be altruist and recipient must exceed the cost in fitness suffered by the altruist. This in a nutshell, was Hamilton's great insight. Living things tend to maximize their *inclusive fitness*: the total of their reproductive success through their offspring *plus* that of their relatives. Of course, in maximizing its inclusive fitness, each living thing is expected to devalue relatives proportionately as they are more distantly related—that is, as they share fewer genes with the would-be altruist. A brother or child 'counts' one-half as much as one's self, a cousin one-eighth, and so on.

Does this mean that genes must be good at elementary algebra? Absolutely not. The fact is that evolution has done the arithmetic during the many long generations of every species' history. In the course of time, some genes have directed their bodies to make bad choices, that is, they made errors in solving the critical equation that includes costs, benefits and relatedness. These error-prone genes have left fewer descendants than those whose calculations were more accurate. The result is that we and everything else that lives might not get A's in arithmetic, but we behave as though we are mathematical geniuses. We are selected to do the right things although we may not know why. We are very calculating creatures: How do I love thee? Let me count thy genes.

Before considering ourselves in some detail, let us look at a few more animal examples of genetically selfish altruism. Imagine you are a prairie dog peacefully nibbling at the edge of your colony. There are other prairie dogs nearby, similarly occupied. Suddenly you see a hawk: what do you do? The safest thing, of course, is to hightail it for the nearest burrow, and, indeed, that is what most prairie dogs do. In addition, however, they often give an alarm call that alerts the others. By doing so, they have conferred a benefit on these others, who now have a greater chance of escaping. However, in alerting the other prairie dogs, the alarmists have suffered a personal cost, since they made themselves more conspicuous to the predator and used time calling that might have been time spent running away.

Imagine two prairie dogs: a caller and a non-caller. The altruistic caller stands a better chance of dying (and therefore not reproducing) than the non-caller, who selfishly keeps quiet and therefore is more likely to survive and reproduce. Doesn't that suggest that calling is therefore selected against? Wouldn't there be fewer callers in succeeding generations? Yet, alarm calling in small rodents is very common. When would we expect natural selection to favor the evolution of such apparent altruism? Clearly, when the benefit is high, the cost is low, and the relatedness between alarmer and hearers is high enough to make the equation give a positive fitness benefit to alarmist genes. We have every reason to believe that this is exactly what happens, and although not all hearers and callers are necessarily related, enough are to permit the system to evolve. In point of fact, though, calling is generally reserved for situations in which relatives are nearby.

Round-tailed ground squirrels are rodents similar in many ways to prairie dogs. The males wander quite a bit, especially in the spring, and if we look at a colony of these animals in the spring, we'll find that the males are likely to be unrelated to their neighbors. What happens when a predator appears? You guessed it: Christopher Dunford of the University of Arizona observed twenty-five alarm-calling episodes, between January and April: of these, twenty-three were performed by females. There is a further test. The young are born later in the year, and by summer those juveniles remaining near their mothers are surrounded by close kin. At this point, more than coincidentally, males are as likely as females to give alarms. Zoologist Paul Sherman of the University of California, Berkeley, has found similar results in an intensive study of another species of ground squirrel. Reproducing females do more alarm calling than those without offspring nearby; those with living relatives nearby do more than those without; residents do more than transients; and females generally do more than males. As you might expect, males in this species live far from their relatives (male animals are often less likely to associate with relatives, probably because males tend to be the more competitive sex), whereas females live nearby. [. . .]

In its most extreme form, the converse of altruism is probably antagonism, resulting in a reduction in the fitness of the victim. Japanese monkeys don't usually hurt each other seriously. But it is significant that, when they do, the aggressor is usually a non-resident and non-relative. Closer to home, pre-industrial human societies are often at war—not the organized full-scale wars of conquest that we practice in our 'advanced' societies, but rather a continuing pattern of feuds and skirmishes. And, no less than among Japanese monkeys, kinship counts. These human hostilities are especially difficult to halt, since they often seek to avenge 'blood debts' incurred in the past. A killing requires revenge, and all relatives on each side must help. Of course, successful revenge demands further revenge from the most recently injured party, and so it continues. Although this system of kin avenging kin is somewhat hard on its victims, it does serve as a damper to massively destructive antagonisms, since everyone concerned knows that injustice visited upon someone else will be a cause for retaliation. Each individual is in a sense protected by his or her own network of relatives. For this reason particularly, young women of many tropical Amazonian tribes are terrified of being married to a man in a distant village—among strangers, they will have no relatives to defend them from their husband's likely brutality.

We all live within a very real and personalized fabric of relatedness, most densely woven near ourselves and progressively thinner as we move away. Accordingly, we expect—and find—the greatest altruism within our immediate family, less among those to whom we are less closely related, and finally perhaps, outright antagonism toward (and from) strangers. We can all recognize this pattern in our daily lives. We *give* Christmas presents to those that are close to us, without reckoning what we get in return; we *exchange* cards with those we know but don't 'love'; and as for a total stranger such as a merchant, we may have little compunction about cheating him—or he us—when either party can get away with it. We are hardly alone in this pattern. University of Michigan anthropologist Marshall Sahlins has shown that among non-industrialized societies, something close to selfless altruism prevails within a household and to a lesser extent among more distant relatives; tit-for-tat holds within the village or the larger ethnic group; and interactions between villages or tribes may be frankly exploitative. The close fit between the expectations of sociobiology and the facts of human social behavior is especially striking when we consider that Sahlins's description was not developed with evolutionary considerations in mind. [. . .]

So the sharing of genes appears to be crucial for certain aspects of social behavior. Although groups of living things can reside together without sharing genes, they are unlikely in such cases to show much in the way of altruistic behavior. On the other hand, when genetic relatedness is high, altruism is to be expected.

My dictionary defines nepotism as 'favoritism shown towards a relative, on the basis of relationship.' Webster and his associates were not sociobiologists and neither are most people, but we are all carriers of genes that have scored well on their evolutionary cost-benefit calculations. This is, in part, probably why nepotism is a virtually universal human trait. Kinship is a basic organizing principle in all human cultures. It is the backbone that supports *Homo sapiens* society, and sociobiology provides a coherent explanation for why: we maximize our inclusive fitness when we treat relatives differently from strangers. Obviously, not every peculiar detail of human social life is determined by the requirements of our inclusive fitness, but biology does provide the underlying matrix—the cake—on top of which human cultural diversity lavishes the icing. What could be more natural?

[*The Whisperings Within* (Harper and Row: New York, 1979), 135–41.]

ii. Reciprocity

FRANS DE WAAL

16   **Chimpanzee Justice**

The influence of the recent past is always overestimated. When we are asked to name the greatest human inventions we tend to think of the telephone, the electric light bulb and the silicon chip rather than the wheel, the plough and the taming of fire. Similarly the origins of modern society are sought in the advent of agriculture, trade and industry, whereas in fact our social history is a thousand times older than these phenomena. It has been suggested that food sharing was a strong stimulus in furthering the evolution of our tendency to reciprocal relations. Would it not be more logical to assume that social reciprocity existed earlier, and that tangible exchanges such as food sharing stem from this phenomenon?

Be this as it may, there are indications of reciprocity in the non-material behaviour of chimpanzees. This is seen, for instance, in their coalitions (A supports B, and vice versa), non-intervention alliances (A remains neutral if B does the same), sexual bargaining (A tolerates B mating after B has groomed A) and reconciliation blackmail (A refuses to have contact with B unless B 'greets' A). It is interesting that reciprocity occurs in both the negative and the positive sense. Nikkie's habit of individually punishing females who a short time before joined forces against him has already been described. In this way he repaid a negative action with another negative action. We regularly see this mechanism in operation before the group separates for the night. This is the time when differences are squared, no matter when these differences may have arisen. For example, one morning a conflict breaks out between Mama and Oor. Oor rushes to Nikkie and with wild gestures and exaggeratedly loud screams persuades him to attack her powerful opponent. Nikkie attacks Mama and Oor wins. That evening, however, a good six hours later, we hear the sound of a scuffle in the sleeping quarters. The keeper later tells me that Mama has attacked Oor in no uncertain manner. Needless to say Nikkie was nowhere in the vicinity. [. . .]

The principle of exchange makes it possible actively to teach someone something: good behaviour is rewarded, bad behaviour is punished. A development in the relationship between Mama and Nikkie demonstrates just how complex such influencing processes can be. Their relationship is ambivalent. There are numerous indications that the two of them are very fond of each other. For example, when Mama returned to the group after an absence of over a month, she spent hours grooming Nikkie, and not Gorilla, Jimmie, Yeroen or any of the other individuals with whom she normally spends her time. And of all the children in the colony Moniek, Mama's daughter, is obviously Nikkie's favourite. But for a while it was the hostile side of their relationship which got the upper hand. This was at the beginning of Nikkie's leadership. Yeroen used to mobilize adult females against the young leader and Mama was his major ally. At the end of such incidents, when Nikkie had been reconciled with Yeroen, he would go over to Mama to punish her for the part she had played. This could take a very long time, because Mama usually punished Nikkie in return by rejecting his subsequent attempts at reconciliation. For instance, Nikkie slaps Mama, but a little later he comes back and sits down by her 'shyly' plucking at some wisps of grass. Mama pretends she has not seen him, gets up and walks off. Nikkie waits a while, then starts all over again, with his hair on end. This was clearly a phase of negative reciprocity.

As Yeroen's resistance to Nikkie decreased, Mama became more favourably inclined towards Nikkie. She still supported Yeroen, but when Nikkie made his peace with her later she no longer took any 'affective revenge' and their conflict remained brief. Later still—a process taking years—Mama reconciled her differences with Nikkie before his conflict with Yeroen had ended. One moment the two older apes were chasing after Nikkie, the next moment Mama affectionately embraced him. The conflict then continued between the two males, but Mama declined to take any further part.

In time the situation became even stranger. Nikkie began kissing Mama before or even during his display against Yeroen. This developed gradually from their reconciliations, until it took place without any preceding conflict. It could be seen as a mark of Mama's neutrality. Nikkie and Mama were showing positive reciprocity.

I have done a statistical study of the bilateral nature of coalitions by comparing how each individual intervenes in the conflicts of the others. In periods of stability such interventions are symmetrical, both in a positive sense (two individuals support each other) and in a negative sense (two individuals support each other's opponents). If we are to get a full picture of reciprocity, however, we will have to analyse more kinds of behaviour. Interventions need not necessarily be offset by other interventions. The receipt of regular support may be answered by greater tolerance towards the supporter, or by grooming. Perhaps we will eventually be able to conduct such an analysis in Arnhem. For the time being I should like to sum up as follows: chimpanzee group life is like a market in power, sex, affection, support, intolerance and hostility. The two basic rules are 'one good turn deserves another' and 'an eye for an eye, a tooth for a tooth'.

The rules are not always obeyed and flagrant disobedience may be punished. This happened once after Puist had supported Luit in chasing Nikkie.

When Nikkie later displayed at Puist she turned to Luit and held out her hand to him in search of support. Luit, however, did nothing to protect her against Nikkie's attack. Immediately Puist turned on Luit, barking furiously, chased him across the enclosure and even hit him. If her fury was in fact the result of Luit's failure to help her after she had helped him, this would suggest that reciprocity among chimpanzees is governed by the same sense of moral rightness and justice as it is among humans.

[*Chimpanzee Politics* (Jonathan Cape: London, 1982), 205–7.]

TONY ASHWORTH

17 Live and Let Live

Live and let live was a truce where enemies stopped fighting by agreement for a period of time: the British let the Germans live provided the Germans let them live in return. Essentially, the term live and let live denoted a process of reciprocal exchange among antagonists, where each diminished the other's risk of death, discomfort and injury by a deliberate restriction of aggressive activity, but only on condition that the other requited the restraint. The 'profound difference' between the quiet sector and the active sector was, therefore, the exchange of peace, according to the rules of live and let live on the former, and the exchange of aggression according to the rules of kill or be killed[1]—the high command policy for normal trench war—upon the latter. The quietness of a sector did not signify either a social void or vacuum between enemies but the replacement of one form of exchange with the enemy by another, which trench fighters found more consistent with their needs.

Truces were usually tacit, but always unofficial and illicit. The agreement between antagonists was unspoken and expressed in certain actions—or non-actions—which were meaningful to front fighters but not always to others. Truces were illegal at all times for they were neither created nor legitimated by authority but explicitly forbidden. The unofficial policy of live and let live was the antithesis of the official kill or be killed.

The size of truces varied considerably. The smallest truce involved only two adversaries, chatting, perhaps, after a chance meeting in no-man's-land, like that described in his diary by an officer of the 24th division:

Visited the sentry posts at 7 a.m. and at the bottom of the largest crater I found Pte Bates . . . who was rather undersized and comical looking . . . fraternising with a German . . . The following was their conversation. Bates: 'What rank are you in

---

[1] Lord Wavell, himself a trench fighter, used the phrase 'kill or be killed' to describe the official trench war policy. See R. H. Kiernan, *Wavell* (George Harrap: London, 1945), 173.

your army?' 'I am a corporal', indicating stripes on his collar. 'What rank are you?'—'Oh', replied Bates, 'I am Company Sergt.-Major'.[1]

On the other hand a truce could implicate hundreds of soldiers: infantry-men, gunners, trench-mortar crews and so forth, and extend along several thousand yards of the front line. Such large-scale truces often surprised new troops on their first trench tour, whose expectations of trench war contrasted with its reality. 'Probably the most outstanding impression gained was the prevailing quietude', remarked an officer of the 41st division. 'It was difficult to believe that there was a war on and that this was really the front line'.[2]

The duration of a truce varied from a few minutes, as with small groups of fraternising trench fighters, to several days, weeks or even months in rare cases where large numbers and areas were involved. Moreover, while the abstract principle of live and let live (exchange) was at all places and times the same in trench warfare, truces assumed a multitude of concrete forms. Clearly, a few soldiers overtly fraternising face to face in a shell crater was a very different situation from one where a large number were covertly involved in a truce and communicating with each other, not directly in a face-to-face situation, but indirectly and over long distances. The former was a definite, explicit agreement between antagonists, whereas the latter was an implicit agreement, comprised of the mutually held assumption of seasoned trench fighters of both sides, that the adversary was in the mood to exchange peace, given a chance. Nevertheless, despite their relatively indefinite form, the influence of large-scale tacit truces was real enough in the trench war, as we will see. [. . .]

[E]xactly how and when were the rules of the game passed on to new troops? In the B.E.F. fresh divisions usually went for an official tour of instruction into trenches held by veterans, and where the line was quiet the newcomers were often instructed in the art of peace as well as war. Such a situation was described by a private of the greenhorn 47th division who with others of his section had been instructed and now were about to take over the trenches from their tutors and, for the first time, hold them alone. The private spoke with the outgoing soldiers:

The man Mike gave some useful hints on trench work. 'It's the Saxons that's across the road' he said, pointing to the enemy lines which were very silent. I had not heard a bullet whistle over since I entered the trench. On the left was an interesting rifle and machine gun fire all the time. 'They're quiet fellows, the Saxons, they don't

---

[1] F. Hitchcock, *Stand to* (Hurst and Blackett: London, 1937), 125 (24th division, 2 / The Leinster Regiment, Nov. 1915, St Eloi, 2nd Army).
[2] R. O. Russel, *The History of the 11th (Lewisham) Battalion The Queen's Own Royal West Kent Regiment* (Lewisham Newspaper Co.: London, 1934), 36 (41st division, 11 / RWK Regt., May 1916, Ploegstreet, 2nd Army).

want to fight any more than we do, so there's a kind of understanding between us. Don't fire at us and we'll not fire at you'.[1]

Likewise a unit of the 29th division took over trenches in France for the first time and was told by an N.C.O. of the garrison relieved that 'Mr Bosche ain't a bad feller. You leave 'im alone: 'e'll leave you alone'.[2]

In much the same way when a single newcomer joined a seasoned unit, he might be told by an old hand both of his official duties and of the unofficial rules guiding their performance. R. C. Sherriff, who served with the 24th division, described such an incident where one officer takes his new colleague around the trenches. Together they crawl along a sap into no-man's-land. A German trench is nearby:

'Yes' said Trotter . . . 'that's the Bosche front line. Bosche looking over this way now, maybe, just as we are—do you play cricket?' he added . . . 'A bit' said Raleigh, 'could you chuck a cricket ball that distance?' 'I think so'. 'Then you could do the same with a Mills Bomb . . . But you won't though' said Trotter . . . 'Come on, let sleeping dogs lie. If we was to throw a bomb you can bet your boots the old Bosche would chuck one back, and Mr Digby and Mr 'Arris (the soldiers occupying the sap) . . . are both married men. Wouldn't be cricket would it?'[3]

One can agree with Trotter: not that it isn't cricket; but neither is it war. [. . .]

A distinction has been drawn between problems of the origin and the persistence of live and let live. In respect of origins, truces emerged before the Christmas of 1914 and first occurred in non-combat activities concerned with the fulfilment of basic needs. Probably these early truces were *ad hoc* and short-lived arrangements but once established they tended to persist and to evolve in accord with a circular process of cause and effect: live and let live entailed indirect or direct communication among enemies, and such communication implied mutual empathy, while empathy encouraged the evolution of live and let live in two ways—firstly, by reinforcing existing truces, and, secondly, by spreading truces into combat activities.

Accordingly, it seems that both sides soon started to make assumptions about each other's behaviour in respect of areas unrelated to war. For example, each side speculated that if we allow the enemy to breakfast in peace, they will allow us the same in return, since like us they are hungry. Mutual empathy was implied in such reasoning and this increased as assumptions were affirmed by events. Moreover the meaning of inertia both as a means of communication and as a mode of live and let live grew less

---

[1] P. MacGill, *The Red Horizon* (Herbert Jenkins: London, 1916), 84 (47th division, 18 / London Regiment, Mar. 1915, N. Festubert, 1st Army).

[2] S. Gillon, *The Story of the 29th Division* (Nelson: London, 1925), 77 (29th division, May 1916, N. Englebelmer, 4th Army). The 29th relieved the 31st division.

[3] R. C. Sherriff and V. Bartlett, *Journey's End* (Corgi: London, 1968), 129–30.

ambiguous as empathy advanced. As a result empathy extended simply and logically to the thought that if we leave the enemy absolutely in peace they will also leave us in peace. When this expectancy was realised, the diffusion of truces from non-combat to combat activities had occurred. The peace within the war now persisted. [. . .]

High command was hostile both to overt and covert truces. Fraternisation was visible, and the authorities quickly and effectively moved against persons involved; in consequence, such truces were not endemic, although they occurred at intervals throughout the war. On the other hand, inertia was a subtle and tacit thing. High command could neither identify nor prove that certain persons at certain places and times had colluded with the enemy. The generals defined inertia as a problem of morale rather than law, but their directives were ineffectual as a counter to inertia which became widespread during the early part of the war. In conclusion, a picture should be emerging by now of soldiers who were not so dominated by events that they were entirely powerless. If they chose, trench fighters could exercise some control over the matter of life and death.

[*Trench Warfare, 1914–1918: The Live and Let Live System* (Macmillan: London, 1980),
19–20, 29–30, 46–7.]

LORNA MARSHALL

18   Reciprocal Gift-Giving among the !Kung

The two rigid requirements in gift-giving are that one must not refuse a proffered gift and that one must give in return. Demi said that even if he might prefer not to be obligated to someone, he would accept and prepare to make his return gift. If a gift were to be refused, he continued, the giver would be terribly angry. He would say, 'Something is very wrong here.' This could involve whole groups in tensions, bad words, taking sides— even a talk might occur—just what the !Kung do not want. Demi said it does not happen: a !Kung never refuses a gift. (I thought of our Christmas giving and how one would feel if one's Christmas gift were refused.) And a !Kung does not fail to give in return. ≠Toma said that would be 'neglecting friendship.' A person would know that others thought him 'far-hearted' and 'this would worry him.'

In reciprocating, one does not give the same object back again but something of comparable value. The interval of time between receiving and reciprocating varies from a few weeks to a few years. Propriety requires that there be no unseemly haste. The giving must not look like trading.

Incidentally, we were not included by the !Kung in their gift-giving patterns. They gave us a few things spontaneously which they thought we would enjoy—python meat for instance—but did not feel obligated to reciprocate for every gift we gave them.

Asking for a first-time gift or asking that a return gift be made after due time has elapsed is within the rules of propriety. People prefer that others give in return without being asked, but ≠ Toma says he does not hesitate to ask if a gift is long overdue. If a person wants a particular object he may ask for it. Asking is also a means by which people play upon each other's feelings. One can test a friendship in this way. One can give vent to jealousy or satisfy it by acquiring some object. And one can make someone else uncomfortable. I thought that / Ti!kay (an intelligent man, but very touchy, self-centered, and—with us—uncooperative) used to ask for gifts in order to play with anger, arousing it for the sake of feeling it, as children do with fear, playing witches in the dark. His remarks one day indicated a mingling of feelings and purposes. He told us that one may ask for anything. He did, he said. He would go to a person's fire and sit and ask. (I could imagine him sitting and asking, his black eyes glancing around.) He would ask usually for only one or two things, but if a person had a lot, he might ask for more. He said he was almost never refused. However, if a man had only one pot and / Ti!kay asked for it, the man might say, 'I am not refusing but it is the only pot I have. If I get another, you may come for this one. I am very sorry but this is the only pot I have.' / Ti!kay said this would not make him angry unless he were refused too many times. To be refused too many times makes a person very angry. But, said / Ti!kay, he himself did not tire of people asking him for gifts. Asking, he claimed, 'formed a love' between people. It meant 'he still loves me, that is why he is asking.' At least it formed a communication of some sort between people, I thought.

I have stressed the mitigation of envy and jealousy as the important value of gift-giving. !Kung informants stressed more the value of making a friendly gesture even if it is only a token gesture. It puts people under the obligation of making a friendly gesture in return. People are quite conscious of this and speak about it. Demi said, 'The worst thing is not giving gifts. If people do not like each other but one gives a gift and the other must accept, this brings a peace between them. We give to one another always. We give what we have. This is the way we live together.'

[*The !Kung of Nyae Nyae* (Harvard University Press: Cambridge, Mass., 1976), 309–11.]

BRUNO MALINOWSKI

19 The Kula Ring

The Kula is a form of exchange, of extensive, inter-tribal character; it is carried on by communities inhabiting a wide ring of islands, which form a closed circuit [. . .] to the North and East of the East end of New Guinea. Along this route, articles of two kinds, and these two kinds only, are constantly travelling in opposite directions. In the direction of the hands of a clock, moves constantly one of these kinds—long necklaces of red shell, called *soulava*. In the opposite direction moves the other kind—bracelets of white shell called *mwali*. Each of these articles, as it travels in its own direction on the closed circuit, meets on its way articles of the other class, and is constantly being exchanged for them. Every movement of the Kula articles, every detail of the transactions is fixed and regulated by a set of traditional rules and conventions, and some acts of the Kula are accompanied by an elaborate magical ritual and public ceremonies.

On every island and in every village, a more or less limited number of men take part in the Kula—that is to say, receive the goods, hold them for a short time, and then pass them on. Therefore every man who is in the Kula, periodically though not regularly, receives one or several *mwali* (armshells), or a *soulava* (necklace of red shell discs), and then has to hand it on to one of his partners, from whom he receives the opposite commodity in exchange. Thus no man ever keeps any of the articles for any length of time in his possession. One transaction does not finish the Kula relationship, the rule being 'once in the Kula, always in the Kula,' and a partnership between two men is a permanent and lifelong affair. Again, any given *mwali* or *soulava* may always be found travelling and changing hands, and there is no question of its ever settling down, so that the principle 'once in the Kula, always in the Kula' applies also to the valuables themselves.

The ceremonial exchange of the two articles is the main, the fundamental aspect of the Kula. But associated with it, and done under its cover, we find a great number of secondary activities and features. Thus, side by side with the ritual exchange of arm- shells and necklaces, the natives carry on ordinary trade. [. . .]

The Kula is not a surreptitious and precarious form of exchange. It is, quite on the contrary, rooted in myth, backed by traditional law, and surrounded with magical rites. All its main transactions are public and ceremonial, and carried out according to definite rules. It is not done on the spur of the moment, but happens periodically, at dates settled in advance, and it is carried on along definite trade routes, which must lead to fixed trysting places. Sociologically, though transacted between tribes differing in language, culture, and probably even in race, it is based on a fixed and permanent status, on a partnership which binds into couples some thousands of individuals. This partnership is a lifelong relationship, it implies various mutual duties and privileges, and constitutes a type of inter-tribal relationship on an enormous scale. As to the economic mechanism of the transactions, this is based on a specific form of credit, which implies a high degree of mutual trust. [. . .]

Men living at hundreds of miles' sailing distance from one another are bound together by direct or intermediate partnership, exchange with each other, know of each other, and on certain occasions meet in a large inter-tribal gathering. Objects given by one, in time reach some very distant indirect partner or other, and not only Kula objects, but various articles of domestic use and minor gifts. It is easy to see that in the long run, not only objects of material culture, but also customs, songs, art motives and general cultural influences travel along the Kula route. It is a vast, inter-tribal net of relationships, a big institution, consisting of thousands of men, all bound together by one common passion for Kula exchange, and secondarily, by many minor ties and interests. [. . .]

As just explained, the armshells and shell-strings always travel in their own respective directions on the ring, and they are never, under any circumstances, traded back in the wrong direction. Also, they never stop. It seems almost incredible at first, but it is the fact, nevertheless, that no one ever keeps any of the Kula valuables for any length of time. Indeed, in the whole of the Trobriands there are perhaps only one or two specially fine armshells and shell-necklaces permanently owned as heirlooms, and these are set apart as a special class, and are once and for all out of the Kula. 'Ownership,' therefore, in Kula, is quite a special economic relation. A man who is in the Kula never keeps any article for longer than, say, a year or two. Even this exposes him to the reproach of being niggardly, and certain districts have the bad reputation of being 'slow' and 'hard' in the Kula. On the other hand, each man has an enormous number of articles passing through his hands during his life time, of which he enjoys a temporary possession, and which he keeps in trust for a time. This possession hardly ever makes him use the articles, and he remains under the obligation soon again to hand them on to one of his partners. But the temporary ownership allows him to draw a great deal of renown, to exhibit his article, to tell how he obtained it, and to plan to whom he is going to give it. And all this forms one of the favourite subjects of tribal conversation and gossip, in which the feats and the glory in Kula of chiefs or commoners are constantly discussed and re-discussed. Thus every article moves in one direction only, never comes back, never permanently stops, and takes as a rule some two to ten years to make the round. [. . .]

This social code, such as we find it among the natives of the Kula is, however, far from weakening the natural desirability of possession; on the contrary, it lays down that to possess is to be great, and that wealth is the indispensable appanage of social rank and attribute of personal virtue. But the important point is that with them to possess is to give—and here the natives differ from us notably. A man who owns a thing is naturally expected to share it, to distribute it, to be its trustee and dispenser. And the higher the rank the greater the obligation. A chief will naturally be expected to give food to any stranger, visitor, even loiterer from another end of the village. He will be expected to share any of the betel-nut or tobacco he has about him. So that a man of rank will have to hide away any surplus of these articles which he wants to preserve for his further use. [. . .] Thus the main symptom of being powerful is to be wealthy, and of wealth is to be generous. Meanness, indeed, is the most despised vice, and the only thing about which the natives have strong moral views, while generosity is the essence of goodness. [. . .]

Thus the fundamental principle of the natives' moral code in this matter makes a man do his fair share in Kula transaction and the more important he is, the more will he desire to shine by his generosity.

[*Argonauts of the Western Pacific* (Routledge and Kegan Paul: London, 1922), 81–97.]

CONFUCIUS

20 A Single Word

Someone said: 'What about "Repay hostility with kindness"?' The Master said: 'How then do you repay kindness? Repay hostility with uprightness and repay kindness with kindness.' [. . .]

Zigong asked: 'Is there a single word such that one could practise it throughout one's life?' The Master said: 'Reciprocity perhaps? Do not inflict on others what you yourself would not wish done to you.'

[*Analects*, trans. Raymond Dawson (Oxford University Press: Oxford, 1993), 58, 62.
Written in 6th–5th cent. BC.]

21 The Law of Hammurabi

196. If a seignior has destroyed the eye of a member of the aristocracy, they shall destroy his eye.

197. If he has broken a(nother) seignior's bone, they shall break his bone.

198. If he has destroyed the eye of a commoner or broken the bone of a commoner, he shall pay one mina of silver.

199. If he has destroyed the eye of a seignior's slave or broken the bone of a seignior's slave, he shall pay one-half his value.

200. If a seignior has knocked out a tooth of a seignior of his own rank, they shall knock out his tooth.

201. If he has knocked out a commoner's tooth, he shall pay one-third mina of silver.

202. If a seignior has struck the cheek of a seignior who is superior to him, he shall be beaten sixty (times) with an oxtail whip in the assembly.

203. If a member of the aristocracy has struck the cheek of a(nother) member of the aristocracy who is of the same rank as himself, he shall pay one mina of silver.

204. If a commoner has struck the cheek of a(nother) commoner, he shall pay ten shekels of silver.

205. If a seignior's slave has struck the cheek of a member of the aristocracy, they shall cut off his ear.

206. If a seignior has struck a(nother) seignior in a brawl and has inflicted an injury on him, that seignior shall swear, 'I did not strike him deliberately'; and he shall also pay for the physician.

207. If he has died because of his blow, he shall swear (as before), and if it was a member of the aristocracy, he shall pay one-half mina of silver.

208. If it was a member of the commonalty, he shall pay one-third mina of silver.

209. If a seignior struck a(nother) seignior's daughter and has caused her to have a miscarriage, he shall pay ten shekels of silver for her fetus.

210. If that woman has died, they shall put his daughter to death.

[*Ancient Near Eastern Texts relating to the Old Testament*, ed. James Pritchard (Princeton University Press: Princeton, NJ, 1969), 175. Written in 1792–1750 BC.]

JESUS

22   Turn the Other Cheek

38. Ye have heard that it hath been said. An eye for an eye, and a tooth for a tooth:

39. But I say unto you, That ye resist not evil: but whosoever shall smite thee on thy right cheek, turn to him the other also.

40. And if any man will sue thee at the law, and take away thy coat, let him have *thy* cloke also.

41. And whosoever shall compel thee to go a mile, go with him twain.

42. Give to him that asketh thee, and from him that would borrow of thee turn not thou away.

43. Ye have heard that it hath been said, Thou shalt love thy neighbour, and hate thine enemy.

44. But I say unto you, Love your enemies, bless them that curse you, do good to them that hate you, and pray for them which despitefully use you, and persecute you;

45. That ye may be the children of your Father which is in heaven: for he maketh his sun to rise on the evil and on the good, and sendeth rain on the just and on the unjust.

46. For if ye love them which love you, what reward have ye? do not even the publicans the same?

47. And if ye salute your brethren only, what do ye more *than others?* do not even the publicans so?

48. Be ye therefore perfect, even as your Father which is in heaven is perfect.

[The Gospel According to St Matthew 5: 38–48, King James Version. Written in *c*.85 AD.]

HILLEL

23 **The Whole Torah, while Standing on One Foot**

On another occasion it happened that a certain heathen came before Shammai and said to him, 'Make me a proselyte, on condition that you teach me the whole Torah while I stand on one foot.' Thereupon he repulsed him with the builder's cubit which was in his hand. When he went before Hillel, he said to him, 'What is hateful to you, do not to your neighbour that is the whole Torah, while the rest is the commentary thereof; go and learn it.'

[*The Babylonian Talmud (Seder Moʻed): Shabbath*, ed. I. Epstein, trans. M. Freedman (The Soncino Press: London, 1938), 140. Written in *c*.30 AD.]

ROBERT TRIVERS

24 **The Evolution of Reciprocal Altruism**

Altruistic behavior can be defined as behavior that benefits another organism, not closely related, while being apparently detrimental to the organism performing the behavior, benefit and detriment being defined in terms of contribution to inclusive fitness. One human being leaping into water, at some danger to himself, to save another distantly related human from drowning may be said to display altruistic behavior. If he were to leap in to save his own child, the behavior would not necessarily be an instance of 'altruism'; he may merely be contributing to the survival of his own genes invested in the child.

Models that attempt to explain altruistic behavior in terms of natural selection are models designed to take the altruism out of altruism. For example, Hamilton has demonstrated that degree of relationship is an important parameter in predicting how selection will operate, and behavior which appears altruistic may, on knowledge of the genetic relationships of the organisms involved, be explicable in terms of natural selection: those genes being selected for that contribute to their own perpetuation, regardless of which individual the genes appear in.[1] The term 'kin selection' will be used in this paper to cover instances of this type—that is, of organisms being selected to help their relatively close kin.

The model presented here is designed to show how certain classes of behavior conveniently denoted as 'altruistic' (or 'reciprocally altruistic') can be selected for even when the recipient is so distantly related to the organism performing the altruistic act that kin selection can be ruled out. The model will apply, for example, to altruistic behavior between members of different species. It will be argued that under certain conditions natural selection favors these altruistic behaviors because in the long run they benefit the organism performing them.

The Model

One human being saving another, who is not closely related and is about to drown, is an instance of altruism. Assume that the chance of the drowning man dying is one-half if no one leaps in to save him, but that the chance that his potential rescuer will drown if he leaps in to save him is much smaller, say, one in twenty. Assume that the drowning man always drowns when his rescuer does and that he is always saved when the rescuer survives the rescue attempt. Also assume that the energy costs involved in rescuing are trivial compared to the survival probabilities. Were this an isolated event, it is clear that the rescuer should not bother to save the drowning man. But if the drowning man reciprocates at some future time, and if the survival chances are then exactly reversed, it will have been to the benefit of each participant to have risked his life for the other. Each participant will have traded a one-half chance of dying for about a one-tenth chance. If we assume that the entire population is sooner or later exposed to the same risk of drowning, the two individuals who risk their lives to save each other will be selected over those who face drowning on their own. Note that the benefits of reciprocity depend on the unequal cost/benefit ratio of the altruistic act, that is, the benefit of the altruistic act to the recipient is greater than the cost of the act to the performer, cost and benefit being defined here as the increase or decrease in chances of the relevant alleles propagating themselves in the population. Note also that, as defined, the benefits and costs depend on the age of the altruist and recipient. (The odds assigned above may not be unrealistic if the drowning man is drowning because of a cramp or if the rescue can be executed by extending a branch from shore.)

---

[1] W. D. Hamilton, 'The Genetical Evolution of Social Behavior', *Journal of Theoretical Biology*, 7 (1964) 1–52.

Why should the rescued individual bother to reciprocate? Selection would seem to favor being saved from drowning without endangering oneself by reciprocating. Why not cheat? ('Cheating' is used throughout this paper solely for convenience to denote failure to reciprocate: no conscious intent or moral connotation is implied.) Selection will discriminate against the cheater if cheating has later adverse affects on his life which outweigh the benefit of not reciprocating. This may happen if the altruist responds to the cheating by curtailing all future possible altruistic gestures to this individual. Assuming that the benefits of these lost altruistic acts outweigh the costs involved in reciprocating, the cheater will be selected against relative to individuals who, because neither cheats, exchange many altruistic acts. [. . .]

If an 'altruistic situation' is defined as any in which one individual can dispense a benefit to a second greater than the cost of the act to himself, then the chances of selecting for altruistic behavior are greatest (1) when there are many such altruistic situations in the lifetime of the altruists, (2) when a given altruist repeatedly interacts with the same small set of individuals, and (3) when pairs of altruists are exposed 'symmetrically' to altruistic situations, that is, in such a way that the two are able to render roughly equivalent benefits to each other at roughly equivalent costs. These three conditions can be elaborated into a set of relevant biological parameters affecting the possibility that reciprocally altruistic behavior will be selected for.

(1) *Length of lifetime.* Long lifetime of individuals of a species maximizes the chance that any two individuals will encounter many altruistic situations, and all other things being equal one should search for instances of reciprocal altruism in long-lived species.

(2) *Dispersal rate.* Low dispersal rate during all or a significant portion of the lifetime of individuals of a species increases the chance that an individual will interact repeatedly with the same set of neighbors, and other things being equal one should search for instances of reciprocal altruism in such species.

(3) *Degree of mutual dependence.* Interdependence of members of a species (to avoid predators, for example) will tend to keep individuals near each other and thus increase the chance they will encounter altruistic situations together. If the benefit of the mutual dependence is greatest when only a small number of individuals are together, this will greatly increase the chance that an individual will repeatedly interact with the same small set of individuals. Individuals in primate troops, for example, are mutually dependent for protection from predation, yet the optimal troop size for foraging is often small.[1] Because they also meet the other conditions outlined here, primates are almost ideal species in which to search for reciprocal altruism. [. . .]

---

[1] J. H. Crook, 'The Socio-Ecology of Primates', in J. H. Crooke (ed.), *Social Behavior in Birds and Mammals* (Academic Press: London, 1969), 103–66.

(4) *Parental care*. A special instance of mutual dependence is that found between parents and offspring in species that show parental care. The relationship is usually so asymmetrical that few or no situations arise in which an offspring is capable of performing an altruistic act for the parents or even for another offspring, but this is not entirely true for some species (such as primates) in which the period of parental care is unusually long. Parental care, of course, is to be explained by Hamilton's model, but there is no reason why selection for reciprocal altruism cannot operate between close kin, and evidence is presented below that such selection has operated in humans.

(5) *Dominance hierarchy*. Linear dominance hierarchies consist by definition of asymmetrical relationships; a given individual is dominant over another but not vice versa. Strong dominance hierarchies reduce the extent to which altruistic situations occur in which the less dominant individual is capable of performing a benefit for the more dominant which the more dominant individual could not simply take at will. [. . .]

(6) *Aid in combat*. No matter how dominance-oriented a species is, a dominant individual can usually be aided in aggressive encounters with other individuals by help from a less dominant individual. Hall and DeVore have described the tendency for baboon alliances to form which fight as a unit in aggressive encounters (and in encounters with predators).[1] Similarly, vervet monkeys in aggressive encounters solicit the aid of other, often less dominant, individuals.[2] Aid in combat is then a special case in which relatively symmetrical relations are possible between individuals who differ in dominance. [. . .]

Human Reciprocal Altruism

Reciprocal altruism in the human species takes place in a number of contexts and in all known culture. Any complete list of human altruism would contain the following types of altruistic behavior:

(1) helping in times of danger (e.g. accidents, predation, intraspecific aggression);
(2) sharing food;
(3) helping the sick, the wounded, or the very young and old;
(4) sharing implements; and
(5) sharing knowledge.

[1] K. R. L. Hall, and I. DeVore, 'Baboon Social Behavior', in I. DeVore (ed.), *Primate Behavior: Field Studies of Monkeys and Apes* (Holt, Rhinehart and Winston: New York, 1965), 53–110.
[2] T. Struhsaker, 'Social Structure among Vervet Monkeys (*Cercopithecus aetiops*)', *Behavior*, 29 (1967), 83–121.

All these forms of behavior often meet the criterion of small cost to the giver and great benefit to the taker.

During the Pleistocene, and probably before, a hominid species would have met the preconditions for the evolution of reciprocal altruism: long lifespan; low dispersal rate; life in small, mutually dependent, stable, social groups;[1] and a long period of parental care. It is very likely that dominance relations were of the relaxed, less linear form characteristic of the living chimpanzee and not of the more rigidly linear form characteristic of the baboon.[2] Aid in intraspecific combat, particularly by kin, almost certainly reduced the stability and linearity of the dominance order in early humans. Lee has shown that in almost all Bushman fights which are initially between two individuals, others have joined in. Mortality, for example, often strikes the secondaries rather than the principals. Tool use has also probably had an equalizing effect on human dominance relations, and the Bushmen have a saying that illustrates this nicely. As a dispute reaches the stage where deadly weapons may be employed, an individual will often declare: 'We are none of us big, and others small; we are all men and we can fight; I'm going to get my arrows.'[3] It is interesting that Van Lawick-Goodall has recorded an instance of strong dominance reversal in chimpanzees as a function of tool use.[4] An individual moved from low in dominance to the top of the dominance hierarchy when he discovered the intimidating effects of throwing a metal tin around. It is likely that a diversity of talents is usually present in a band of hunter-gatherers such that the best maker of a certain type of tool is not often the best maker of a different sort or the best user of the tool. This contributes to the symmetry of relationships, since altruistic acts can be traded with reference to the special talents of the individuals involved.

To analyze the details of the human reciprocal-altruistic system, several distinctions are important and are discussed here.

(1) *Kin selection.* The human species also met the preconditions for the operation of kin selection. Early hominid hunter-gatherer bands almost certainly (like today's hunter-gatherers) consisted of many close kin, and kin selection must often have operated to favor the evolution of some types of altruistic behavior.[5] In general, in attempting to discriminate be-

[1] R. Lee and I. DeVore, *Man the Hunter* (Aldine: Chicago, 1968). B. Campbell, *Human Evolution*, (Aldine: Chicago, 1966).

[2] J. Van Lawick-Goodall, 'A Preliminary Report on Expressive Movements and Communication in the Gombe Stream Chimpanzees', P. Jay (ed.), *Primates*, (Holt, Rhinehart and Winston: New York, 1968), 313–74; Hall and DeVore, 'Baboon social behavior', 53–110.

[3] R. Lee, '!Kung Bushman violence', paper presented at a meeting of American Anthropological Association, Nov. 1969.

[4] Van Lawick-Goodall, 'A Preliminary Report on the Gombe Stream Chimpanzees'.

[5] J. B. S. Haldane, 'Population Genetics', *New Biology*, 18 (1955), 34–51; Hamilton, 'The Genetical Evolution of Social Behavior; 'Selection of Selfish and Altruistic Behavior in Some Extreme Models', paper presented at 'Man and Beast Symposium' Smithsonian Institution, 1969.

tween the effects of kin selection and what might be called reciprocal-altruistic selection, one can analyze the form of the altruistic behaviors themselves. For example, the existence of discrimination against non-reciprocal individuals cannot be explained on the basis of kin selection, in which the advantage accruing to close kin is what makes the altruistic behavior selectively advantageous, not its chance of being reciprocated. [. . .]

(2) *Reciprocal altruism among close kin.* If both forms of selection have operated, one would expect some interesting interactions. One might expect, for example, a lowered demand for reciprocity from kin than from nonkin, and there is evidence to support this. The demand that kin show some reciprocity suggests, however, that reciprocal-altruistic selection has acted even on relations between close kin.[1] [. . .]

(3) *Gross and subtle cheating.* Two forms of cheating can be distinguished, here denoted as gross and subtle. In *gross cheating* the cheater fails to reciprocate at all, and the altruist suffers the costs of whatever altruism he has dispensed without any compensating benefits. [. . .]

Clearly, selection will strongly favor prompt discrimination against the gross cheater. *Subtle cheating*, by contrast, involves reciprocating, but always attempting to give less than one was given, or more precisely, to give less than the partner would give if the situation were reversed. In this situation, the altruist still benefits from the relationship but not as much as he would if the relationship were completely equitable. The subtle cheater benefits more than he would if the relationship were equitable. [. . .]

Because human altruism may span huge periods of time, a lifetime even, and because thousands of exchanges may take place, involving many different 'goods' and with many different cost/benefit ratios, the problem of computing the relevant totals, detecting imbalances, and deciding whether they are due to chance or to small-scale cheating is an extremely difficult one. Even then, the altruist is in an awkward position, symbolized by the folk saying, 'half a loaf is better than none,' for if attempts to make the relationship equitable lead to the rupture of the relationship, the altruist, assuming other things to be equal, will suffer the loss of the substandard altruism of the subtle cheater. It is the subtlety of the discrimination necessary to detect this form of cheating and the awkward situation that ensues that permit some subtle cheating to be adaptive. This sets up a dynamic tension in the system that has important repercussions, as discussed below. [. . .]

---

[1] L. K. Marshall, 'Sharing, Talking and Giving: Relief of Social Tension among !Kung Bushmen', *Africa*, 31 (1969) 231–49; A. Balikci, 'Development of Basic Socio-Economic Units in Two Eskimo Communities', *National Museum of Canada Bulletin*, 202, (1964).

The Psychological System underlying Human Reciprocal Altruism

Anthropologists have recognized the importance of reciprocity in human behavior, but when they have ascribed functions to such behavior they have done so in terms of group benefits, reciprocity cementing group relations and encouraging group survival. The individual sacrifices so that the group may benefit. Recently psychologists have studied altruistic behavior in order to show what factors induce or inhibit such behavior. No attempt has been made to show what function such behavior may serve, nor to describe and interrelate the components of the psychological system affecting altruistic behavior. The purpose of this section is to show that the above model for the natural selection of reciprocally altruistic behavior can readily explain the function of human altruistic behavior and the details of the psychological system underlying such behavior. The psychological data can be organized into functional categories, and it can be shown that the components of the system complement each other in regulating the expression of altruistic and cheating impulses to the selective advantage of individuals. No concept of group advantage is necessary to explain the function of human altruistic behavior.

There is no direct evidence regarding the degree of reciprocal altruism practiced during human evolution nor its genetic basis today, but given the universal and nearly daily practice of reciprocal altruism among humans today, it is reasonable to assume that it has been an important factor in recent human evolution and that the underlying emotional dispositions affecting altruistic behavior have important genetic components. To assume as much allows a number of predictions.

(1) *A complex, regulating system.* The human altruistic system is a sensitive, unstable one. Often it will pay to cheat: namely, when the partner will not find out, when he will not discontinue his altruism even if he does find out, or when he is unlikely to survive long enough to reciprocate adequately. And the perception of subtle cheating may be very difficult. Given this unstable character of the system, where a degree of cheating is adaptive, natural selection will rapidly favor a complex psychological system in each individual regulating both his own altruistic and cheating tendencies and his responses to these tendencies in others. As selection favors subtler forms of cheating, it will favor more acute abilities to detect cheating. The system that results should simultaneously allow the individual to reap the benefits of altruistic exchanges, to protect himself from gross and subtle forms of cheating, and to practice those forms of cheating that local conditions make adaptive. Individuals will differ not in being altruists or cheaters but in the degree of altruism they show and in the conditions under which they will cheat. [. . .]

(2) *Friendship and the emotions of liking and disliking.* The tendency to like others, not necessarily closely related, to form friendships and to act altruist-

ically toward friends and toward those one likes will be selected for as the immediate emotional rewards motivating altruistic behavior and the formation of altruistic partnerships. (Selection may also favor helping strangers or disliked individuals when they are in particularly dire circumstances). Selection will favor a system whereby these tendencies are sensitive to such parameters as the altruistic tendencies of the liked individual. In other words, selection will favor liking those who are themselves altruistic. [. . .]

(3) *Moralistic aggression.* Once strong positive emotions have evolved to motivate altruistic behavior, the altruist is in a vulnerable position because cheaters will be selected to take advantage of the altruist's positive emotions. This in turn sets up a selection pressure for a protective mechanism. Moralistic aggression and indignation in humans was selected for in order

(a) to counteract the tendency of the altruist, in the absence of any reciprocity, to continue to perform altruistic acts for his own emotional rewards;

(b) to educate the unreciprocating individual by frightening him with immediate harm or with the future harm of no more aid; and

(c) in extreme cases, perhaps, to select directly against the unreciprocating individual by injuring, killing, or exiling him.

Much of human aggression has moral overtones. Injustice, unfairness, and lack of reciprocity often motivate human aggression and indignation. Lee has shown that verbal disputes in Bushmen usually revolve around problems of gift-giving, stinginess, and laziness.[1] DeVore (pers. commun.) reports that a great deal of aggression in hunter-gatherers revolves around real or imagined injustices—inequities, for example, in food-sharing.[2] A common feature of this aggression is that it often seems out of all proportion to the offenses committed. Friends are even killed over apparently trivial disputes. But since small inequities repeated many times over a lifetime may exact a heavy toll in relative fitness, selection may favor a strong show of aggression when the cheating tendency is discovered. [. . .]

(4) *Gratitude, sympathy, and the cost/benefit ratio of an altruistic act.* If the cost/benefit ratio is an important parameter in determining the adaptiveness of reciprocal altruism, then humans should be selected to be sensitive to the cost and benefit of an altruistic act, both in deciding whether to perform one and in deciding whether, or how much, to reciprocate. I suggest that the emotion of gratitude has been selected to regulate human response to altruistic acts and that the emotion is sensitive to the cost/benefit

[1] Lee, '!Kung Bushman violence'.
[2] E. M. Thomas, *The Harmless People*, (Random House: New York, 1958); Balikci, 'Development of Socio-Economic Units in Eskimo communites'; Marshall, 'Sharing, talking and giving'.

ratio of such acts. I suggest further that the emotion of sympathy has been selected to motivate altruistic behavior as a function of the plight of the recipient of such behavior; crudely put, the greater the potential benefit to the recipient, the greater the sympathy and the more likely the altruistic gesture, even to strange or disliked individuals. If the recipient's gratitude is indeed a function of the cost / benefit ratio, then a sympathetic response to the plight of a disliked individual may result in considerable reciprocity. [. . .]

(5) *Guilt and reparative altruism.* If an organism has cheated on a reciprocal relationship and this fact has been found out, or has a good chance of being found out, by the partner and if the partner responds by cutting off all future acts of aid, then the cheater will have paid dearly for his misdeed. It will be to the cheater's advantage to avoid this, and, providing that the cheater makes up for his misdeed and does not cheat in the future, it will be to his partner's benefit to avoid this, since in cutting off future acts of aid he sacrifices the benefits of future reciprocal help. The cheater should be selected to make up for his misdeed and to show convincing evidence that he does not plan to continue his cheating sometime in the future. In short, he should be selected to make a reparative gesture. It seems plausible, furthermore, that the emotion of guilt has been selected for in humans partly in order to motivate the cheater to compensate his misdeed and to behave reciprocally in the future, and thus to prevent the rupture of reciprocal relationships. [. . .]

(6) *Subtle cheating: the evolution of mimics.* Once friendship, moralistic aggression, guilt, sympathy, and gratitude have evolved to regulate the altruistic system, selection will favor mimicking these traits in order to influence the behavior of others to one's own advantage. Apparent acts of generosity and friendship may induce genuine friendship and altruism in return. Sham moralistic aggression when no real cheating has occurred may nevertheless induce reparative altruism. Sham guilt may convince a wronged friend that one has reformed one's ways even when the cheating is about to be resumed. Likewise, selection will favor the hypocrisy of pretending one is in dire circumstances in order to induce sympathy-motivated altruistic behavior. Finally, mimicking sympathy may give the appearance of helping in order to induce reciprocity, and mimicking gratitude may mislead an individual into expecting he will be reciprocated. It is worth emphasizing that a mimic need not necessarily be conscious of the deception; selection may favor feeling genuine moralistic aggression even when one has not been wronged if so doing leads another to reparative altruism. [. . .]

(7) *Detection of the subtle cheater: trustworthiness, trust, and suspicion.* Selection should favor the ability to detect and discriminate against subtle cheaters. Selection will clearly favor detecting and countering sham moralistic aggression. The argument for the others is more complex. Selection may

favor distrusting those who perform altruistic acts without the emotional basis of generosity or guilt because the altruistic tendencies of such individuals may be less reliable in the future. One can imagine, for example, compensating for a misdeed without any emotional basis but with a calculating, self-serving motive. Such an individual should be distrusted because the calculating spirit that leads this subtle cheater now to compensate may in the future lead him to cheat when circumstances seem more advantageous (because of unlikelihood of detection, for example, or because the cheated individual is unlikely to survive). Guilty motivation, in so far as it evidences a more enduring commitment to altruism, either because guilt teaches or because the cheater is unlikely not to feel the same guilt in the future, seems more reliable. A similar argument can be made about the trustworthiness of individuals who initiate altruistic acts out of a calculating rather than a generous-hearted disposition or who show either false sympathy or false gratitude. Detection on the basis of the underlying psychological dynamics is only one form of detection. In many cases, unreliability may more easily be detected through experiencing the cheater's inconsistent behavior. [. . .]

(8) *Developmental plasticity.* The conditions under which detection of cheating is possible, the range of available altruistic trades, the cost/benefit ratios of these trades, the relative stability of social groupings, and other relevant parameters should differ from one ecological and social situation to another and should differ through time in the same small human population. Under these conditions one would expect selection to favor developmental plasticity of those traits regulating altruistic and cheating tendencies and responses to these tendencies in others. For example, developmental plasticity may allow the growing organism's sense of guilt to be educated, perhaps partly by kin, so as to permit those forms of cheating that local conditions make adaptive and to discourage those with more dangerous consequences. One would not expect any simple system regulating the development of altruistic behavior. To be adaptive, altruistic behavior must be dispensed with regard to many characteristics of the recipient (including his degree of relationship, emotional makeup, past behavior, friendships, and kin relations), of other members of the group, of the situation in which the altruistic behavior takes place, and of many other parameters, and no simple developmental system is likely to meet these requirements. [. . .]

The above review of the evidence has only begun to outline the complexities of the human altruistic system. [. . .] For example, once moralistic aggression has been selected for to protect against cheating, selection favors sham moralistic aggression as a new form of cheating. This should lead to selection for the ability to discriminate the two and to guard against the latter. The guarding can, in turn, be used to counter real moralistic aggression: one can, in effect, *impute* cheating motives to another person in order to protect one's own cheating. And so on. Given the psychological and cognitive complexity the system rapidly acquires, one may wonder to what extent the importance of altruism in human evolution set up a selection pressure for psychological and cognitive powers which partly contributed to the large increase in hominid brain size during the Pleistocene.

['The Evolution of Reciprocal Altruism', *Quarterly Review of Biology*, 46 (1971), 35–57.]

ROBERT AXELROD

25 Tit for Tat

Under what conditions will cooperation emerge in a world of egoists without central authority? This question has intrigued people for a long time. And for good reason. We all know that people are not angels, and that they tend to look after themselves and their own first. Yet we also know that cooperation does occur and that our civilization is based upon it. But, in situations where each individual has an incentive to be selfish, how can cooperation ever develop?

The answer each of us gives to this question has a fundamental effect on how we think and act in our social, political, and economic relations with others. And the answers that others give have a great effect on how ready they will be to cooperate with us.

The most famous answer was given over three hundred years ago by Thomas Hobbes. It was pessimistic. He argued that before governments existed, the state of nature was dominated by the problem of selfish individuals who competed on such ruthless terms that life was 'solitary, poor, nasty, brutish, and short'. In his view, cooperation could not develop without a central authority, and consequently a strong government was necessary. Ever since, arguments about the proper scope of government have often focused on whether one could, or could not, expect cooperation to emerge in a particular domain if there were not an authority to police the situation. [. . .]

This basic problem occurs when the pursuit of self-interest by each leads to a poor outcome for all. To make headway in understanding the vast array of specific situations which have this property, a way is needed to represent what is common to these situations without becoming bogged down in the details unique to each. Fortunately, there is such a representation available: the famous *Prisoner's Dilemma* game.[1]

---

[1] The Prisoner's Dilemma game was invented in about 1950 by Merrill Flood and Melvin Dresher, and formalized by A. W. Tucker shortly thereafter.

In the Prisoner's Dilemma game, there are two players. Each has two choices, namely cooperate or defect. Each must make the choice without knowing what the other will do. No matter what the other does, defection yields a higher payoff than cooperation. The dilemma is that if both defect, both do worse than if both had cooperated. This simple game will provide the basis for the entire analysis used in this book.

The way the game works is shown in figure 1. One player chooses a row, either cooperating or defecting. The other player simultaneously chooses a column, either cooperating or defecting. Together, these choices result in one of the four possible outcomes shown in that matrix. If both players cooperate, both do fairly well. Both get R, the *reward for mutual cooperation*. In the concrete illustration of figure 1 the reward is 3 points. This number might, for example, be a payoff in dollars that each player gets for that outcome. If one player cooperates but the other defects, the defecting player gets the *temptation to defect*, while the cooperating player gets the *sucker's payoff*. In the example, these are 5 points and 0 points respectively. If both defect, both get 1 point, the *punishment for mutual defection*.

FIGURE 1 *The Prisoner's Dilemma*

| | | Column Player | |
		Cooperate	Defect
Row Player	Cooperate	$R = 3, R = 3$ Reward for mutual cooperation	$S = 0, T = 5$ Sucker's payoff, and temptation to defect
	Defect	$T = 5, S = 0$ Temptation to defect and sucker's payoff	$P = 1, P = 1$ Punishment for mutual defection

NOTE: The payoffs to the row chooser are listed first.

What should you do in such a game? Suppose you are the row player, and you think the column player will cooperate. This means that you will get one of the two outcomes in the first column of figure 1. You have a choice. You can cooperate as well, getting the 3 points of the reward for mutual cooperation. Or you can defect, getting the 5 points of the temptation payoff. So it pays to defect if you think the other player will cooperate. But now suppose that you think the other player will defect. Now you are in the second column of figure 1, and you have a choice between cooperating, which would make you a sucker and give you 0 points, and defecting, which would result in mutual punishment giving you 1 point. So it pays to defect if you think the other player will defect. This means that it is better to defect if you think the other player will cooperate, *and* it is better to defect if you think the other player will defect. So no matter what the other player does, it pays for you to defect.

So far, so good. But the same logic holds for the other player too. Therefore, the other player should defect no matter what you are expected to do. So you should both defect. But then you both get 1 point which is worse than the 3 points of the reward that you both could have gotten had you both cooperated. Individual rationality leads to a worse outcome for both than is possible. Hence the dilemma.

The Prisoner's Dilemma is simply an abstract formulation of some very common and very interesting situations in which what is best for each person individually leads to mutual defection, whereas everyone would have been better off with mutual cooperation. [. . .]

I have explored the emergence of cooperation through a study of what is a good strategy to employ if confronted with an iterated Prisoner's Dilemma. This exploration has been done in a novel way, with a computer tournament. Professional game theorists were invited to submit their favorite strategy, and each of these decision rules was paired off with each of the others to see which would do best overall. Amazingly enough, the winner was the simplest of all strategies submitted. This was TIT FOR TAT, the strategy which cooperates on the first move and then does whatever the other player did on the previous move. A second round of the tournament was conducted in which many more entries were submitted by amateurs and professionals alike, all of whom were aware of the results of the first round. The result was another victory for TIT FOR TAT! The analysis of the data from these tournaments reveals four properties which tend to make a decision rule successful: avoidance of unnecessary conflict by cooperating as long as the other player does, provocability in the face of an uncalled for defection by the other, forgiveness after responding to a provocation, and clarity of behavior so that the other player can adapt to your pattern of action.

These results from the tournaments demonstrate that under suitable conditions, cooperation can indeed emerge in a world of egoists without central authority. [. . .] They show that cooperation can get started by even a small cluster of individuals who are prepared to reciprocate cooperation, even in a world where no one else will cooperate. The analysis also shows that the two key requisites for cooperation to thrive are that the cooperation be based on reciprocity, and that the shadow of the future is important enough to make this reciprocity stable. But once cooperation based on reciprocity is established in a population, it can protect itself from invasion by uncooperative strategies.

It is encouraging to see that cooperation can get started, can thrive in a variegated environment, and can protect itself once established. But what is most interesting is how little had to be assumed about the individuals or the social setting to establish these results. The individuals do not have to be rational: the evolutionary process allows the successful strategies to thrive, even if the players do not know why or how. Nor do the players have to exchange messages or commitments: they do not need words, because their deeds speak for them. Likewise, there is no need to assume trust between the players: the use of reciprocity can be enough to make defection unproductive. Altruism is not needed: successful strategies can elicit cooperation even from an egoist. Finally, no central authority is needed: cooperation based on reciprocity can be self-policing.

The emergence, growth, and maintenance of cooperation do require some assumptions about the individuals and the social setting. They require an individual to be able to recognize another player who has been dealt with before. They also require that one's prior history of interactions with this player can be remembered, so that a player can be responsive. Actually, these requirements for recognition and recall are not as strong as they might seem. Even bacteria can fulfill them by interacting with only one other organism and using a strategy (such as TIT FOR TAT) which responds only to the recent behavior of the other player. And if bacteria can play games, so can people and nations.

For cooperation to prove stable, the future must have a sufficiently large shadow. This means that the importance of the next encounter between the same two individuals must be great enough to make defection an unprofitable strategy when the other player is provocable. It requires that the players have a large enough chance of meeting again and that they do not discount the significance of their next meeting too greatly. For example, what made cooperation possible in the trench warfare of World War I was the fact that the same small units from opposite sides of no- man's-land would be in contact for long periods of time, so that if one side broke the tacit understandings, then the other side could retaliate against the same unit.

Finally, the evolution of cooperation requires that successful strategies can thrive and that there be a source of variation in the strategies which are being used. These mechanisms can be classical Darwinian survival of the fittest and mutation, but they can also involve more deliberate processes such as imitation of successful patterns of behavior and intelligently designed new strategic ideas.

In order for cooperation to get started in the first place, one more condition is required. The problem is that in a world of unconditional defection, a single individual who offers cooperation cannot prosper unless others are around who will reciprocate. On the other hand, cooperation can emerge from small clusters of discriminating individuals as long as these individuals have even a small proportion of their interactions with each other. So there must be some clustering of individuals who use strategies with two properties: the strategies will be the first to cooperate, and they will discriminate between those who respond to the cooperation and those who do not.

The conditions for the evolution of cooperation tell what is necessary, but do not, by themselves, tell what strategies will be most successful. For this question, the tournament approach has offered striking evidence in favor of the robust success of the simplest of all discriminating strategies: TIT FOR TAT. By cooperating on the first move, and then doing whatever the other player did on the previous move, TIT FOR TAT managed to do well with a wide variety of more or less sophisticated decision rules. It not only won the first round of the Computer Prisoner's Dilemma Tournament when facing entries submitted by professional game theorists, but it also won the second round which included over sixty entries designed by people who were able to take the results of the first round into account. It was also the winner in five of the six major variants of the second round (and second in the sixth variant). And most impressive, its success was not based only upon its ability to do well with strategies which scored poorly for themselves. This was shown by an ecological analysis of hypothetical future rounds of the tournament. In this simulation of hundreds of rounds of the tournament, TIT FOR TAT again was the most successful rule, indicating that it can do well with good and bad rules alike.

TIT FOR TAT's robust success is due to being nice, provocable, forgiving, and clear. Its niceness means that it is never the first to defect, and this property prevents it from getting into unnecessary trouble. Its retaliation discourages the other side from persisting whenever defection is tried. Its forgiveness helps restore mutual cooperation. And its clarity makes its behavioral pattern easy to recognize; and once recognized, it is easy to perceive that the best way of dealing with TIT FOR TAT is to cooperate with it. [. . .]

If a nice strategy, such as TIT FOR TAT, does eventually come to be adopted by virtually everyone, then individuals using this nice strategy can afford to be generous in dealing with any others. In fact, a population of nice rules can also protect itself from clusters of individuals using any other strategy just as well as they can protect themselves against single individuals.

These results give a chronological picture for the evolution of cooperation. Cooperation can begin with small clusters. It can thrive with rules that are nice, provocable, and somewhat forgiving. And once established in a population, individuals using such discriminating strategies can protect themselves from invasion. The overall level of cooperation tends to go up and not down. In other words, the machinery for the evolution of cooperation contains a ratchet.

[*The Evolution of Cooperation* (Basic Books: New York, 1984), 3–9, 19–21, 173–7.]

iii Sexual Morality

JANE GOODALL

26 **Incest Avoidance among Chimpanzees**

In Japanese macaques, rhesus monkeys and olive baboons, mating between close kin who remain together as adults is rare. The same is true for chimpanzees.

Incestuous matings between sexually mature males and their mothers are extremely uncommon. Figan and Faben, who were with their mother for at least some part of her five periods of estrus, were never observed even *trying* to mate her—during her 1963 and 1967 periods of estrus they were the only males of any age who did not do so. In fact, they never showed the slightest sign of sexual arousal in her presence. The same was true of Evered and his mother, Olly.

Tutin observed Satan copulating with his mother, Sprout. She tried to escape from him but he followed her to the top of a tall tree. Although she submitted, she screamed loudly throughout and leaped away prior to ejaculation. Goblin quite frequently showed sexual interest in his mother, Melissa, when he was nineteen years old. His first observed copulation was during her first postpartum cycle after the birth of the twins, two or three days before deflation. When he summoned her she refused to approach; eventually, after repeated branch shaking and two short bouts of chasing, Goblin stamped on her back three times and soon afterward gave up. The following day he was again observed to chase his mother. This time she stopped, screaming, and crouched for copulation; but after he had delivered a few thrusts she leaped away before he had ejaculated. Another mild attack resulted, but she escaped, hitting out at him as she did so, then took refuge up a tree. He gazed up and shook branches at her, but she climbed very high and after a further minute he gave up. During Melissa's next period of swelling Goblin was once more observed as he summoned her, but he did not persist when she ran from him.

The following year, after a miscarriage, Melissa resumed cycling. She was followed daily during both her periods of swelling. Goblin was observed to summon her only once during the first estrus and he quickly gave up when she avoided him. A month later, however, he copulated with her, apparently successfully, after displaying and chasing her up a tree.

Over the years we have collected data on the sexual relationships of five late-adolescent or mature females with their elder known or assumed brothers: Miff with Pepe, Gilka with Evered, Gigi with Willy Wally, and

Fifi with both Figan and Faben. Copulations between these brother–sister pairs were observed very infrequently. On the one occasion that Miff was seen copulating with her elder brother she was quite calm; mostly, he showed no sexual interest in her. Gigi once attacked her presumed elder brother, Willy Wally, when he persisted in trying to mate with her, but another time she accepted him without fuss. Gilka was never seen to be mated by her brother, Evered, despite the fact that, when swollen, she was followed extensively. Three times he showed low-key sexual interest in her, but did not follow when she moved away. Pusey has shown that these three females all associated significantly less often with their brothers after first estrus.[1]

Fifi was mated by all late-adolescent and mature males during her first full swelling *except* her two brothers, Figan and Faben. Figan (aged thirteen) was not observed to show interest in her at this stage, but Faben (about nineteen) was twice seen to approach her with hair and penis erect. Each time Fifi hurried away, screaming, although she was eager to respond to the sexual advances of most suitors.[2] During her eighth period of estrus, however, both Figan and Faben were seen copulating with her (Figan once, Faben twice). She did not try to escape from Faben, but when Figan approached and courted, she screamed and tried to jump from the tree. Figan pursued her and caught up, but she did not present; he copulated, as best he could, as she hung, screaming, from a branch. During the two years of Fifi's adolescent sterility, Figan was seen to mate with her only four times, Faben seven.

After giving birth and after five years of lactational anestrus Fifi once more began to cycle. She was observed during parts of four periods of estrus: Figan (still alpha) was seen to copulate or try to copulate with her on seventeen different occasions. Five times she resisted these courtships so persistently that he gave up. Twice, even though she refused to cooperate, he persisted until he did in fact achieve intromission. Once this was after courting her vigorously for over a minute, during which time he swayed the vegetation so wildly that at the end she was virtually imprisoned beneath a layer of branches; these he held down over her back during mating! Fifi was not observed to reject any other male in this way.

The relationship between the sixth sibling pair, Goblin and Gremlin, was unusual. He was the second mature male seen to copulate with her during her first adult swelling; she responded to his courtship with the typical crouch-present and showed no signs of protest. Over the next seven months, during which Gremlin cycled regularly, Goblin was seen to mate his sister an additional twenty-five times. On twenty-one of these occasions she

[1] A. E. Pusey, 'Inbreeding Avoidance in Chimpanzees, *Animal Behavior*, 28 (1980), 543–52.
[2] J. Goodall, *In the Shadow of Man* (Collins: London, 1971).

accepted him calmly, as she had the first day, but four times she became very upset, screaming and trying to avoid his sexual advances. Once he managed to copulate regardless, but only after chasing and attacking her quite severely (one of the few instances of 'rape,' and similar to his behavior when he tried to mate with his mother). The other three times Gremlin managed to avoid him. Gremlin also resisted some of the sexual advances of other males, but not so frequently: she resisted (though not always successfully) 30.8 percent of Goblin's copulation attempts as compared with 12.0 percent of Satan's; and she resisted the advances of Evered and Jomeo once each. [. . .]

Copulations between fathers and daughters and between paternal siblings are unlikely to be inhibited, for the individuals concerned do not 'know' their relationship. There is no close bonding between them and they do not achieve the high level of familiarity that presumably underlies incest avoidance between mothers and sons and maternal siblings.

[*The Chimpanzees of Gombe* (Harvard University Press: Cambridge, Mass, 1986), 466–9.]

EDWARD WESTERMARCK

27 The Horror of Incest

It seems that the horror of incest is wellnigh universal in the human race, and that the few cases in which this feeling is said to be absent can only be regarded as abnormalities. But the degrees of kinship within which marriage is forbidden are by no means the same everywhere. It is most, and almost universally, abominated between parents and children. It is also held in general abhorrence between brothers and sisters who are children of the same mother as well as of the same father. Most of the exceptions to this rule refer to royal persons, for whom it is considered improper to contract marriage with individuals of less exalted birth. [. . .] As a rule, the prohibited degrees are more numerous among peoples unaffected by modern civilisation than they are in more advanced communities, the prohibitions in a great many cases referring even to all the members of the tribe or clan; and the violation of these rules is regarded as a most heinous crime. [. . .]

Not less intense is the horror of incest among nations that have passed beyond savagery and barbarism. Among the Chinese incest with a grand-uncle, a father's first cousin, a brother, or a nephew, is punishable by death, and a man who marries his mother's sister is strangled; nay, punishment is inflicted even on him who marries a person with the same surname as his own, sixty blows being the penalty. So also incest was held in the utmost horror by the so-called Aryan peoples in ancient times. In the 'Institutes of

Vishnu' it is said that sexual intercourse with one's mother or daughter or daughter-in-law is a crime of the highest degree, for which there is no other atonement than to proceed into the flames.

Various theories have been set forth to account for the prohibition of marriage between near kin. [. . .] [T]here is an innate aversion to sexual intercourse between persons living very closely together from early youth, and as such persons are in most cases related by blood, this feeling would naturally display itself in custom and law as a horror of intercourse between near kin. Indeed, an abundance of ethnographical facts seem to indicate that it is not in the first place by the degree of consanguinity, but by the close living together, that prohibitory laws against intermarriage are determined. Thus many peoples have a rule of 'exogamy' which does not depend on kinship at all, but on purely local considerations, all the members of a horde or village, though not related by blood, being forbidden to intermarry. The prohibited degrees are very differently defined in the customs or laws of different nations, and it appears that the extent to which relatives are prohibited from intermarrying is nearly connected with their close living together. Very often the prohibitions against incest are more or less one-sided, applying more extensively either to the relatives on the father's side or to those on the mother's, according as descent is reckoned through men or women. Now, since the line of descent is largely connected with local relationships, we may reasonably infer that the same local relationships exercise a considerable influence on the table of prohibited degrees. However, in a large number of cases prohibitions of intermarriage are only indirectly influenced by the close living together. Aversion to the intermarriage of persons who live in intimate connection with one another has called forth prohibitions of the intermarriage of relations; and, as kinship is traced by means of a system of names, the name comes to be considered identical with relationship. This system is necessarily one-sided. Though it will keep up the record of descent either on the male or female side, it cannot do both at once; and the line which has not been kept up by such means of record, even where it is recognised as a line of relationship, is naturally more or less neglected and soon forgotten. Hence the prohibited degrees frequently extend very far on the one side—to the whole clan—but not on the other. [. . .] Generally speaking, the feeling that two persons are intimately connected in some way or other may, through an association of ideas, gives rise to the notion that marriage or sexual intercourse between them is incestuous. Hence the prohibitions of marriage between relations by alliance and by adoption.

[*The Origin and Development of the Moral Ideas* (Macmillan: London, 1906), ii. 364–9.]

Dandy is the youngest and lowest ranking of the four grown males. The other three, and in particular the alpha male, do not tolerate any sexual intercourse between Dandy and the adult females. Nevertheless every now and again he does succeed in mating with them, after having made a 'date'. When this happens the female and Dandy pretend to be walking in the same direction by chance, and if all goes well they meet behind a few tree trunks. These 'dates' take place after the exchange of a few glances and in some cases brief physical contact.

This kind of furtive mating is frequently associated with signal suppression and concealment. I can remember the first time I noticed it very vividly indeed, because it was such a comical sight. Dandy and a female were courting each other surreptitiously. Dandy began to make advances to the female, whilst at the same time restlessly looking around to see if any of the other males were watching. Male chimpanzees start their advances by sitting with their legs wide apart revealing their erection. Precisely at the point when Dandy was exhibiting his sexual urge in this way, Luit, one of the older males, unexpectedly came round the corner. Dandy immediately dropped his hands over his penis concealing it from view.

On another occasion Luit was making advances to a female while Nikkie, the alpha male, was lying in the grass about 50 metres away. When Nikkie looked up and got to his feet, Luit slowly shifted a few paces away from the female and sat down, once again with his back to Nikkie. Nikkie slowly moved towards Luit, picking up a heavy stone on his way. His hair was standing slightly on end. Now and then Luit looked round to watch Nikkie's progress and then he looked back at his own penis, which was gradually losing its erection. Only when his penis was no longer visible did Luit turn around and walk towards Nikkie. He briefly sniffed at the stone Nikkie was holding, then he wandered off leaving Nikkie with the female.

Females sometimes give away their clandestine mating sessions by emitting a special, high scream at the point of climax. As soon as the alpha male hears this he runs towards the hidden couple to interrupt them. An adolescent female, Oor, used to scream particularly loudly at the end of her matings. However, by the time she was almost adult she still screamed at the end of mating sessions with the alpha male, but hardly ever during her 'dates'. During a 'date' she adopted the facial expressions which go with screaming (bared teeth, open mouth) and uttered a kind of noiseless scream (blowing from the back of the throat).

In all these examples sexual signals are either concealed or suppressed. Oor's noiseless scream gives the impression of violent emotions which are only controlled with the greatest of effort. The males are faced with the problem that the evidence of their sexual arousal cannot disappear to order, but they too have their solutions. [. . .]

There is, generally speaking, a definite link between the rank of a male and his copulation frequency, although it is by no means a rigid law but rather a rule to which exceptions are possible. It is not that high-ranking males are more virile, but that they are incredibly intolerant and chase lower-ranking rivals away from oestrus females. If they catch another male mating, they intervene by attacking either him or his mate. The females are also clearly aware of this risk. Sometimes a female consistently refuses to accept invitations to mate from certain males, as if she is just not interested in them. Then, when the colony goes indoors in the evening, opportunities suddenly present themselves for undisturbed mating and it turns out that the female is perfectly willing to mate with males she has cold-shouldered during the day. We have even seen females rush to the cages of the males to copulate quickly through the bars. This only happens, of course, when the alpha male is still outside or separated from them in another part of the system of passages. If the alpha male happens to spot what is going on, he immediately reacts by hooting and bluffing but he is powerless to intervene.

What is the reason for this intolerance? Why are the males unable to leave each other alone? Jealousy is once again only half the explanation. The problem of its function remains. Jealousy would have disappeared from the earth a long time ago if the tensions and risks involved did not have some positive function. The biological explanation for sexual rivalry between males is as follows. A female can only be fertilized by one male. By keeping other males away from her a male increases the certainty that he will be the father of her child. Consequently children will more often be sired by jealous than by tolerant males. If jealousy is hereditary—and that is what this theory assumes—more and more children will be born with this characteristic, and later they in turn will attempt to exclude other members of the same sex from the reproductive act.

Whereas the males fight for the right to fertilize as many females as possible, the situation for the female is completely different. Whether she copulates with one or one hundred males, it will not alter the number of children she will give birth to. Jealousy among females is therefore less marked. The struggle among females for the attentions of the male occurs almost exclusively in pair-forming species, and then it concerns the long-term tie with the male rather than the sexual contact. [. . .]

One problem remains. If I had to say which of the males is the most ambitious and jealous, I would say Yeroen. And with respect to protectiveness I would also say, after wavering between Yeroen and Luit, Yeroen. These characteristics are assumed to be associated with successful reproduction. It is, therefore, all the more remarkable that Yeroen wins on both counts when we know that despite frequent copulation (often with ejaculation) his physical deficiency makes him unable to fertilize any female. All his efforts are in vain. At first sight his case appears to disprove the theory.

In fact it does not do so, because Yeroen does not know the ultimate goal of fatherhood. He does not know that males can reproduce, because animals are not aware of the link between sex and procreation. They mate only for pleasure and are ambitious, jealous and protective without knowing that this can benefit their offspring. Even though the function of their behaviour is to aid their offspring and the reason for its evolution, they themselves only recognize certain *sub*goals: a high rank, more mating than other group members and a safe environment for all the children in the group. They unconsciously serve the *main* goal of all living creatures. The fact that even an impotent male such as Yeroen does this illustrates the blindness of the urge to reproduce. [. . .]

The oldest children in our colony were fathered in Yeroen's heyday, which means that he cannot have had a complete sexual monopoly. Lower-ranking group members always find ways, although this often means being secretive. Mariëtte van der Weel studied the openness with which the group members mated by recording which of the other males could see the act. She found that Nikkie and Dandy were concerned about their mating sessions being visible to others, whereas Yeroen and Luit were not unduly worried. We would have expected this of Luit, because he was the alpha male at the time, but not of Yeroen. I have never once seen Yeroen make a 'date' with a female: he either mates openly or not at all. Perhaps this has something to do with the females. A conspiracy is needed to set up a mating session removed from the others. Perhaps the females, who accept Yeroen's direct invitations, are not prepared to walk a long way for sexual contact which, in Yeroen's case, is unsatisfactory.

The female is free to choose whether or not to have sex. Although I have heard of isolated instances of rape among chimpanzees in laboratory cages, I have never seen this happen in our colony. If the female does not want to mate, then that is the end of the matter. Persistent males run the risk of being chased by the female they approached and some of the other females too. Puist, who normally sides with the males in a conflict, always supports the oestrus female in such cases. Hence the link between dominance and sexual rights, which exists among the males, is only half the story. Another important factor is the individual preference of the female, and this does not always tally with the rank of the male. Consequently it is the females who largely engineer the evasion of the rules which exist among males.

That everyone knows these social rules is clear not only from the furtiveness of certain contacts but also from the phenomenon of *telling tales*. Two examples serve to illustrate this. In the first, Dandy sees Luit paying court to Spin while the leader, Yeroen, is sitting a long way off and cannot see what is going on. Barking excitedly Dandy runs to Yeroen and attracts his attention. He then leads Yeroen to the spot where the two are in the middle of mating.

The second example dates from the period of Luit's leadership. While Luit has his back turned Yeroen and Nikkie both seize the opportunity to invite Gorilla to have sexual intercourse. She ignores Yeroen and presents to Nikkie. At once Yeroen begins to hoot at Luit, who turns round. Nikkie remains rooted to the spot and then wanders away as nonchalantly as possible.

[*Chimpanzee Politics* (Jonathan Cape: London, 1982, 48–50, 168–75.]

LORNA MARSHALL

29   Adultery among the !Kung

!Kung society has an overall prohibition against any sexual relations outside of marriage, with one exception. [. . .] Premarital unchastity, unchastity of widows, and prostitution are not among their social conventions. But /*kamheri*, though not required, is either fully permitted or tolerated as not a very bad thing; I never reached certainty as to which of these attitudes the society adopted.

/*Kamheri* means that two men may agree to exchange wives temporarily, provided the wives consent. This is regarded as a concern of the couples involved rather than a concern of society as a whole. One man said, 'If you want to sleep with someone's wife, you get him to sleep with yours, then neither of you goes after the other with poisoned arrows.'

No actual instance of /kamheri came to our attention, and we failed to find out if it is now practiced. One man in /Gam lent his first wife to an unmarried friend, one of the gossips told us, because he was in love with his second and did not care any longer for the first; but this was a mere deviation from the rules, not an instance of /kamheri.

We heard of several instances of adultery, in addition to the irregular sexual union mentioned above. No instances of rape were recounted. Fornication must be very rare, because there is practically no one with whom to commit it. Almost all females are married, except for very young girls and leathery old grandmothers. Adultery is the usual form for irregular unions to take. Adultery, however, is sharply limited by several deterrents.

One deterrent is the incest taboo, which forbids extramarital sexual relations with tabooed categories of kin as it does marriage with persons to
whom the taboo is extended. [. . .]

Ease of divorce must exert a modifying influence on adulterous unions.
If a married couple really want to change mates, nothing need deter them
but the general difficulty of extricating themselves from the web of responsibilities that marriage entails.

In a sense, the impossibility of maintaining secrecy exerts a control over
extramarital relations. There is no privacy in a !Kung encampment, and the
vast veld is not a cover. The very life of these people depends on their being
trained from childhood to look sharply at things and to take into their
attention what they see. They must observe the most minute marks on
vegetation to distinguish from the matted grasses the almost hair-thin
brown vine stems that come up from the edible roots. Hunters memorize
visual impressions and are able to follow the tracks of an individual animal
in the midst of a large herd in a way that seems to us miraculous. They
register every person's footprints in their minds, more vividly I am sure than
we do faces, and read in the sand who walked where and how long ago.

The !Kung value control of anger. They uphold self-control as an ideal,
train themselves to exercise it, and reward it with approval. Despite this,
volatile tempers sometimes flare and burst out of all control. And always at
hand are the little poisoned arrows. They are formidable weapons. There
is no antidote for the poison; at least our !Kung informants said they know
none, and they told us of tragic deaths from the poison which would have
been averted had they had an antidote.

Adultery, so exceedingly provocative of anger and vengeance, could be
very dangerous under these conditions. Anger turns upon the adulterer.
We were never told about a woman who had been killed or even very
severely punished, but a husband is considered to be quite within his rights
by !Kung rules of conduct if he kills a man who sleeps with his wife.
However, the adulterer may fight back. With poisoned arrows both men
might be killed. Fighting is so dangerous it is feared by the !Kung with a
pervading dread.

Nevertheless, although prudence counsels against it and anxiety may
attend it, adultery does occur. During the years from 1951 to 1958, five
instances in our sample came to our knowledge. When it did occur, the
most clearly observable behavior was the attempt on the part of related
persons and other members of the band to help resolve the situation in
order to avoid fighting and discord, for fighting, like fire, may spread and
consume much before it is quenched.

A husband and a young widower had quarreled and almost fought over
the young widower's attentions to the wife. The fight had been averted by
the husband's running away. He came to Gautscha where we were with

Band 1. When I saw him handling his weapons, his face contorted with emotion, visions possessed me of the two men, both angry and afraid, shooting each other in nervous self- defense, writhing, bleeding, and dying in agony, and I was as filled with the fear of fighting as any Bushman. But before sundown that day the affair was resolved in the following fashion. Toma, a relative of the young widower, undertook to use his influence and went and brought the young widower and the wife to Gautscha. Toma had two motives. He wanted peace, as everybody does, and he wanted no disgrace in his family, which the affair would bring, for the young widower and the wife were sexually taboo to each other, albeit in the mildest and most extended way. Toma is an able man, and he succeeded. The pair agreed to his behests. When they arrived at Gautscha the wife went directly to her husband and, to our surprise, in a few minutes they left the encampment with their child and came over to our camp, where they settled themselves right in our cleared camp space. Presently the young widower came too, with his three children, and settled himself beside the others. Under our wings they had less fear of each other's flares of temper, and tensions relaxed. In a day or so the young widower left. Peace prevailed. The wife was still with her husband in 1958. We did not see them after that.

(*The !Kung of Nyae Nyae* (Harvard University Press: Cambridge, Mass., 1976), 279–81.)

THE BIBLE

30 Incest and Adultery

6 ¶ None of you shall approach to any that is near of kin to him, to uncover *their* nakedness: I *am* the LORD.

7 The nakedness of thy father, or the nakedness of thy mother, shalt thou not uncover: she *is* thy mother; thou shalt not uncover her nakedness.

8 The nakedness of thy father's wife shalt thou not uncover: it *is* thy father's nakedness.

9 The nakedness of thy sister, the daughter of thy father, or daughter of thy mother, *whether she be* born at home, or born abroad, *even* their nakedness thou shalt not uncover.

10 The nakedness of thy son's daughter, or of thy daughter's daughter, *even* their nakedness thou shalt not uncover: for their's *is* thine own nakedness.

11 The nakedness of thy father's wife's daughter, begotten of thy father, she is thy sister, thou shalt not uncover her nakedness.

12 Thou shalt not uncover the nakedness of thy father's sister: she *is* thy father's near kinswoman.

13 Thou shalt not uncover the nakedness of thy mother's sister: for she *is* thy mother's near kinswoman.

14 Thou shalt not uncover the nakedness of thy father's brother, thou shalt not approach to his wife: she *is* thine aunt.

15 Thou shalt not uncover the nakedness of thy daughter in law: she *is* thy son's wife; thou shalt not uncover her nakedness.

16 Thou shalt not uncover the nakedness of thy brother's wife: it *is* thy brother's nakedness.

17 Thou shalt not uncover the nakedness of a woman and her daughter, neither shalt thou take her son's daughter, or her daughter's daughter, to uncover her nakedness; *for* they *are* her near kinswomen: it *is* wickedness.

18 Neither shalt thou take a wife to her sister, to vex *her*, to uncover her nakedness, beside the other in her life *time*.

19 Also thou shalt not approach unto a woman to uncover her nakedness, as long as she is put apart for her uncleanness.

20 Moreover thou shalt not lie carnally with thy neighbour's wife, to defile thyself with her.

21 And thou shalt not let any of thy seed pass through *the fire* to Molech, neither shalt thou profane the name of thy God: I *am* the LORD.

22 Thou shalt not lie with mankind, as with womankind: it *is* abomination.

23 Neither shalt thou lie with any beast to defile thyself therewith: neither shall any woman stand before a beast to lie down thereto: it *is* confusion.

24 Defile not ye yourselves in any of these things: for in all these the nations are defiled which I cast out before you:

25 And the land is defiled: therefore I do visit the iniquity thereof upon it, and the land itself vomiteth out her inhabitants.

26 Ye shall therefore keep my statutes and my judgments, and shall not commit *any* of these abominations; *neither* any of your own nation, nor any stranger that sojourneth among you:

27 (For all these abominations have the men of the land done, which *were* before you, and the land is defiled;)

28 That the land spue not you out also, when ye defile it, as it spued out the nations that *were* before you.

29 For whosoever shall commit any of these abominations, even the souls that commit *them* shall be cut off from among their people.

30 Therefore shall ye keep mine ordinance, that *ye* commit not *any one* of these abominable customs, which were committed before you, and that ye defile not yourselves therein: I *am* the LORD your God.

* * * * * *

27 Ye have heard that it was said by them of old time, Thou shalt not commit adultery:

28 But I say unto you, That whosoever looketh on a woman to lust after her hath committed adultery with her already in his heart.

29 And if thy right eye offend thee, pluck it out, and cast *it* from thee: for it is profitable for thee that one of thy members should perish, and not *that* thy whole body should be cast into hell.

30 And if thy right hand offend thee, cut it off, and cast *it* from thee: for it is profitable for thee that one of thy members should perish, and not *that* thy whole body should be cast into hell.

31 It hath been said, Whosoever shall put away his wife, let him give her a writing of divorcement:

32 But I say unto you, That whosoever shall put away his wife, saving for the cause of fornication, causeth her to commit adultery: and whosoever shall marry her that is divorced committeth adultery.

[Leviticus 18: 6–30. Compiled in 6th–5th cent. BC from more ancient material; The Gospel According to St Matthew 5: 27–32. Written in *c*. 85 AD.]

MARTIN LUTHER

31 **A Commentary on the Sixth Commandment**

The Sixth Commandment: 'You shall not commit adultery'

Explicit injunction is here given against injury [to the neighbor] by the disgrace of his wife. Adultery is particularly mentioned, because among the Jewish people marriage was obligatory. Young people were advised to marry at the earliest age possible. Virginity was not particularly commended; harlots and libertines were never tolerated. There was no form of unchastity more common than that of the breaking of the marriage vow. But since there is among us such a shameful and vile mixture of all forms of vice and lewdness, this commandment is directed against every form of unchastity, under any name. Not only the actual deed is forbidden, but also every prompting and incentive to it. Heart, lips, and the whole body must be chaste and give no occasion, no help or suggestion to unchastity. Further, we are to restrain, protect, and rescue where there is need. We are to assist our neighbors to maintain their honor. In brief, the requirement of this commandment is chastity for one's self and the endeavor to secure it for the neighbor.

But since particular attention is here called to the married state, let us carefully note, first, how God especially honors and commends wedded life, since he confirms and protects it with a special command. Hence he requires us to honor, guard, and observe it as a divine and blessed estate. Significantly he established it as the first of all institutions, and with it in view he did not create man and woman alike. God's purpose, as is plain, was not that they should live a life of wickedness, but that they might be true to each other, beget children, and nourish and rear them to his glory. Therefore God blessed this institution above all others and made everything on earth serve and spring from it, so that it might be well and amply provided for. It is not an exceptional estate but the most universal and the noblest, pervading all Christendom, yea, extending through the whole world.

Remember that marriage is not only an honorable but also a necessary estate, earnestly commanded by God, so that in general men and women of all conditions, created for it, should be found in it. Yet there are some exceptions, although few, whom God has especially exempted, either because they are unfit for wedded life or because, by reason of extraordinary gifts, they have become free to live chaste lives unmarried. To unaided human nature, as God created it, chastity apart from matrimony is an impossibility. For flesh and blood remain flesh and blood, and the natural inclination and excitement run their course without let or hindrance, as everyone's observation and experience testify. Therefore that man might more easily keep his evil lust in bounds, God commanded marriage, that each may have his proper portion and be satisfied; although God's grace is still needed for the heart to be pure.

This commandment requires man not only to live chaste in act, word, and thought in his station, and especially in his married life, but also to love and appreciate the consort God has given him. For love and harmony between husband and wife are above all things essential to conjugal chastity. Heart confidence and perfect fidelity must obtain. They are of chief importance, for thereby is created love and the desire for chastity. From such a condition chastity always follows spontaneously, without commandment.

> [Luther's 'Ten Sermons on the Catechism', in his *Works*, Li, trans. J. W. Doberstein (Muhlenberg Press, Philadelphia, 1959), 153–5. First published in 1528.]

DONALD SYMONS

32 The Double Standard

Consider the following statements concerning men's feelings about adultery:

(a) 'The men believe it is a good thing for them to have many lovers, but bad for women and especially bad for their wives'.[1]

---

[1] T. Gregor, 'Privacy and Extra-Marital Affairs in a Tropical Forest Community', in D. R. Gross (ed.), *Peoples and Cultures of Native South America* (The Natural History Press: New York, 1973), 247, on the Mehinacu of Brazil.

(b) 'While men conventionally regard any woman outside the prohibited range, married or not, as a potential sexual partner, their own wives, they consider, should remain faithful to them'.[1]

(c) 'Men constantly attempt to seduce the wives of their village mates and take extreme offense when their own wives, in turn, are seduced'.[2]

(d) 'Even those males who disapprove of extra-marital coitus for their own wives may be interested in securing such contacts for themselves, and this in most instances means securing coitus with the wives of other males'.[3]

While women's views on adultery may typically differ from men's views, I would expect women's feelings to be no less self-interested than men's. These statements suggest that the most fundamental, most universal double standard is not male versus female but each individual human versus everyone else. In a proximate sense, using male adultery as an example, this double standard results from such banal facts as that one's own orgasms feel substantially better to oneself than anyone else's orgasms do, and imagining one's wife copulating with another man is substantially more painful and threatening than imagining someone else's wife committing adultery (if the imagined accessory is oneself, the image may be pleasant rather than painful). In an ultimate sense, this double standard results from the fact that, among sexually reproducing organisms, every conspecific is to a greater or lesser extent one's reproductive competitor.

The word 'promiscuous,' in the sense of nonselective sexual intercourse, is pejorative in English and generally is applied to women;[4] this also is true of the equivalent word in the Trobriand Islands, Western Arnhem Land, and highland New Guinea.[5] Similarly, Marshall writes of Mangaia: 'Traditionally, a male goes from female to female—leaving one for another when he tires of the first or hears that she has gone with another man. People admire the boy who has had many girls, comparing him to "a strong man, like a bull, going from woman to woman." . . . But they do not admire the girl who has many boys, comparing her to a pig.'[6] I suggest this represents,

[1] R. M. Berndt, *Excess and Restraint* (University of Chicago Press: Chicago, 1962), 127–8, on New Guinea.

[2] N. A. Chagnon, 'Yanomamö social organization and warfare', in M. Fried, M. Harris, and R. Murphy (eds.), *War: The Anthropology of Armed Conflict and Aggression*, (The Natural History Press: New York, 1968), 131, on the Yanomanö.

[3] A. C. Kinsey, W. B. Pomeroy, C. E. Martin, and P. H. Gebhard, *Sexual Behaviour in the Human Female*, (W. B. Saunders: Philadelphia, 1953), 415, on the United States.

[4] J. T. Hurber, 'Discussion', in G. D. Goldman and D. S. Milman (eds.), *Modern Woman: Her Psychology and Sexuality* (Charles C. Thomas: Springfield, Ill., 1969).

[5] B. Malinowski, *The Sexual Life of Savages in North-Western Melanesia* (Halcyon House: New York, 1929); R. M. Berndt, and C. H. Berndt, *Sexual Behaviour in Western Arnhem Land* (Viking Fund: New York, 1951); R. M. Berndt, *Excess and Restraint* (University of Chicago Press: Chicago, 1962).

[6] D. S. Marshall, 'Sexual Behavior on Mangaia', in D. S. Marshall and R. C. Suggs (eds.), *Human Sexual Behavior*, (Basic Books: New York, 1971), 150.

not culture causing the sexual double standard, but the cumulative history of individuals attempting to influence one another through language. It seems likely that parents (and perhaps other elder kin) have systematically attempted to inculcate one set of sexual attitudes in their daughters and another in their sons, since copulation exposes males and females to very different risks. [. . .]

[T]he emotional bases of adultery are similar everywhere. [T]hese emotional bases can be illuminated by considering male–female differences. In brief, I shall suggest that a woman's sexual desire for a man other than her husband results largely from a comparison between the potential partner and her husband, and indicates either that she perceives the potential partner as being in some way superior to her husband, or that she is sexually or emotionally dissatisfied with her husband, or both. While men too make these comparisons, a man's sexual desire for a woman to whom he is not married is largely the result of her not being his wife. In addition, I shall suggest that a wife's experience of sexual jealousy varies with the degree of threat to herself that she perceives in her husband's adultery, whereas a husband's experience of sexual jealousy is relatively invariant, his wife's adultery almost always being perceived as threatening. [. . .]

With respect to the desire for sexual variety, the data on adultery can be interpreted as follows. For both sexes, adultery is without doubt influenced both by ontogenetic experiences and by immediate circumstances: people who have been taught that adultery is bad or dangerous are less likely to engage in it than are people who have been taught differently; adultery is more common when its costs—in terms of time, energy, and risk—are low than it is when its costs are high. But although human beings are complex, the determinants of human behavior various and interacting, and the human condition one of mixed emotion, the persistent hint of male–female differences holds out some promise of regularity within diversity.

Women do not generally seem to experience a pervasive, autonomous sexual desire for men to whom they are not married; a woman is most likely to experience desire for extramarital sex when she perceives another man as somehow superior to her husband or when she is in some way dissatisfied with her marriage (while investigators have most often considered emotional and sexual dissatisfactions, economic dissatisfaction may also be important). A woman about to embark on an affair may not be thinking of her husband or her marriage at all, but simply be experiencing sexual desire for her intended lover; yet from the standpoint of ultimate causation, her sexual desire may function primarily as part of the process by which women trade up in the husband market. [. . .] Adultery may also function to increase the genetic quality of a woman's offspring, but this probably is a minor (or rare) function, since it seems unlikely that the detectable genetic differences among males are often great enough to repay the investment of time, energy, and risk that adultery entails.

A male obviously stands to benefit genetically from adultery in that he may sire offspring at almost no cost to himself in terms of time and energy, even when he cannot obtain or support additional wives. Males can be expected to experience a persistent, autonomous desire for extramarital sex because this desire functions to create low-cost reproductive opportunities. As suggested above, human communities probably have always been complex enough that reproductive opportunities could occur at almost any time to almost any adult male; if the desire for variety were satisfied even once in a lifetime, it might pay off reproductively. Adultery does, of course, often entail substantial risk, including risk to marital happiness. For males, then, the occurrence of a low-risk opportunity probably is the most important determinant of adultery. [. . .]

The male desire for sexual variety may also pay off reproductively if it results in obtaining additional wives, especially young wives, and the strength of the sexual desire for young women may vary with male age. It seems likely that throughout human history in early middle age married men often became able to obtain and to support an additional wife or wives, and hence the sexual desire for young women would be especially adaptive at this age. This desire could be adaptive regardless of a male's circumstance if it functioned to motivate the economic and political effort that might make its fulfillment possible. That the desire for prestige, status, and power are autonomous and important male motives and that possession of women is often a sign of status do not negate the importance of sexual motives for economic, political, or sexual behavior. In the West—where polygyny is illegal—affairs involving young women and middle-aged men, which are usually attributed to such factors as 'male menopause,' and which not infrequently result in a man's divorcing an aging wife and beginning a second family with a young wife, might have resulted in polygyny in times past. [. . .]

Sex differences are also apparent in the occurrence of sexual jealousy over a spouse's adultery. In cross-cultural perspective there is no doubt that husbands typically are more concerned about their wives' fidelity than wives are about their husbands' fidelity.[1] Among the Turu of Tanzania, marriages are made for economic rather than emotional reasons and, since marriage is almost exclusively a business enterprise, women are lonely and may initiate extramarital affairs, although most commonly men initiate

---

[1] C. S. Ford, *A Comparative Study of Human Reproduction* (Yale University Press: New Haven, 1945); A. C. Kinsey, W. B. Pomeroy, and C. E. Martin, *Sexual Behavior in the Human Male*, (W. B. Saunders: Philadelphia, 1948); Kinsey *et al.*, *Sexual Behavior in the Human Female*; C. Safilios-Rothschild, 'Attitudes of Greek Spouses toward Marital Infidelity', in G. Neubeck (ed.), *Extramarital Relations*, (Prentice-Hall: Englewood Cliffs, NJ, 1969), 77–93.

them.[1] (According to Schneider, women attempt to establish a kind of relationship missing in their marriage and do not appear to seek sexual variety *per se*.) But although extramarital affairs are common, most Turu husbands want their wives to be faithful; the Turu have an extremely high divorce rate and one of the highest assault and murder rates in Tanzania, primarily owing to wives' extramarital affairs. Kinsey *et al.* (1953) note that men, twice as often as women, said that their spouses' extramarital activities was the main factor precipitating divorce.[2] Kinsey *et al.* write: 'Wives at every social level, more often accept the non-marital activities of their husbands. Husbands are much less inclined to accept the non-marital activities of their wives. It has been so since the dawn of history. The biology and psychology of this difference need more careful analysis than the available data yet afford.'[3]

In Philip Roth's *Portnoy's Complaint*, Alex Portnoy fantasizes giving his father the following pep talk should the latter be discovered in adultery: 'What after all does it consist of? You put your dick some place and moved it back and forth and stuff came out the front. So, Jake, what's the big deal?' Why adultery so often is a big deal, and why it is especially likely to be a big deal to men, can be explained in a straightforward manner by evolutionary biology. As a man never can be certain of paternity, a cuckold risks investing in the offspring of, and having his wife's reproductive efforts tied up by, a reproductive competitor; as a woman always is certain of maternity, and as her husband's adultery does not diminish his capacity to inseminate her, a wife may risk little if her husband engages in extramarital sex.[4] This also explains why having an affair is a more effective female than male tactic in marital skirmishing and why even modern, sophisticated males may be ambivalent about the desirability of libidinousness in a wife.

Charlie Citrine, the protagonist of Saul Bellow's novel *Humboldt's Gift*, says of his lover: 'as a carnal artist she was disheartening as well as thrilling, because, thinking of her as wife-material, I had to ask myself where she had learned all this and whether she had taken the PhD once and for all.' Sex researchers often seem to consider the male tendency to divide women into 'whores' and 'madonnas' (a tendency which reaches ludicrous extremes in some societies) to constitute a sort of perverse contradiction in the male psyche. From an evolutionary perspective, however, a wife's most important sexual attribute by far is fidelity, and this male tendency is less paradoxical.

---

[1] H. K. Schneider, 'Romantic Love among the Turu', in Marshall and Suggs (eds.), *Human Sexual Behavior*, 59–70.

[2] Kinsey *et al.*, *Sexual Behavior in the Human Female*.

[3] Kinsey *et al.*, *Sexual Behavior in the Human Male*, 592.

[4] D. P. Barash, 'Sociobiology and Rape in Mallards (*Anas platyrhynchos*): Responses of the Mated Male', *Science*, 197 (1977), 788–9.

Needless to say, the hypothesis that the ultimate function of male sexual jealousy is to increase the probability that one's wife will conceive one's own rather than someone else's child does not imply that this is a conscious male motive, any more than it is a motive of any sexually jealous male animal. The often vitriolic debate in the literature over whether the members of any human group are really ignorant of the male's role in procreation is fascinating; the reader of this debate gradually abandons the naïve notion that a given people either are or are not ignorant of paternity, and ultimately confronts the questions: What constitutes ignorance or awareness of paternity? and, How can ignorance or awareness be determined?[1] The most likely candidate for a people lacking awareness of paternity are the Trobriand Islanders, among whom male sexual jealousy is pronounced.[2] Indeed, over a very long period of time the existence of reasonably accurate knowledge of the male's role in procreation might actually promote the reduction of male sexual jealousy by natural selection. If the primary function of male jealousy is to reduce the probability that one's wife will be impregnated by another man, and if husbands are able to predict with some accuracy their wives' fertile periods, selection might favor males who are emotionally committed to the goal of siring their wives' offspring (that is, males among whom the ultimate goal had become the proximate, conscious goal) but who rely more on intellect than on 'blind' sexual jealousy to achieve this goal. Such men could be more emotionally flexible on the issue of their wives' extramarital activities and hence could more easily engage in adaptive wife exchanges and could profit from gifts bestowed on their wives in exchange for sexual favors.

In modern Western societies it seems fairly clear that some, perhaps even many, married men can learn to overcome sexual jealousy in order to participate in spouse exchanges and group sex. These sexual arrangements are carefully structured to minimize romantic involvements that might disrupt marriages, and the possibility of conception is eliminated by modern contraceptive technology. But in the few non-Western cases in which male sexual jealousy is alleged to be minimal, it is also stated or implied that paternity is uncertain and unproblematic. One such example was discussed in detail—the Siriono of Bolivia—and it was pointed out that in one of the eight births Holmberg witnessed the woman's husband maintained that the infant was not his; he refused to accept it, and subsequently he would have nothing to do with his wife or her child. Moreover, Holmberg notes that quarrels and fights over sex are common. It was suggested that biological paternity may be more certain, and more important to

[1] E. Leach, 'Virgin Birth', *Proceedings of the Royal Anthropological Institute of Great Britain and Ireland* (1966), 39–49; M. E. Spiro, 'Virgin Birth, Parthenogenesis and Physiological Paternity: An Essay in Cultural Interpretation', *Man*, 3 (1968) 242–61.

[2] Malinowski, *The Sexual Life of Savages in North-Western Melanesia*.

Siriono males, than Holmberg implies, and that there may be substantially less 'sexual freedom' among the Siriono than Holmberg was led to believe.[1]

A second ethnographic example of sexual freedom is that of the Kuikuru of the Brazilian Mato Grosso.[2] According to Carneiro, all adult Kuikuru participate in an elaborate system of extramarital relations: each person has one or more extramarital partners (*ajoi*) who are known to everyone, including spouses, and 'adultery, as a crime, cannot be said to exist in Kuikuru society'.[3] The number of *ajois* a person has is said to vary with his or her attractiveness. Although Carneiro indicates that extramarital liaisons are conducted clandestinely, and that husbands and wives may quarrel and even scratch and bruise one another in disputes over extramarital adventures, no fights among males are recorded, and only one man is reported to have divorced a wife because of her affairs (he subsequently married a less attractive, but harder working, woman who had only one *ajoi*).

An unmarried Kuikuru woman who becomes pregnant attempts abortion; if this fails, she kills the infant at birth. But

if a married woman is going to have a child which she believes has been fathered by an *ajoi* rather than by her legal husband, she goes to the village plaza and makes a public declaration of this fact. The men of the village are then supposed to beat the man allegedly responsible for making her pregnant. This, at any rate, is the idealized procedure. We could learn of no instance in which any such public denunciation had actually been made. In practice, of course, the average Kuikuru wife would ordinarily have no way of knowing just who the biological father of her child was. But at least in this way the Kuikuru can preserve the myth that whether he be wise or not, every man knows his own father.[4]

Ajoi relationships are the subject of a great deal of gossip, joking, and teasing. Carneiro writes:

The Kuikuru did not at first reveal to us the existence of their system of extra-marital sex partners. But once they knew that we had become aware of it, they lost no time in trying to bring us into the system, in name if not in fact. This attempt, indeed, became the basis of a good deal of friendly humor between the tribe and ourselves. They jokingly assigned 5 or 6 *ajois* to my wife and to me, and soon everyone in the village knew the names of our alleged *ajois* as well as they knew the actual tribal ones. They never tired of trying to get us to name our supposed sex partners, and enjoyed it immensely when we counted them off on our fingers, Kuikuru style.

[1] A. R. Holmberg, *Nomads of the Long Bow: The Siriono of Eastern Bolivia* (United States Government Printing Office: Washington, DC, 1950).

[2] R. Carneiro, 'Extra-Marital Sex Freedom among the Kuikuru Indians of Mato Grosso', *Revista do Museu Paulista, São Paulo*, 10 (1958), 137.

[3] Ibid. 141–2.

[4] Ibid. 140.

The chief's wife was said to be one of my *ajois*, and one day when I was in her house an elderly man came up to me and with a perfectly straight face asked me for my red plaid shirt in payment for favors purportedly granted to me by this woman. She was his classificatory daughter.[1]

Now Carneiro does not claim to have ever witnessed an actual act of extramarital intercourse; like all ethnographers, he inferred their existence from the information provided him, information which apparently seemed to be internally consistent and consonant with other aspects of Kuikuru culture. Yet in the single instance in which he had independent evidence— namely himself—the number of publicly known *ajois* was five or six, but the number of actual *ajois*, according to Carneiro, was zero. In a second instance—Carneiro's wife—the actual number of *ajois* also was believed by Carneiro to be zero. Thus it seems reasonable to entertain some skepticism concerning Carneiro's conclusion that biological paternity among the Kuikuru is essentially unknowable.

Uncertain paternity and lack of male jealousy are easily accounted for sociobiologically: where paternity is uncertain, it need only be assumed that men invest in their sisters', rather than their wives', offspring (although this does not appear to be the case among the Kuikuru). Uncertain paternity and lack of male jealousy can be accounted for even more easily by cultural determinism since, in this view, it is the persistence of social systems that is important, and human emotion is largely the product of these systems, rather than the other way around. Biological paternity eliminations on a series of Kuikuru infants would be helpful in resolving this matter; as things stand, the issue remains an open one. Nevertheless, the evidence presently available seems to me not to rule out the following hypotheses: (1) men everywhere prefer their wives to be sexually faithful; and (2) there is not now, and never has been, a society in which confidence in paternity is so low that men are typically more closely related genetically to their sisters' than to their wives' offspring. Happily promiscuous, non-possessive, Rousseauian chimpanzees turned out not to exist; I am not convinced by the available evidence that such human beings exist either.

[*The Evolution of Human Sexuality* (Oxford University Press: New York, 1979), 229–44.]

Section C

The Role of Reason

INTRODUCTION

This section covers the most fundamental of all the issues that can be raised about—rather than within—ethics. If ethics is to have an objective basis, it must be because of the role that reasoning can play in ethical argument. If there is no role, or only a minor role, for reason in ethics, then it will not be possible to resolve ethical disputes between people with clashing emotional attitudes or different customary values. Perhaps that is the tough reality that we face, and we should simply accept it. Certainly it is not easy to see how entrenched opponents can resolve their differences over a matter like abortion, for example. But among many of us the hope remains strong that there is, at least in principle, a way out of such disagreements. This would mean that if those who favour and those who oppose abortion understood the nature of ethics and the rational basis of ethical argument, and could agree on all the relevant facts, they would be able to reach the same conclusion about the justifiability of abortion. Of course, it is difficult to put this hope to the test, since agreement on all the relevant facts is usually impossible to obtain—especially when, as in this example, the 'facts' may be as intangible as whether the foetus has an immortal soul.

On contentious issues like abortion, agreement is often beyond reach in practice, and difficult to imagine even in theory. In other cases, however, we shudder to think that both sides in a dispute stand on an equal footing with regard to the ultimate justification—or lack of it—for their views. The Nazi holocaust, or the murderous policies of Pol Pot in Cambodia are the obvious examples. No doubt most decent people disagree with Hitler and Pol Pot on many matters of fact as well as ethics, but it seems likely that, even if the factual differences were cleared away, some utterly fundamental ethical differences would remain. Are we then content to say that there is no further basis for judging between us and the Nazis or the Khmer Rouge? Is there no sense in which our opposition to the murder of millions of people is, when compared to any possible defence of such policies, better grounded, more rational, more defensible, more justifiable—in one word, *right*?

That is what is at stake in the section that follows. David Hume sets up the modern debate, by arguing that reason has only a very limited role to play in influencing what we decide to do. It is not contrary to reason, he insists, to prefer the destruction of the whole world to the scratching of one's little finger; or, conversely, to choose one's own ruin for some small benefit to a total stranger. Since reason has so limited a role to play in our practical decisions, Hume argues, it is not possible for reason to determine what is good or evil—for to recognize that something is good or evil must influence our actions, otherwise ethics would have no point. Hence Hume concludes that the distinction between good and evil must derive from our feelings, not from our capacity to reason. To this he then appends, almost as an afterthought, a remark on the difficulty of deriving an 'ought' judgement from a series of 'is' statements. This concise exposition of the fallacy of deducing values from facts has become one of the most frequently cited passages of modern meta-ethics.

Kant is undoubtedly the greatest opponent of Hume's view of the role of reason in ethics. In the first of the two passages presented here, drawn from *The Foundations of the Metaphysics of Morals*, he indicates the extent to which he excludes all feelings as moral motives. To help others because one has kindly feelings towards them is, Kant states, of no moral worth; an act has moral worth only in so far as it is done out of a sense of duty—that is, out of respect for the pure moral law in itself. He then argues that when we abstract all feelings, we are left with only the pure form of the rational moral law, which, since it holds for all rational beings, must be universal in its form. Thus Kant reaches his famous categorical imperative: 'Act only on that maxim through which you can at the same time will that it should become a universal law.' (For a continuation of Kant's argument here, and the substantive ethical conclusions that he draws from it, see also the extract from this work in Part IIB.)

Kant's argument for the categorical imperative does, however, leave one important question unanswered. For Kant, although human beings take part in the world of reason, through their intellectual capacities, they must act in the physical world, ruled by cause and effect. Even if we grant, therefore, that reason alone leads us to the categorical imperative as the standard by which all moral action must be judged, there remains a puzzle about how this judgement of reason can ever lead human beings to act. Is reason alone a motive, or can it—as Hume argued—only give rise to action if it shows us how to achieve what we already want? In the passage reprinted here from *The Critique of Practical Reason*, Kant tries to overcome this problem by suggesting that our recognition of the moral law *necessarily* leads to a special feeling of respect that serves as an incentive to us to follow the moral law. Hence a feeling does serve as the basis of our actions, but, uniquely among feelings, it is one that all rational beings must have.

Kant's attempt to show that reason alone can guide us to do what is right has had an enormous impact on later thinkers, especially on the European continent; but it was not long before Hegel, the greatest German philosopher of the generation that grew up in the shadow of Kant, raised doubts about its success. Hegel's dialectical method in philosophy was always to show that each step forward leads to contradictions that produce its opposite, or antithesis, and both aspects of the contradiction must play a role in a satisfactory solution to it. So Kant's morality of duty was, Hegel said, so abstract that it had no real content. 'Duty for duty's sake' is an empty formula that can give no guidance until it is filled with substantive ethical principles, which must come from somewhere else—in Hegel's view, from our absorption in the real ethical life of our own community. Hegel would like to reconcile Kant's morality of abstract universal reason with the more substantive ethical standards given by one's own community; the difficulty is to show how this reconciliation is possible, without abandoning reason in favour of blind obedience to custom.

Other extracts in this section show a variety of positions on the role of reason in ethics. Henry Sidgwick, the last of the great nineteenth-century English utilitarians, sought axioms on which to base his moral philosophy. He called these axioms 'intuitions', but they were not the kind of intuition for which we need some special sense. Rather, they were principles that we can see, when we consider them carefully, to be self-evidently true. Edward Westermarck, writing his encyclopaedic study *The Origin and Development of the Moral Ideas* shortly after Sidgwick had published *The Methods of Ethics*, was certain that people from different cultures would not share Sidgwick's judgement that these axioms are self-evidently true. For him, there was no objective moral truth, only custom—sharing some patterns of development, it is true, but ultimately based on emotion, and varying from one society to the next.

Ludwig Wittgenstein wrote very little that was explicitly on ethics; the lecture reprinted here, which was given in Cambridge in 1929 but not published until many years later, is an exception. The lecture displays Wittgenstein's unique style of philosophy, including his focus on language. Both this and the following reading, from A. J. Ayer's *Language, Truth and Logic*, work out, in different ways, the implications of logical positivism for ethics. A central tenet of this philosophical movement, so influential in the first half of the present century, is that there is a sharp distinction between scientific statements, which describe the state of the world and are, at least in principle, verifiable, and all other utterances, which tell us nothing about the world. These other statements are either truths of logic, in which case they are tautologies, or else, strictly speaking, they are nonsense. This means, for Wittgenstein, that they cannot be uttered intelligibly, and so, about topics like ethics, it is better to remain silent. Ayer, on the other hand, interprets ethical judgements as expressions of emotions, rather like 'hurray' and 'boo'. On neither account is there a role for reason in ethics.

Ayer's 'emotivist' account of ethics became the dominant philosophical view in the English-speaking world after World War II. In France this period was the heyday of existentialism, which led to equally sceptical conclusions about the role of reason. In the selection from *Existentialism is a Humanism*, Jean-Paul Sartre explains that if there is no God, we are not made according to any plan, nor have any objective values been laid down for us. We are free to choose, and there are no rules to help us in our quandaries—a point that Sartre makes with the help of the example of the young Frenchman who, during the war, had to choose between joining the Free French Forces in England or staying with his mother, who lived only for him. Memorable as this oft-cited example is, however, it may prove less than Sartre thinks. Even those who think that ethics has an objective basis could readily accept the difficulty of making decisions in such circumstances, when the probable outcome of each course of action is so unclear.

Thomas Nagel is a contemporary American philosopher who, for many years, has been developing arguments against Hume's view of the very limited role that reason can play in our practical decisions. The passage reprinted here gives a brief and simplified account of one of these arguments; Nagel tries to show that the sufferings of others are bad and that, from a general point of view, they matter, irrespective of how we might feel about them. If he is right, then Hume must have been wrong when he said that it was not contrary to reason for me to choose the destruction of the whole world in order to avoid scratching my little finger. Because such a choice would give no weight to the sufferings of others, it would, in Nagel's view, be contrary to reason, irrespective of how little I cared for everyone else in the world. Here Nagel's idea of reason is closer to that of Kant's categorical imperative than to Hume's view of reason as the slave of the passions. For J. L. Mackie, however, there is something 'queer' about such a reason. Mackie sides with Hume, and adds another buttress to his position by pointing out that if there is something that is good, in an objective sense, for everyone, it would have to have 'to-be-pursuedness' built into it. Just what in the world this could be, remains quite mysterious. At this point it is appropriate to note that the boundary between meta-ethics and normative ethics is sometimes hard to draw, and one essay in Part IIB of this anthology could equally well have been placed here, in the present section. In 'The Structure of Ethics and Morals' R. M. Hare presents an account of reasoning in ethics that leads to a form of utilitarianism. The effect of the kind of ethical reasoning that Hare defends is rather like that of Nagel, but by relying on what he believes to be inherent in the moral concepts, rather than on any notion of objective reason, Hare avoids difficulties about the possibility of objective goodness or 'to-be-pursuedness'. The question is whether, in so doing, he limits the application of his view to those who accept a particular set of moral concepts.

Colin McGinn is one of a small number of philosophers who have tried to use our growing knowledge of social evolution to provide a better understanding of the nature of ethics. In 'Evolution and the Basis of Morality' he develops a novel argument against Hume and his supporters. How, McGinn asks, can we explain the very existence of morality in our species, given what we know about the way in which the process of evolution would deselect altruists who assist strangers when there is no prospect of any reciprocity? His answer is: only if we assume that ethics has a rational basis. Then we could argue that there were evolutionary advantages in the development of our reasoning powers, and when evolution selected for reason, it had to take morality as part of the package.

The rise of feminist ways of thinking has added a new twist to the long debate about reason in ethics. Some women have argued that the ideal of an ethic derived from some universal law of reason is a male vision which is not universal at all, because it leaves out the way in which half the human population thinks about ethics. This claim is disturbing to a male who believes, as I do, that reasoning is the best way of getting closer to resolving the ethical controversies that we face. In this section Virginia Held considers whether male bias has led to a greater emphasis on the role played by reason, rather than emotion, in ethics; and she asks what a genuinely gender-neutral moral theory would be like.

Michael Smith's essay brings up to date the discussion of the role of reason in ethics. In philosophy departments today, these long-standing issues are being fought out in the form of a debate over 'moral realism', or, as Smith puts it, 'the metaphysical view that there exist moral facts'. In the light of Mackie's argument from queerness, however, modern moral realists like Smith see moral facts as nothing more mysterious than the desires we would have if we were to reflect on our desires under special circumstances. Smith's essay makes a fitting conclusion to the debate between Hume and Kant, because his notion of idealized desires as reasons for action suggests a possible convergence between desire-based and reason-based theories.

Of the Influencing Motives of the Will

Nothing is more usual in philosophy, and even in common life, than to talk of the combat of passion and reason, to give the preference to reason, and to assert that men are only so far virtuous as they conform themselves to its dictates. Every rational creature, 'tis said, is oblig'd to regulate his actions by reason; and if any other motive or principle challenge the direction of his conduct, he ought to oppose it, 'till it be entirely subdu'd, or at least brought to a conformity with that superior principle. On this method of thinking the greatest part of moral philosophy, ancient and modern, seems to be founded; nor is there an ampler field, as well for metaphysical arguments, as popular declamations, than this suppos'd pre-eminence of reason above passion. The eternity, invariableness, and divine origin of the former have been display'd to the best advantage: The blindness, unconstancy and deceitfulness of the latter have been as strongly insisted on. In order to shew the fallacy of all this philosophy, I shall endeavour to prove *first*, that reason alone can never be a motive to any action of the will; and *secondly*, that it can never oppose passion in the direction of the will.

The understanding exerts itself after two different ways, as it judges from demonstration or probability; as it regards the abstract relations of our ideas, or those relations of objects, of which experience only gives us information. I believe it scarce will be asserted, that the first species of reasoning alone is ever the cause of any action. As its proper province is the world of ideas, and as the will always places us in that of realities, demonstration and volition seem, upon that account, to be totally remov'd, from each other. Mathematics, indeed, are useful in all mechanical operations, and arithmetic in almost every art and profession: But 'tis not of themselves they have any influence. Mechanics are the art of regulating the motions of bodies *to some design'd end or purpose*; and the reason why we employ arithmetic in fixing the proportions of numbers, is only that we may discover the proportions of their influence and operation. A merchant is desirous of knowing the sum total of his accounts with any person: Why? but that he may learn what sum will have the same *effects* in paying his debt, and going to market, as all the particular articles taken together. Abstract or demonstrative reasoning, therefore, never influences any of our actions, but only as it directs our judgment concerning causes and effects; which leads us to the second operation of the understanding.

'Tis obvious, that when we have the prospect of pain or pleasure from any object, we feel a consequent emotion of aversion or propensity, and are carry'd to avoid or embrace what will give us this uneasiness or satisfaction. 'Tis also obvious, that this emotion rests not here, but making us cast our view on every side, comprehends whatever objects are connected with its original one by the relation of cause and effect. Here then reasoning takes place to discover this relation; and according as our reasoning varies, our actions receive a subsequent variation. But 'tis evident in this case, that the impulse arises not from reason, but is only directed by it. 'Tis from the prospect of pain or pleasure that the aversion or propensity arises towards any object: And these emotions extend themselves to the causes and effects of that object, as they are pointed out to us by reason and experience. It can never in the least concern us to know, that such objects are causes, and such others effects, if both the causes and effects be indifferent to us. Where the objects themselves do not affect us, their connexion can never give them any influence; and 'tis plain, that as reason is nothing but the discovery of this connexion, it cannot be by its means that the objects are able to affect us.

Since reason alone can never produce any action, or give rise to volition, I infer, that the same faculty is as incapable of preventing volition, or of disputing the preference with any passion or emotion. This consequence is necessary. 'Tis impossible reason cou'd have the latter effect of preventing volition, but by giving an impulse in a contrary direction to our passion; and that impulse, had it operated alone, would have been able to produce volition. Nothing can oppose or retard the impulse of passion, but a contrary impulse; and if this contrary impulse ever arises from reason, that latter faculty must have an original influence on the will, and must be able to cause, as well as hinder any act of volition. But if reason has no original influence, 'tis impossible it can withstand any principle, which has such an efficacy, or ever keep the mind in suspense a moment. Thus it appears, that the principle, which opposes our passion, cannot be the same with reason, and is only call'd so in an improper sense. We speak not strictly and philosophically when we talk of the combat of passion and of reason. Reason is, and ought only to be the slave of the passions, and can never pretend to any other office than to serve and obey them. As this opinion may appear somewhat extraordinary, it may not be improper to confirm it by some other considerations.

A passion is an original existence, or, if you will, modification of existence, and contains not any representative quality, which renders it a copy of any other existence or modification. When I am angry, I am actually possest with the passion, and in that emotion have no more a reference to any other object, than when I am thirsty, or sick, or more than five foot high. 'Tis impossible, therefore, that this passion can be oppos'd by, or be contradictory to truth and reason; since this contradiction consists in the disagreement of ideas, consider'd as copies, with those objects, which they represent.

What may at first occur on this head, is, that as nothing can be contrary to truth or reason, except what has a reference to it, and as the judgments of our understanding only have this reference, it must follow, that passions can be contrary to reason only so far as they are *accompany'd* with some judgment or opinion. According to this principle, which is so obvious and natural, 'tis only in two senses, that any affection can be call'd unreasonable. First, When a passion, such as hope or fear, grief or joy, despair or security, is founded on the supposition of the existence of objects, which really do not exist. Secondly, When in exerting any passion in action, we chuse means insufficient for the design'd end, and deceive ourselves in our judgment of causes and effects. Where a passion is neither founded on false suppositions, nor chuses means insufficient for the end, the understanding can neither justify nor condemn it. 'Tis not contrary to reason to prefer the destruction of the whole world to the scratching of my finger. 'Tis not contrary to reason for me to *chuse* my total ruin, to prevent the least uneasiness of an *Indian* or person wholly unknown to me. 'Tis as little contrary to reason to prefer even my own acknowledg'd lesser good to my greater, and have a more ardent affection for the former than the latter. A trivial good may, from certain circumstances, produce a desire superior to what arises from the greatest and most valuable enjoyment; nor is there any thing more extraordinary in this, than in mechanics to see one pound weight raise up a hundred by the advantage of its situation. In short, a passion must be accompany'd with some false judgment, in order to its being unreasonable; and even then 'tis not the passion, properly speaking, which is unreasonable, but the judgment.

The consequences are evident. Since a passion can never, in any sense, be call'd unreasonable, but when founded on a false supposition, or when it chuses means insufficient for the design'd end, 'tis impossible, that reason and passion can ever oppose each other, or dispute for the government of the will and actions. The moment we perceive the falshood of any supposition, or the insufficiency of any means our passions yield to our reason without any opposition. I may desire any fruit as of an excellent relish; but whenever you convince me of my mistake, my longing ceases. I may will the performance of certain actions as means of obtaining any desir'd good; but as my willing of these actions is only secondary, and founded on the supposition, that they are causes of the propos'd effect; as soon as I discover the falshood of that supposition, they must become indifferent to me.

'Tis natural for one, that does not examine objects with a strict philosophic eye, to imagine, that those actions of the mind are entirely the same, which produce not a different sensation, and are not immediately distinguishable to the feeling and perception. Reason, for instance, exerts itself without producing any sensible emotion; and except in the more sublime disquisitions of philosophy, or in the frivolous subtilties of the schools, scarce ever conveys any pleasure or uneasiness. Hence it proceeds, that every action of the mind, which operates with the same calmness and tranquillity, is confounded with reason by all those, who judge of things from the first view and appearance. Now 'tis certain, there are certain calm desires and tendencies, which, tho' they be real passions, produce little emotion in the mind, and are more known by their effects than by the immediate feeling or sensation. These desires are of two kinds; either certain instincts originally implanted in our natures, such as benevolence and resentment, the love of life, and kindness to children; or the general appetite to good, and aversion to evil, consider'd merely as such. When any of these passions are calm, and cause no disorder in the soul, they are very readily taken for the determinations of reason, and are suppos'd to proceed from the same faculty, with that, which judges of truth and falshood. Their nature and principles have been suppos'd the same, because their sensations are not evidently different.

Beside these calm passions, which often determine the will, there are certain violent emotions of the same kind, which have likewise a great influence on that faculty. When I receive any injury from another, I often feel a violent passion of resentment, which makes me desire his evil and punishment, independent of all considerations of pleasure and advantage to myself. When I am immediately threaten'd with any grievous ill, my fears, apprehension, and aversions rise to a great height, and produce a sensible emotion.

The common error of metaphysicians has lain in ascribing the direction of the will entirely to one of these principles, and supposing the other to have no influence. Men often act knowingly against their interest: For which reason the view of the greatest possible good does not always influence them. Men often counter-act a violent passion in prosecution of their interests and designs: 'Tis not therefore the present uneasiness alone, which determines them. In general we may observe, that both these principles operate on the will; and where they are contrary, that either of them prevails, according to the *general* character or *present* disposition of the person. What we call strength of mind, implies the prevalence of the calm passions above the violent; tho' we may easily observe, there is no man so constantly possess'd of this virtue, as never on any occasion to yield to the sollicitations of passion and desire. From these variations of temper proceeds the great difficulty of deciding concerning the actions and resolutions of men, where there is any contrariety of motives and passions. [. . .]

Moral Distinctions Not Deriv'd from Reason

[U]pon the whole, 'tis impossible, that the distinction betwixt moral good and evil, can be made by reason; since that distinction has an influence upon our actions, of which reason alone is incapable. Reason and judgment may, indeed, be the mediate cause of an action, by prompting, or by directing a passion: But it is not pretended, that a judgment of this kind, either in its truth or falshood, is attended with virtue or vice. And as to the judgments, which are caused by our judgments, they can still less bestow those moral qualities on the actions, which are their causes. [. . .]

But can there be any difficulty in proving, that vice and virtue are not matters of fact, whose existence we can infer by reason? Take any action allow'd to be vicious: Wilful murder, for instance. Examine it in all lights, and see if you can find that matter of fact, or real existence, which you call *vice*. In which-ever way you take it. you find only certain passions, motives, volitions and thoughts. There is no other matter of fact in the case. The vice entirely escapes you, as long as you consider the object. You never can find it, till you turn your reflexion into your own breast, and find a sentiment of disapprobation, which arises in you, towards this action. Here is a matter of fact; but 'tis the object of feeling, not of reason. It lies in yourself, not in the object. So that when you pronounce any action or character to be vicious, you mean nothing, but that from the constitution of your nature you have a feeling or sentiment of blame from the contemplation of it. Vice and virtue, therefore, may be compar'd to sounds, colours, heat and cold, which, according to modern philosophy, are not qualities in objects, but perceptions in the mind: And this discovery in morals, like that other in physics, is to be regarded as a considerable advancement of the speculative sciences; tho', like that too, it has little or no influence on practice. Nothing can be more real, or concern us more, than our own sentiments of pleasure and uneasiness; and if these be favourable to virtue, and unfavourable to vice, no more can be requisite to the regulation of our conduct and behaviour.

I cannot forbear adding to these reasonings an observation, which may, perhaps, be found of some importance. In every system of morality, which I have hitherto met with, I have always remark'd, that the author proceeds for some time in the ordinary way of reasoning, and establishes the being of a God, or makes observations concerning human affairs; when of a sudden I am surpriz'd to find, that instead of the usual copulations of propositions, *is*, and *is not*, I meet with no proposition that is not connected with an *ought*, or an *ought not*. This change is imperceptible; but is, however, of the last consequence. For as this *ought* or *ought not*, expresses some new relation or affirmation, 'tis necessary that it shou'd be observ'd and explain'd; and at the same time that a reason should be given, for what seems altogether inconceivable, how this new relation can be a deduction from others, which are entirely different from it. But as authors do not commonly use this precaution, I shall presume to recommend it to the readers; and am persuaded, that this small attention would subvert all the vulgar systems of morality, and let us see, that the distinction of vice and virtue is not founded merely on the relations of objects, nor is perceiv'd by reason.

Moral Distinctions Deriv'd from a Moral Sense

Thus the course of the argument leads us to conclude, that since vice and virtue are not discoverable merely by reason, or the comparison of ideas, it must be by means of some impression or sentiment they occasion, that we are able to mark the difference betwixt them. Our decisions concerning moral rectitude and depravity are evidently perceptions; and as all perceptions are either impressions or ideas, the exclusion of the one is a convincing argument for the other. Morality, therefore, is more properly felt than judg'd of; tho' this feeling or sentiment is commonly so soft and gentle, that we are apt to confound it with an idea, according to our common custom of taking all things for the same, which have any near resemblance to each other.

[*A Treatise on Human Nature*, ed. L. A. Selby-Bigge (Clarendon Press: Oxford, 1888), 413–18, 462–3, 468–70. First published in 1739–40.]

IMMANUEL KANT

34 **Pure Practical Reason and the Moral Law**

Nothing in the world—indeed nothing even beyond the world—can possibly be conceived which could be called good without qualification except a *good will*. Intelligence, wit, judgment, and the other talents of the mind, however they may be named, or courage, resoluteness, and perseverence as qualities of temperament are doubtless in many respects good and desirable. But they can become extremely bad and harmful if the will, which is to make use of these gifts of nature and which in its special constitution is called character, is not good. It is the same with the gifts of fortune. Power, riches, honor, even health, general well-being, and the contentment with one's condition which is called happiness make for pride and even arrogance if there is not a good will to correct their influence on the mind and on its principles of action, so as to make it universally conformable to its end. It need hardly be mentioned that the sight of a being adorned with no feature of a pure and good will yet enjoying uninterrupted prosperity can never give pleasure to a rational impartial observer. Thus the good will seems to constitute the indispensable condition even of worthiness to be happy.

Some qualities seem to be conducive to this good will and can facilitate its action, but, in spite of that, they have no intrinsic unconditional worth.

They rather presuppose a good will, which limits the high esteem which one otherwise rightly has for them and prevents their being held to be absolutely good. Moderation in emotions and passions, self-control, and calm deliberation not only are good in many respects but even seem to constitute a part of the inner worth of the person. But however unconditionally they were esteemed by the ancients, they are far from being good without qualification. For, without the principles of a good will, they can become extremely bad, and the coolness of a villain makes him not only far more dangerous but also more directly abominable in our eyes than he would have seemed without it.

The good will is not good because of what it effects or accomplishes or because of its adequacy to achieve some proposed end; it is good only because of its willing, i.e. it is good of itself. And, regarded for itself, it is to be esteemed incomparably higher than anything which could be brought about by it in favor of any inclination or even of the sum total of all inclinations. Even if it should happen that, by a particularly unfortunate fate or by the niggardly provision of a stepmotherly nature, this will should be wholly lacking in power to accomplish its purpose, and if even the greatest effort should not avail it to achieve anything of its end, and if there remained only the good will (not as a mere wish but as the summoning of all the means in our power), it would sparkle like a jewel with its own light, as something that had its full worth in itself. Usefulness or fruitlessness can neither diminish nor augment this worth. Its usefulness would be only its setting, as it were, so as to enable us to handle it more conveniently in commerce or to attract the attention of those who are not yet connoisseurs, but not to recommend it to those who are experts or to determine its worth.

But there is something so strange in this idea of the absolute worth of the will alone, in which no account is taken of any use, that, notwithstanding the agreement even of common sense, the suspicion must arise that perhaps only high-flown fancy is its hidden basis, and that we may have misunderstood the purpose of nature in its appointment of reason as the ruler of our will. We shall therefore examine this idea from this point of view.

In the natural constitution of an organized being, i.e. one suitably adapted to life, we assume as an axiom that no organ will be found for any purpose which is not the fittest and best adapted to that purpose. Now if its preservation, welfare—in a word, its happiness—were the real end of nature in a being having reason and will, then nature would have hit upon a very poor arrangement in appointing the reason of the creature to be the executor of this purpose. For all the actions which the creature has to perform with this intention, and the entire rule of its conduct, would be dictated much more exactly by instinct, and that end would be far more certainly attained by instinct than it ever could be by reason. And if, over and above this, reason should have been granted to the favored creature, it would have served only to let it contemplate the happy constitution of its nature, to admire it, to rejoice in it, and to be grateful for it to its beneficent cause. But reason would not have been given in order that the being should subject its faculty of desire to that weak and delusive guidance and to meddle with the purpose of nature. In a word, nature would have taken care that reason did not break forth into practical use nor have the presumption, with its weak insight, to think out for itself the plan of happiness and the means of attaining it. Nature would have taken over not only the choice of ends but also that of the means and with wise foresight would have intrusted both to instinct alone.

And, in fact, we find that the more a cultivated reason deliberately devotes itself to the enjoyment of life and happiness, the more the man falls short of true contentment. From this fact there arises in many persons, if only they are candid enough to admit it, a certain degree of misology, hatred of reason. This is particularly the case with those who are most experienced in its use. After counting all the advantages which they draw—I will not say from the invention of the arts of common luxury—from the sciences (which in the end seem to them to be also a luxury of the understanding), they nevertheless find that they have actually brought more trouble on their shoulders instead of gaining in happiness; they finally envy, rather than despise, the common run of men who are better guided by mere natural instinct and who do not permit their reason much influence on their conduct. And we must at least admit that a morose attitude or ingratitude to the goodness with which the world is governed is by no means always found among those who temper or refute the boasting eulogies which are given of the advantages of happiness and contentment with which reason is supposed to supply us. Rather their judgment is based on the idea of another and far more worthy purpose of their existence for which, instead of happiness, their reason is properly intended, this purpose, therefore, being the supreme condition to which the private purposes of men must for the most part defer.

Reason is not, however, competent to guide the will safely with regard to its objects and the satisfaction of all our needs (which it in part multiplies), and to this end an innate instinct would have led with far more certainty. But reason is given to us as a practical faculty, i.e. one which is meant to have an influence on the will. As nature has elsewhere distributed capacities suitable to the functions they are to perform, reason's proper function must be to produce a will good in itself and not one good merely as a means, for to the former reason is absolutely essential. This will must indeed not be the sole and complete good but the highest good and the condition of all others, even of the desire for happiness. In this case it is entirely compatible with the wisdom of nature that the cultivation of reason, which is required for the former unconditional purpose, at least in this life restricts in many ways—indeed can reduce to less than nothing—the achievement of the latter conditional purpose, happiness. For one perceives that nature here does not proceed unsuitably to its purpose, because reason, which recognizes its highest practical vocation in the establishment of a good will, is capable only of a contentment of its own kind, i.e. one that springs from the attainment of a purpose, which in turn is determined by reason, even though this injures the ends of inclination.

We have, then, to develop the concept of a will which is to be esteemed as good of itself without regard to anything else. It dwells already in the natural sound understanding and does not need so much to be taught as only to be brought to light. In the estimation of the entire worth of our actions it always takes first place and is the condition of everything else. In order to show this, we shall take the concept of duty. It contains that of a good will, though with certain subjective restrictions and hindrances; but these are far from concealing it and making it unrecognizable, for they rather bring it out by contrast and make it shine forth all the brighter.

I here omit all actions which are recognized as opposed to duty, even though they may be useful in one respect or another, for with these the question does not arise at all as to whether they may be done *from* duty, since they conflict with it. I also pass over the actions which are really in accordance with duty and to which one has no direct inclination, rather doing them because impelled to do so by another inclination. For it is easily decided whether an action in accord with duty is done from duty or for some selfish purpose. It is far more difficult to note this difference when the action is in accordance with duty and, in addition, the subject has a direct inclination to do it. For example, it is in fact in accordance with duty that a dealer should not overcharge an inexperienced customer, and wherever there is much business the prudent merchant does not do so, having a fixed price for everyone, so that a child may buy of him as cheaply as any other. Thus the customer is honestly served. But this is far from sufficient to justify the belief that the merchant has behaved in this way from duty and principles of honesty. His own advantage required this behavior; but it cannot be assumed that over and above that he had a direct inclination to the purchaser and that, out of love, as it were, he gave none an advantage in price over another. Therefore the action was done neither from duty nor from direct inclination but only for a selfish purpose.

On the other hand, it is a duty to preserve one's life, and moreover everyone has a direct inclination to do so. But, for that reason, the often anxious care which most men take of it has no intrinsic worth, and the maxim of doing so has no moral import. They preserve their lives according to duty, but not from duty. But if adversities and hopeless sorrow completely take away the relish for life; if an unfortunate man, strong in soul, is indignant rather than despondent or dejected over his fate and wishes for death, and yet preserves his life without loving it and from neither inclination nor fear but from duty—then his maxim has a moral import.

To be kind where one can is duty, and there are, moreover, many persons so sympathetically constituted that without any motive of vanity or selfishness they find an inner satisfaction in spreading joy and rejoice in the contentment of others which they have made possible. But I say that, however dutiful and amiable it may be, that kind of action has no true moral worth. It is on a level with other inclinations, such as the inclination to honor, which, if fortunately directed to what in fact accords with duty and is generally useful and thus honorable, deserve praise and encouragement but no esteem. For the maxim lacks the moral import of an action done not from inclination but from duty. But assume that the mind of that friend to mankind was clouded by a sorrow of his own which extinguished all sympathy with the lot of others and that he still had the power to benefit others in distress, but that their need left him untouched because he was preoccupied with his own need. And now suppose him to tear himself, unsolicited by inclination, out of this dead insensibility and to do this action only from duty and without any inclination—then for the first time his action has genuine moral worth. Furthermore, if nature has put little sympathy in the heart of a man, and if he, though an honest man, is by temperament cold and indifferent to the sufferings of others perhaps because he is provided with special gifts of patience and fortitude, and expects or even requires that others should have the same—and such a man would certainly not be the meanest product of nature—would not he find in himself a source from which to give himself a far higher worth than he could have got by having a good-natured temperament? This is unquestionably true even though nature did not make him philanthropic, for it is just here that the worth of the character is brought out, which is morally and incomparably the highest of all: he is beneficent not from inclination but from duty.

To secure one's own happiness is at least indirectly a duty, for discontent with one's condition under pressure from many cares and amid unsatisfied wants could easily become a great temptation to transgress duties. But, without any view to duty, all men have the strongest and deepest inclination to happiness, because in this idea all inclinations are summed up. But the precept of happiness is often so formulated that it definitely thwarts some inclinations, and men can make no definite and certain concept of the sum of satisfaction of all inclinations, which goes under the name of happiness. It is not to be wondered at, therefore, that a single inclination, definite as to what it promises and as to the time at which it can be satisfied, can outweigh a fluctuating idea, and that, for example, a man with the gout can choose to enjoy what he likes and to suffer what he may, because according to his calculations at least on this occasion he has not sacrificed the enjoyment of the

present moment to a perhaps groundless expectation of a happiness supposed to lie in health. But, even in this case, if the universal inclination to
happiness did not determine his will, and if health were not at least for him a
necessary factor in these calculations, there yet would remain, as in all other
cases, a law that he ought to promote his happiness, not from inclination but
from duty. Only from this law would his conduct have true moral worth.

It is in this way, undoubtedly, that we should understand those passages
of Scripture which command us to love our neighbor and even our enemy,
for love as an inclination cannot be commanded. But beneficence from
duty, also when no inclination impels it and even when it is opposed by a
natural and unconquerable aversion, is practical love, not pathological love;
it resides in the will and not in the propensities of feeling, in principles of
action and not in tender sympathy; and it alone can be commanded.

[Thus the first proposition of morality is that to have moral worth an
action must be done from duty.] The second proposition is: An action done
from duty does not have its moral worth in the purpose which is to be
achieved through it but in the maxim by which it is determined. Its moral
value, therefore, does not depend on the reality of the object of the action
but merely on the principle of volition by which the action is done without
any regard to the objects of the faculty of desire. From the preceding
discussion it is clear that the purposes we may have for our actions and their
effects as ends and incentives of the will cannot give the actions any
unconditional and moral worth. Wherein, then, can this worth lie, if it is
not in the will in relation to its hoped-for effect? It can lie nowhere else than
in the principle of the will irrespective of the ends which can be realized by
such action. For the will stands, as it were, at the crossroads halfway
between its a priori principle which is formal and its a posteriori incentive
which is material. Since it must be determined by something, if it is done
from duty, it must be determined by the formal principle of volition as
such, since every material principle has been withdrawn from it.

The third principle, as a consequence of the two preceding, I would
express as follows: Duty is the necessity of an action done from respect for
the law. I can certainly have an inclination to the object as an effect of the
proposed action, but I can never have respect for it precisely because it is a
mere effect and not an activity of a will. Similarly, I can have no respect for
any inclination whatsoever, whether my own or that of another; in the
former case I can at most approve of it and in the latter I can even love it,
i.e. see it as favorable to my own advantage. But that which is connected
with my will merely as ground and not as consequence, that which does
not serve my inclination but overpowers it or at least excludes it from being
considered in making a choice—in a word, the law itself—can be an object
of respect and thus a command. Now as an act from duty wholly excludes
the influence of inclination and therewith every object of the will, nothing

remains which can determine the will objectively except the law and subjectively except pure respect for this practical law. This subjective element is the maxim that I should follow such a law even if it thwarts all my inclinations.

Thus the moral worth of an action does not lie in the effect which is expected from it or in any principle of action which has to borrow its motive from this expected effect. For all these effects (agreeableness of condition, indeed even the promotion of the happiness of others) could be brought about through other causes and would not require the will of a rational being, while the highest and unconditional good can be found only in such a will. Therefore, the pre-eminent good can consist only in the conception of the law in itself (which can be present only in a rational being) so far as this conception and not the hoped-for effect is the determining ground of the will. This pre-eminent good, which we call moral, is already present in the person who acts according to this conception, and we do not have to expect it first in the result.

But what kind of a law can that be, the conception of which must determine the will without reference to the expected result? Under this condition alone the will can be called absolutely good without qualification. Since I have robbed the will of all impulses which could come to it from obedience to any law, nothing remains to serve as a principle of the will except universal conformity of its action to law as such. That is, I should never act in such a way that I could not will that my maxim should be a universal law. Mere conformity to law as such (without assuming any particular law applicable to certain actions) serves as the principle of the will, and it must serve as such a principle if duty is not to be a vain delusion and chimerical concept. The common reason of mankind in its practical judgments is in perfect agreement with this and has this principle constantly in view.

* * * * * *

What is essential in the moral worth of actions is that the moral law should directly determine the will. If the determination of the will occurs in accordance with the moral law but only by means of a feeling of any kind whatsoever, which must be presupposed in order that the law may become a determining ground of the will, and if the action thus occurs not for the sake of the law, it has legality but not morality. [. . .]

Any further motives which would make it possible for us to dispense with that of moral law must not be sought, for they would only produce hypocrisy without any substance. Even to let other motives (such as those toward certain advantages) co-operate with the moral law is risky. Therefore, for the purpose of giving the moral law influence on the will, nothing remains but to determine carefully in what way the moral law becomes an incentive and, since the moral law is such an incentive, to see what happens to the human faculty of desire as a consequence of this determining ground. For how a law in itself can be the direct determining ground of the will (which is the essence of morality) is an insoluble problem for the human reason. It is identical with the problem of how a free will is possible. Therefore, we shall not have to show a priori why the moral law supplies an incentive but rather what it effects (or better, must effect) in the mind, so far as it is an incentive.

The essential point in all determination of the will through the moral law is this: as a free will, and thus not only without co-operating with sensuous impulses but even rejecting all of them and checking all inclinations so far as they could be antagonistic to the law, it is determined merely by the law. Thus far, the effect of the moral law as an incentive is only negative, and as such this incentive can be known a priori. For all inclination and every sensuous impulse is based on feeling, and the negative effect on feeling (through the check on the inclinations) is itself feeling. Consequently, we can see a priori that the moral law as a ground of determination of the will, by thwarting all our inclinations, must produce a feeling which can be called pain. Here we have the first and perhaps the only case wherein we can determine from a priori concepts the relation of a cognition (here a cognition of pure practical reason) to the feeling of pleasure or displeasure. All inclinations taken together (which can be brought into a fairly tolerable system, whereupon their satisfaction is called happiness) constitute self-regard (*solipsismus*). This consists either of self-love, which is a predominant benevolence toward one's self (*philautia*) or of self-satisfaction (*arrogantia*). The former is called, more particularly, selfishness; the latter, self-conceit. Pure practical reason merely checks selfishness, for selfishness, as natural and active in us even prior to the moral law, is restricted by the moral law to agreement with the law; when this is done, selfishness is called rational self-love. But it strikes self-conceit down, since all claims of self-esteem which precede conformity to the moral law are null and void. For the certainty of a disposition which agrees with this law is the first condition of any worth of the person (as will soon be made clear), and any presumption [to worth] prior to this is false and opposed to the law. Now the propensity to self-esteem, so long as it rests only on the sensibility, is one of the inclinations which the moral law checks. Therefore, the moral law strikes down self-conceit. [...]

If anything checks our self-conceit in our own judgment, it humiliates. Therefore, the moral law inevitably humbles every man when he compares the sensuous propensity of his nature with the law. Now if the idea of something as the determining ground of the will humiliates us in our self-consciousness, it awakens respect for itself so far as it is positive and the ground of determination. The moral law, therefore, is even subjectively a cause of respect. [...]

Fontanelle says, 'I bow to a great man, but my mind does not bow.' I can add: to a humble plain man, in whom I perceive righteousness in a higher degree than I am conscious of in myself, *my mind bows* whether I choose or not, and however high I carry my head that he may not forget my superior position. Why? His example holds a law before me which strikes down my self-conceit when I compare my own conduct with it; that it is a law which can be obeyed, and consequently is one that can actually be put into practice, is proved before my eyes by the act. I may even be conscious of a like degree of righteousness in myself, and yet respect remains. In men all good is defective, but the law made visible in an example always humbles my pride, since the man whom I see before me provides me with a standard, by clearly appearing to me in a more favorable light regardless of his imperfections, which, though perhaps always with him, are not so well known to me as are my own. Respect is a tribute we cannot refuse to pay to merit whether we will or not; we can indeed outwardly withhold it, but we cannot help feeling it inwardly. [...]

Respect for the moral law is therefore the sole and undoubted moral incentive, so far as this feeling is directed to no object except on this basis. First, the moral law determines the will directly and objectively in the judgment of reason. Freedom, the causality of which is determinable merely through the law, consists, however, only in the fact that it limits all inclinations, including self-esteem, to the condition of obedience to its pure law. This limitation exerts an effect on feeling and produces the sensation of displeasure, which can be known a priori from the moral law. Since, however, it is so far a merely negative effect, originating from the influence of pure practical reason, it checks the activity of the subject to the extent that inclinations are its grounds of determination, and consequently it checks also the opinion of his personal worth, which is nothing without accordance with the moral law. Thus the effect of this law on feeling is merely humiliation, which we thus see a priori, though we cannot know the force of the pure practical law as incentive but only the resistance to the incentives of sensibility. The same law, however, is objectively, i.e. in the conception of pure reason, a direct determining ground of the will. Hence this humiliation occurs proportionately to the purity of the law; for that reason the lowering of the pretensions of moral self-esteem (humiliation) on the sensuous side is an elevation of the moral, i.e. practical, esteem for the law on the intellectual side. In a word, respect for the law is thus by virtue of its intellectual cause a positive feeling that can be known a priori.

[*The Foundations of the Metaphysics of Morals* and *Critique of Practical Reason*, in *The Philosophy of Immanuel Kant*, trans. L. W. Beck (University of Chicago Press: Chicago, 1949), 55–63, 180–6. First published in 1785 and 1788 respectively.]

35   Adding Ethical Substance to Kant's Empty Formalism

Duty itself in the moral self-consciousness is the essence or the universality of that consciousness, the way in which it is inwardly related to itself alone; all that is left to it, therefore, is abstract universality, and for its determinate character it has identity without content, or the abstractly positive, the indeterminate.

However essential it is to give prominence to the pure unconditioned self-determination of the will as the root of duty, and to the way in which knowledge of the will, thanks to Kant's philosophy, has won its firm foundation and starting-point for the first time owing to the thought of its infinite autonomy, still to adhere to the exclusively moral position, without making the transition to the conception of ethics, is to reduce this gain to an empty formalism, and the science of morals to the preaching of duty for duty's sake. From this point of view, no immanent doctrine of duties is possible; of course, material may be brought in from outside and particular duties may be arrived at accordingly, but if the definition of duty is taken to be the absence of contradiction, formal correspondence with itself—which is nothing but abstract indeterminacy stabilized—then no transition is possible to the specification of particular duties nor, if some such particular content for acting comes under consideration, is there any criterion in that principle for deciding whether it is or is not a duty. On the contrary, by this means any wrong or immoral line of conduct may be justified.

Kant's further formulation, the possibility of visualizing an action as a *universal* maxim, does lead to the more concrete visualization of a situation, but in itself it contains no principle beyond abstract identity and the 'absence of contradiction' already mentioned.

The absence of property contains in itself just as little contradiction as the non-existence of this or that nation, family, &c., or the death of the whole human race. But if it is already established on other grounds and presupposed that property and human life are to exist and be respected, then indeed it is a contradiction to commit theft or murder; a contradiction must be a contradiction of something, i.e. of some content presupposed from the start as a fixed principle. It is to a principle of that kind alone, therefore, that an action can be related either by correspondence or contradiction. But if duty is to be willed simply for duty's sake and not for the sake of some content, it is only a formal identity whose nature it is to exclude all content and specification. [. . .]

Virtue is the ethical order reflected in the individual character so far as that character is determined by its natural endowment. When virtue displays itself solely as the individual's simple conformity with the duties of the station to which he belongs, it is rectitude.

In an *ethical* community, it is easy to say what man must do, what are the duties he has to fulfil in order to be virtuous: he has simply to follow the well-known and explicit rules of his own situation. Rectitude is the general character which may be demanded of him by law or custom. But from the standpoint of *morality*, rectitude often seems to be something comparatively inferior, something beyond which still higher demands must be made on oneself and others, because the craving to be something special is not satisfied with what is absolute and universal; it finds consciousness of peculiarity only in what is exceptional.

The various facets of rectitude may equally well be called virtues, since they are also properties of the individual, although not specially of him in contrast with others. Talk about virtue, however, readily borders on empty rhetoric, because it is only about something abstract and indeterminate; and furthermore, argumentative and expository talk of the sort is addressed to the individual as to a being of caprice and subjective inclination. In an existing ethical order in which a complete system of ethical relations has been developed and actualized, virtue in the strict sense of the word is in place and actually appears only in exceptional circumstances or when one obligation clashes with another. The clash, however, must be a genuine one, because moral reflection can manufacture clashes of all sorts to suit its purpose and give itself a consciousness of being something special and having made sacrifices. It is for this reason that the phenomenon of virtue proper is commoner when societies and communities are uncivilized, since in those circumstances ethical conditions and their actualization are more a matter of private choice or the natural genius of an exceptional individual. For instance, it was especially to Hercules that the ancients ascribed virtue. In the states of antiquity, ethical life had not grown into this free system of an objective order self-subsistently developed, and consequently it was by the personal genius of individuals that this defect had to be made good. It follows that if a 'doctrine of virtues' is not a mere 'doctrine of duties', and if therefore it embraces the particular facet of character, the facet grounded in natural endowment, it will be a natural history of mind. [. . .]

But when individuals are simply identified with the actual order, ethical life appears as their general mode of conduct, i.e. as custom, while the habitual practice of ethical living appears as a second nature which, put in the place of the initial, purely natural will, is the soul of custom permeating it through and through, the significance and the actuality of its existence. It is mind living and present as a world, and the substance of mind thus exists now for the first time as mind.

In this way the ethical substantial order has attained its right, and its right its validity. That is to say, the self-will of the individual has vanished together with his private conscience which had claimed independence and opposed itself to the ethical substance. [. . .]

The right of individuals to be subjectively destined to freedom is fulfilled when they belong to an actual ethical order, because their conviction of their freedom finds its truth in such an objective order, and it is in an ethical order that they are actually in possession of their own essence or their own inner universality.

When a father inquired about the best method of educating his son in ethical conduct, a Pythagorean replied: 'Make him a citizen of a state with good laws.'

[*The Philosophy of Right*, trans. T. M. Knox (Clarendon Press: Oxford, 1952), 89–90, 107–9. First published in 1821.]

HENRY SIDGWICK

36   The Axioms of Ethics

Can we then, between this Scylla and Charybdis of ethical inquiry, avoiding on the one hand doctrines that merely bring us back to common opinion with all its imperfections, and on the other hand doctrines that lead us round in a circle, find any way of obtaining self-evident moral principles of real significance? It would be disheartening to have to regard as altogether illusory the strong instinct of Common Sense that points to the existence of such principles, and the deliberate convictions of the long line of moralists who have enunciated them. At the same time, the more we extend our knowledge of man and his environment, the more we realise the vast variety of human natures and circumstances that have existed in different ages and countries, the less disposed we are to believe that there is any definite code of absolute rules, applicable to all human beings without exception. And we shall find, I think, that the truth lies between these two conclusions. There are certain absolute practical principles, the truth of which, when they are explicitly stated, is manifest; but they are of too abstract a nature, and too universal in their scope, to enable us to ascertain by immediate application of them what we ought to do in any particular case; particular duties have still to be determined by some other method.

One such principle was given [earlier, when] I pointed out that whatever action any of us judges to be right for himself, he implicitly judges to be right for all similar persons in similar circumstances. Or, as we may otherwise put it, 'if a kind of conduct that is right (or wrong) for me is not right (or wrong) for some one else, it must be on the ground of some difference between the two cases, other than the fact that I and he are different persons.' A corresponding proposition may be stated with equal truth in respect of what ought to be done *to*—not *by*—different individuals. These principles have been most widely recognised, not in their most abstract and universal form, but in their special application to the situation of two (or more) individuals similarly related to each other: as so applied, they appear in what is popularly known as the Golden Rule, 'Do to others as you would have them do to you.' This formula is obviously unprecise in statement; for one might wish for another's co-operation in sin, and be willing to reciprocate it. Nor is it even true to say that we ought to do to others only what we think it right for them to do to us; for no one will deny that there may be differences in the circumstances—and even in the natures—of two individuals, A and B, which would make it wrong for A to treat B in the way in which it is right for B to treat A. In short the self-evident principle strictly stated must take some such negative form as this; 'it cannot be right for A to treat B in a manner in which it would be wrong for B to treat A, merely on the ground that they are two different individuals, and without there being any difference between the natures or circumstances of the two which can be stated as a reasonable ground for difference of treatment.' Such a principle manifestly does not give complete guidance—indeed its effect, strictly speaking, is merely to throw a definite *onus probandi* on the man who applies to another a treatment of which he would complain if applied to himself; but Common Sense has amply recognised the practical importance of the maxim: and its truth, so far as it goes, appears to me self-evident.

A somewhat different application of the same fundamental principle that individuals in similar conditions should be treated similarly finds its sphere in the ordinary administration of Law, or (as we say) of 'Justice.' Accordingly I drew attention [earlier] to 'impartiality in the application of general rules,' as an important element in the common notion of Justice; indeed, there ultimately appeared to be no other element which could be intuitively known with perfect clearness and certainty. Here again it must be plain that this precept of impartiality is insufficient for the complete determination of just conduct, as it does not help us to decide what kind of rules should be thus impartially applied; though all admit the importance of excluding from government, and human conduct generally, all conscious partiality and 'respect of persons.'

The principle just discussed, which seems to be more or less clearly implied in the common notion of 'fairness' or 'equity,' is obtained by considering the similarity of the individuals that make up a Logical Whole or Genus. There are others, no less important, which emerge in the consideration of the similar parts of a Mathematical or Quantitative Whole. Such a Whole is presented in the common notion of the Good—or, as is sometimes said, 'good on the whole'—of any individual human being. The proposition 'that one ought to aim at one's own good' is sometimes given as the maxim of Rational Self-love or Prudence: but as so stated it does not clearly avoid tautology; since we may define 'good' as 'what one ought to aim at.' If, however, we say 'one's good on the whole,' the addition suggests a principle which, when explicitly stated, is, at any rate, not tautological. I have already referred to this principle as that 'of impartial concern for all parts of our conscious life':—we might express it concisely by saying 'that Hereafter *as such* is to be regarded neither less nor more than Now.' It is not, of course, meant that the good of the present may not reasonably be preferred to that of the future on account of its greater certainty: or again, that a week ten years hence may not be more important to us than a week now, through an increase in our means or capacities of happiness. All that the principle affirms is that the mere difference of priority and posteriority in time is not a reasonable ground for having more regard to the consciousness of one moment than to that of another. The form in which it practically presents itself to most men is 'that a smaller present good is not to be preferred to a greater future good' (allowing for difference of certainty): since Prudence is generally exercised in restraining a present desire (the object or satisfaction of which we commonly regard as *pro tanto* 'a good'), on account of the remoter consequences of gratifying it. The commonest view of the principle would no doubt be that the present *pleasure* or *happiness* is reasonably to be foregone with the view of obtaining greater pleasure or happiness hereafter: but the principle need not be restricted to a hedonistic application; it is equally applicable to any other interpretation of 'one's own good,' in which good is conceived as a mathematical whole, of which the integrant parts are realised in different parts or moments of a lifetime. And therefore it is perhaps better to distinguish it here from the principle 'that Pleasure is the sole Ultimate Good,' which does not seem to have any logical connexion with it.

So far we have only been considering the 'Good on the Whole' of a single individual: but just as this notion is constructed by comparison and integration of the different 'goods' that succeed one another in the series of our conscious states, so we have formed the notion of Universal Good by comparison and integration of the goods of all individual human—or sentient—existences. And here again, just as in the former case, by considering the relation of the integrant parts to the whole and to each other, I obtain the self-evident principle that the good of any one individual is of no more importance, from the point of view (if I may say so) of the Universe, than the good of any other; unless, that is, there are special grounds for believing that more good is likely to be realised in the one case than in the other. And it is evident to me that as a rational being I am bound to aim at good generally,—so far as it is attainable by my efforts,—not merely at a particular part of it.

From these two rational intuitions we may deduce, as a necessary inference, the maxim of Benevolence in an abstract form: viz. that each one is morally bound to regard the good of any other individual as much as his own, except in so far as he judges it to be less, when impartially viewed, or less certainly knowable or attainable by him. I before observed that the duty of Benevolence as recognised by common sense seems to fall some-what short of this. But I think it may be fairly urged in explanation of this that *practically* each man, even with a view to universal Good, ought chiefly to concern himself with promoting the good of a limited number of human beings, and that generally in proportion to the closeness of their connexion with him. I think that a 'plain man,' in a modern civilised society, if his conscience were fairly brought to consider the hypothetical question, whether it would be morally right for him to seek his own happiness on any occasion if it involved a certain sacrifice of the greater happiness of some other human being,—without any counterbalancing gain to any one else,—would answer unhesitatingly in the negative.

I have tried to show how in the principles of Justice, Prudence, and Rational Benevolence as commonly recognised there is at least a self-evid-ent element, immediately cognisable by abstract intuition; depending in each case on the relation which individuals and their particular ends bear as parts to their wholes, and to other parts of these wholes. I regard the apprehension, with more or less distinctness, of these abstract truths, as the permanent basis of the common conviction that the fundamental precepts of morality are essentially reasonable. No doubt these principles are often placed side by side with other precepts to which custom and general consent have given a merely illusory air of self-evidence: but the distinction between the two kinds of maxims appears to me to become manifest by merely reflecting upon them. I know by direct reflection that the proposi-tions, 'I ought to speak the truth,' 'I ought to keep my promises'—however true they may be—are not self-evident to me; they present themselves as propositions requiring rational justification of some kind. On the other hand, the propositions, 'I ought not to prefer a present lesser good to a future greater good,' and 'I ought not to prefer my own lesser good to the greater good of another,' do present themselves as self-evident; as much (*e.g.*) as the mathematical axiom that 'if equals be added to equals the wholes are equal.'

[*The Methods of Ethics*, 7th edn. (Macmillan: London, 1907), 379–83.]

EDWARD WESTERMARCK

37   Society the School, Custom the Headmaster

Society is the school in which men learn to distinguish between right and wrong. The headmaster is Custom, and the lessons are the same for all. The first moral judgments were pronounced by public opinion; public indignation and public approval are the prototypes of the moral emotions. As regards questions of morality, there was, in early society, practically no difference of opinion; hence a character of universality, or objectivity, was from the very beginning attached to all moral judgments. And when, with advancing civilisation, this unanimity was to some extent disturbed by individuals venturing to dissent from the opinions of the majority, the disagreement was largely due to facts which in no way affected the moral principle, but had reference only to its application.

Most people follow a very simple method in judging of an act. Particular modes of conduct have their traditional labels, many of which are learnt with language itself; and the moral judgment commonly consists simply in labelling the act according to certain obvious characteristics which it presents in common with others belonging to the same group. But a conscientious and intelligent judge proceeds in a different manner. He carefully examines all the details connected with the act, the external and internal conditions under which it was performed, its consequences, its motive; and, since the moral estimate in a large measure depends upon the regard paid to these circumstances, his judgment may differ greatly from that of the man in the street, even though the moral standard which they apply be exactly the same. But to acquire a full insight into all the details which are apt to influence the moral value of an act is in many cases anything but easy, and this naturally increases the disagreement. There is thus in every advanced society a diversity of opinion regarding the moral value of certain modes of conduct which results from circumstances of a purely intellectual character—from the knowledge or ignorance of positive facts,—and involves no discord in principle.

Now it has been assumed by the advocates of various ethical theories that all the differences of moral ideas originate in this way, and that there is some ultimate standard which must be recognised as authoritative by everybody who understands it rightly. [. . .] [A]ll disagreement as to questions of morals is attributed to ignorance or misunderstanding.

The influence of intellectual considerations upon moral judgments is certainly immense. We shall find that the evolution of the moral consciousness to a large extent consists in its development from the unreflecting to the reflecting, from the unenlightened to the enlightened. All higher emotions are determined by cognitions, they arise from 'the presentation of determinate objective conditions'; and moral enlightenment implies a true and comprehensive presentation of those objective conditions by which the moral emotions, according to their very nature, are determined. Morality may thus in a much higher degree than, for instance, beauty be a subject of instruction and of profitable discussion, in which persuasion is carried by the representation of existing data. But although in this way many differences may be accorded, there are points in which unanimity cannot be reached even by the most accurate presentation of facts or the subtlest process of reasoning.

Whilst certain phenomena will almost of necessity arouse similar moral emotions in every mind which perceives them clearly, there are others with which the case is different. The *emotional constitution of man* does not present the same uniformity as the human intellect. Certain cognitions inspire fear in nearly every breast; but there are brave men and cowards in the world, independently of the accuracy with which they realise impending danger. Some cases of suffering can hardly fail to awaken compassion in the most pitiless heart; but the sympathetic dispositions of men vary greatly, both in regard to the beings with whose sufferings they are ready to sympathise, and with reference to the intensity of the emotion. The same holds good for the moral emotions. The existing diversity of opinion as to the rights of different classes of men, and of the lower animals, which springs from emotional differences, may no doubt be modified by a clearer insight into certain facts, but no perfect agreement can be expected as long as the conditions under which the emotional dispositions are formed remain unchanged. Whilst an enlightened mind *must* recognise the complete or relative irresponsibility of an animal, a child, or a madman, and *must* be influenced in its moral judgment by the motives of an act—no intellectual enlightenment, no scrutiny of facts, can decide how far the interests of the lower animals should be regarded when conflicting with those of men, or how far a person is bound, or allowed, to promote the welfare of his nation, or his own welfare, at the cost of that of other nations or other individuals. Professor Sidgwick's well-known moral axiom, 'I ought not to prefer my own lesser good to the greater good of another,' would, if explained to a Fuegian or a Hottentot, be regarded by him, not as self-evident, but as simply absurd; nor can it claim general acceptance even among ourselves. Who is that 'Another' to whose greater good I ought not to prefer my own lesser good? A fellow-countryman, a savage, a criminal, a bird, a fish—all without distinction? It will, perhaps, be argued that on this, and on all other points of morals, there would be general agreement, if only the moral consciousness of men were sufficiently developed. But then, when speaking of a 'sufficiently developed' moral consciousness (beyond insistence upon a full insight into the governing facts of each case), we practically mean nothing else than agreement with our own moral convictions. The expression is faulty and deceptive, because, if intended to mean anything more, it presupposes an objectivity of the moral judgments which they do not possess, and at the same time seems to be proving what it presupposes. We may speak of an intellect as sufficiently developed to grasp a certain truth, because truth is objective; but it is not proved to be objective by the fact that it is recognised as true by a 'sufficiently developed' intellect. The objectivity of truth lies in the recognition of facts as true by all who understand them *fully*, whilst the appeal to a *sufficient* knowledge assumes their objectivity. To the verdict of a perfect intellect, that is, an intellect which knows everything existing, all would submit; but we can form no idea of a moral consciousness which could lay claim to a similar authority. If the believers in an all-good God, who has revealed his will to mankind, maintain that they in this revelation possess a perfect moral standard, and that, consequently, what is in accordance with such a standard must be objectively right, it may be asked what they mean by an 'all-good' God. And in their attempt to answer this question, they would inevitably have to assume the objectivity they wanted to prove. [. . .]

The presumed objectivity of moral judgments thus being a chimera, there can be no moral truth in the sense in which this term is generally understood. The ultimate reason for this is, that the moral concepts are based upon emotions, and that the contents of an emotion fall entirely outside the category of truth.

[*The Origin and Development of the Moral Ideas* (Macmillan: London, 1906), 9–17.]

LUDWIG WITTGENSTEIN

38   A Lecture on Ethics

Before I begin to speak about my subject proper let me make a few introductory remarks. I feel I shall have great difficulties in communicating my thoughts to you and I think some of them may be diminished by mentioning them to you beforehand. The first one, which almost I need not mention, is that English is not my native tongue and my expression therefore often lacks that precision and subtlety which would be desirable if one talks about a difficult subject. All I can do is to ask you to make my task easier by trying to get at my meaning in spite of the faults which I will constantly be committing against the English grammar. The second difficulty I will mention is this, that probably many of you come up to this lecture of mine with slightly wrong expectations. And to set you right in this point I will say a few words about the reason for choosing the subject I have chosen: When your former secretary honoured me by asking me to read a paper to your society, my first thought was that I would certainly do it and my second thought was that if I was to have the opportunity to speak to you I should speak about something which I am keen on communicating to you and that I should not misuse this opportunity to give you a lecture about, say, logic. I call this a misuse, for to explain a scientific matter to you it would need a course of lectures and not an hour's paper. Another alternative would have been to give you what's called a popular-scientific lecture, that is a lecture intended to make you believe that you understand a thing which actually you don't understand, and to gratify what I believe to be one of the lowest desires of modern people, namely the superficial curiosity about the latest discoveries of science. I rejected these alternatives and decided to talk to you about a subject which seems to me to be of general importance, hoping that it may help to clear up your thoughts about this subject (even if you should entirely disagree with what I will say about it). My third and last difficulty is one which, in fact, adheres to most lengthy philosophical lectures and it is this, that the hearer is incapable of seeing both the road he is led and the goal which it leads to. That is to say: he either thinks: 'I understand all he says, but what on earth is he driving at' or else he thinks 'I see what he's driving at, but how on earth is he going to get there.' All I can do is again to ask you to be patient and to hope that in the end you may see both the way and where it leads to.

I will now begin. My subject, as you know, is Ethics and I will adopt the explanation of that term which Professor Moore has given in his book *Principia Ethica*. He says: 'Ethics is the general enquiry into what is good.' Now I am going to use the term Ethics in a slightly wider sense, in a sense in fact which includes what I believe to be the most essential part of what is generally called Aesthetics. And to make you see as clearly as possible what I take to be the subject matter of Ethics I will put before you a number of more or less synonymous expressions each of which could be substituted for the above definition, and by enumerating them I want to produce the same sort of effect which Galton produced when he took a number of photos of different faces on the same photographic plate in order to get the picture of the typical features they all had in common. And as by showing to you such a collective photo I could make you see what is the typical— say—Chinese face; so if you look through the row of synonyms which I will put before you, you will, I hope, be able to see the characteristic features they all have in common and these are the characteristic features of Ethics. Now instead of saying 'Ethics is the enquiry into what is good' I could have said Ethics is the enquiry into what is valuable, or, into what is really important, or I could have said Ethics is the enquiry into the meaning of life, or into what makes life worth living, or into the right way of living. I believe if you look at all these phrases you will get a rough idea as to what it is that Ethics is concerned with. Now the first thing that strikes one about all these expressions is that each of them is actually used in two very different senses. I will call them the trivial or relative sense on the one hand and the ethical or absolute sense on the other. If for instance I say that this is a *good* chair this means that the chair serves a certain predetermined purpose and the word good here has only meaning so far as this purpose has been previously fixed upon. In fact the word good in the relative sense simply means coming up to a certain predetermined standard. Thus when we say that this man is a good pianist we mean that he can play pieces of a certain degree of difficulty with a certain degree of dexterity. And similarly if I say that it is *important* for me not to catch cold I mean that catching a cold produces certain describable disturbances in my life and if I say that this is the *right* road I mean that it's the right road relative to a certain goal. Used in this way these expressions don't present any difficult or deep problems. But this is not how Ethics uses them. Supposing that I could play tennis and one of you saw me playing and said 'Well, you play pretty badly' and suppose I answered 'I know, I'm playing badly but I don't want to play any better,' all the other man could say would be 'Ah then that's all right.' But suppose I had told one of you a preposterous lie and he came up to me and said 'You're behaving like a beast' and then I were to say 'I know I behave badly, but then I don't want to behave any better,' could he then say 'Ah, then that's all right'? Certainly not; he would say 'Well, you *ought* to want to behave better.' Here you have an absolute judgment of value, whereas the first instance was one of a relative judgment. The essence of this difference seems to be obviously this: Every judgment of relative value is a mere statement of facts and can therefore be put in such a form that it loses all the appearance of a judgment of value: Instead of saying 'This is the right way to Granchester,' I could equally well have said, 'This is the right way you have to go if you want to get to Granchester in the shortest time'; 'This man is a good runner' simply means that he runs a certain number of miles in a certain number of minutes, etc. Now what I wish to contend is that, although all judgments of relative value can be shown to be mere statements of facts, no statement of fact can ever be, or imply, a judgment of absolute value. Let me explain this: Suppose one of you were an omniscient person and therefore knew all the movements of all the bodies in the world dead or alive and that he also knew all the states of mind of all human beings that ever lived, and suppose this man wrote all he knew in a big book, then this book would contain the whole description of the world; and what I want to say is, that this book would contain nothing that we would call an *ethical* judgment or anything that would logically imply such a judgment. It would of course contain all relative judgments of value and all true scientific propositions and in fact all true propositions that can be made. But all the facts described would, as it were, stand on the same level and in the same way all propositions stand on the same level. There are no propositions which, in any absolute sense, are sublime, important, or trivial. Now perhaps some of you will agree to that and be reminded of Hamlet's words: 'Nothing is either good or bad, but thinking makes it so.' But this again could lead to a misunderstanding. What Hamlet says seems to imply that good and bad, though not qualities of the world outside us, are attributes to our states of mind. But what I mean is that a state of mind, so far as we mean by that a fact which we can describe, is in no ethical sense good or bad. If for instance in our world-book we read the description of a murder with all its details physical and psychological, the mere description of these facts will contain nothing which we could call an *ethical* proposition. The murder will be on exactly the same level as any other event, for instance the falling of a stone. Certainly the reading of this description might cause us pain or rage or any other emotion, or we might read about the pain or rage caused by this murder in other people when they heard of it, but there will simply be facts, facts, and facts but no Ethics. And now I must say that if I contemplate what Ethics really would have to be if there were such a science, this result seems to me quite obvious. It seems to me obvious that nothing we could ever think or say should be *the* thing. That we cannot write a scientific book, the subject matter of which could be intrinsically sublime and above all other subject matters. I can only describe my feeling by the metaphor, that, if a man could write a book on Ethics which really was a book on Ethics, this book would, with an explosion, destroy all the other books in the world. Our words used as we use them in science, are vessels capable only of containing and conveying meaning and sense, *natural* meaning and sense. Ethics, if it is anything, is supernatural and our words will only express facts; as a teacup will only hold a teacup full of water and if I were to pour out a gallon over it. I said that so far as facts and propositions are concerned there is only relative value and relative good, right, etc. And let me, before I go on, illustrate this by a rather obvious example. The right road is the road which leads to an arbitrarily predetermined end and it is quite clear to us all that there is no sense in talking about the right road apart from such a predetermined goal. Now let us see what we could possibly mean by the expression, '*the* absolutely right road.' I think it would be the road which *everybody* on seeing it would, *with logical necessity*, have to go, or be ashamed for not going. And similarly the *absolute good*, if it is a describable state of affairs, would be one which everybody, independent of his tastes and inclinations, would *necessarily* bring about or feel guilty for not bringing about. And I want to say that such a state of affairs is a chimera. No state of affairs has, in itself, what I would like to call the coercive power of an absolute judge. Then what have all of us who, like myself, are still tempted to use such expressions as 'absolute good,' 'absolute value,' etc., what have we in mind and what do we try to express? Now whenever I try to make this clear to myself it is natural that I should recall cases in which I would certainly use these expressions and I am then in the situation in which you would be if, for instance, I were to give you a lecture on the psychology of pleasure. What you would do then would be to try and recall some typical situation in which you always felt pleasure. For, bearing this situation in mind, all I should say to you would become concrete and, as it were, controllable. One man would perhaps choose as his stock example the sensation when taking a walk on a fine summer's day. Now in this situation I am, if I want to fix my mind on what I mean by absolute or ethical value. And there, in my case, it always happens that the idea of one particular experience presents itself to me which therefore is, in a sense, my experience *par excellence* and this is the reason why, in talking to you now, I will use this experience as my first and foremost example. (As I have said before, this is an entirely personal matter and others would find other examples more striking.) I will describe this experience in order, if possible, to make you recall the same or similar experiences, so that we may have a common ground for our investigation. I believe the best way of describing it is to say that when I have it *I wonder at the existence of the world*. And I am then inclined to use such phrases as 'how extraordinary that anything should exist' or 'how extraordinary that the world should exist.' I will mention another experience straight away which I also know and which others of you might be acquainted with: it is, what one might call, the experience of feeling *absolutely* safe. I mean the state of mind in which one is inclined to say 'I am safe, nothing can injure me whatever happens.' Now let me consider these experiences, for, I believe, they exhibit the very characteristics we try to get clear about. And there the first thing I have to say is, that the verbal expression which we give to these experiences is nonsense! If I say 'I wonder at the existence of the world' I am misusing language. Let me explain this: It has a perfectly good and clear sense to say that I wonder at something being the case, we all understand what it means to say that I wonder at the size of a dog which is bigger than anyone I have ever seen before or at any thing which, in the common sense of the word, is extraordinary. In every such case I wonder at something being the case which I *could* conceive *not* to be the case. I wonder at the size of this dog because I could conceive of a dog of another, namely the ordinary size, at which I should not wonder. To say 'I wonder at such and such being the case' has only sense if I can imagine it not to be the case. In this sense one can wonder at the existence of, say, a house when one sees it and has not visited it for a long time and has imagined that it had been pulled down in the meantime. But it is nonsense to say that I wonder at the existence of the world, because I cannot imagine it not existing. I could of course wonder at the world round me being as it is. If for instance I had this experience while looking into the blue sky, I could wonder at the sky being blue as opposed to the case when it's clouded. But that's not what I mean. I am wondering at the sky being *whatever it is*. One might be tempted to say that what I am wondering at is a tautology, namely at the sky being blue or not blue. But then it's just nonsense to say that one is wondering at a tautology. Now the same applies to the other experience which I have mentioned, the experience of absolute safety. We all know what it means in ordinary life to be safe. I am safe in my room, when I cannot be run over by an omnibus. I am safe if I have had whooping cough and cannot therefore get it again. To be safe essentially means that it is physically impossible that certain things should happen to me and therefore it's nonsense to say that I am safe *whatever* happens. Again this is a misuse of the word 'safe' as the other example was of a misuse of the word 'existence' or 'wondering.' Now I want to impress on you that a certain characteristic misuse of our language runs through *all* ethical and religious expressions. All these expressions *seem*, prima facie, to be just *similes*. Thus it seems that when we are using the word *right* in an ethical sense, although, what we mean, is not right in its trivial sense, it's something similar, and when we say 'This is a good fellow,' although the word good here doesn't mean what it means in the sentence 'This is a good football player' there seems to be some similarity. And when we say 'This man's life was valuable' we don't mean it in the same sense in which we would speak of some valuable jewelry but there seems to be some sort of analogy. Now all religious terms seem in this sense to be used as similes or allegorically. For when we speak of God and that he sees everything and when we kneel and pray to him all our terms and actions seem to be parts of a great and elaborate allegory which represents him as a human being of great power whose grace we try to win, etc., etc. But this allegory also describes the experiences which I have just referred to. For the first of them is, I believe, exactly what people were referring to when they said that God had created the world; and the experience of absolute safety has been described by saying that we feel safe in the hands of God. A third experience of the same kind is that of feeling guilty and again this was described by the phrase that God disapproves of our conduct. Thus in ethical and religious language we seem constantly to be using similes. But a simile must be the simile for *something*. And if I can describe a fact by means of a simile I must also be able to drop the simile and to describe the facts without it. Now in our case as soon as we try to drop the simile and simply to state the facts which stand behind it, we find that there are no such facts. And so, what at first appeared to be a simile now seems to be mere nonsense. Now the three experiences which I have mentioned to you (and I could have added others) seem to those who have experienced them, for instance to me, to have in some sense an intrinsic, absolute value. But when I say they are experiences, surely, they are facts; they have taken place then and there, lasted a certain definite time and consequently are describable. And so from what I have said some minutes ago I must admit it is nonsense to say that they have absolute value. And I will make my point still more acute by saying 'It is the paradox that an experience, a fact, should seem to have supernatural value.' Now there is a way in which I would be tempted to meet this paradox. Let me first consider, again, our first experience of wondering at the existence of the world and let me describe it in a slightly different way; we all know what in ordinary life would be called a miracle. It obviously is simply an event the like of which we have never yet seen. Now suppose such an event happened. Take the case that one of you suddenly grew a lion's head and began to roar. Certainly that would be as extraordinary a thing as I can imagine. Now whenever we should have recovered from our surprise, what I would suggest would be to fetch a doctor and have the case scientifically investigated and if it were not for hurting him I would have him vivisected. And where would the miracle have got to? For it is clear that when we look at it in this way everything miraculous has disappeared; unless what we mean by this term is merely that a fact has not yet been explained by science which again means that we have hitherto failed to group this fact with others in a scientific system. This shows that it is absurd to say 'Science has proved that there are no miracles.' The truth is that the scientific way of looking at a fact is not the way to look at it as a miracle. For imagine whatever fact you may, it is not in itself miraculous in the absolute sense of that term. For we see now that we have been using the word 'miracle' in a relative and an absolute sense. And I will now describe the experience of wondering at the existence of the world by saying: it is the experience of seeing the world as a miracle. Now I am tempted to say that the right expression in language for the miracle of the existence of the world, though it is not any proposition *in* language, is the existence of language itself. But what then does it mean to be aware of this miracle at some times and not at other times? For all I have said by shifting the expression of the miraculous from an expression *by means of* language to the expression *by the existence* of language, all I have said is again that we cannot express what we want to express and that all we *say* about the absolute miraculous remains nonsense. Now the answer to all this will seem perfectly clear to many of you. You will say: Well, if certain experiences constantly tempt us to attribute a quality to them which we call absolute or ethical value and importance, this simply shows that by these words we *don't* mean nonsense, that after all what we mean by saying that an experience has absolute value *is just a fact like other facts* and that all it comes to is that we have not yet succeeded in finding the correct logical analysis of what we mean by our ethical and religious expressions. Now when this is urged against me I at once see clearly, as it were in a flash of light, not only that no description that I can think of would do to describe what I mean by absolute value, but that I would reject every significant description that anybody could possibly suggest, *ab initio*, on the ground of its significance. That is to say: I see now that these nonsensical expressions were not nonsensical because I had not yet found the correct expressions, but that their nonsensicality was their very essence. For all I wanted to do with them was just *to go beyond* the world and that is to say beyond significant language. My whole tendency and I believe the tendency of all men who ever tried to write or talk Ethics or Religion was to run against the boundaries of language. This running against the walls of our cage is perfectly, absolutely hopeless. Ethics so far as it springs from the desire to say something about the ultimate meaning of life, the absolute good, the absolutely valuable, can be no science. What it says does not add to our knowledge in any sense. But it is a document of a tendency in the human mind which I personally cannot help respecting deeply and I would not for my life ridicule it.

[A lecture delivered at Cambridge University in Nov. 1929, first published in the *Philosophical Review*, 74/1 (Jan. 1965).]

A. J. AYER

39   Ethics for Logical Positivists

We begin by admitting that the fundamental ethical concepts are unanalysable, inasmuch as there is no criterion by which one can test the validity of the judgements in which they occur. So far we are in agreement with the absolutists. But, unlike the absolutists, we are able to give an explanation of this fact about ethical concepts. We say that the reason why they are unanalysable is that they are mere pseudo-concepts. The presence of an ethical symbol in a proposition adds nothing to its factual content. Thus if I say to someone, 'You acted wrongly in stealing that money,' I am not stating anything more than if I had simply said, 'You stole that money.' In adding that this action is wrong I am not making any further statement about it. I am simply evincing my moral disapproval of it. It is as if I had said, 'You stole that money,' in a peculiar tone of horror, or written it with the addition of some special exclamation marks. The tone, or the exclamation marks, adds nothing to the literal meaning of the sentence. It merely serves to show that the expression of it is attended by certain feelings in the speaker.

If now I generalise my previous statement and say, 'Stealing money is wrong,' I produce a sentence which has no factual meaning—that is, expresses no proposition which can be either true or false. It is as if I had written 'Stealing money!!'—where the shape and thickness of the exclamation marks show, by a suitable convention, that a special sort of moral disapproval is the feeling which is being expressed. It is clear that there is nothing said here which can be true or false. Another man may disagree with me about the wrongness of stealing, in the sense that he may not have the same feelings about stealing as I have, and he may quarrel with me on account of my moral sentiments. But he cannot, strictly speaking, contradict me. For in saying that a certain type of action is right or wrong, I am not making any factual statement, not even a statement about my own state of mind. I am merely expressing certain moral sentiments. And the man who is ostensibly contradicting me is merely expressing his moral sentiments. So that there is plainly no sense in asking which of us is in the right. For neither of us is asserting a genuine proposition.

What we have just been saying about the symbol 'wrong' applies to all normative ethical symbols. Sometimes they occur in sentences which record ordinary empirical facts besides expressing ethical feeling about those facts: sometimes they occur in sentences which simply express ethical feeling about a certain type of action, or situation, without making any statement of fact. But in every case in which one would commonly be said to be making an ethical judgement, the function of the relevant ethical word is purely 'emotive.' It is used to express feeling about certain objects, but not to make any assertion about them.

It is worth mentioning that ethical terms do not serve only to express feeling. They are calculated also to arouse feeling, and so to stimulate action. Indeed some of them are used in such a way as to give the sentences in which they occur the effect of commands. Thus the sentence 'It is your duty to tell the truth' may be regarded both as the expression of a certain sort of ethical feeling about truthfulness and as the expression of the command 'Tell the truth.' The sentence 'You ought to tell the truth' also involves the command 'Tell the truth,' but here the tone of the command is less emphatic. In the sentence 'It is good to tell the truth' the command has become little more than a suggestion. And thus the 'meaning' of the word 'good,' in its ethical usage, is differentiated from that of the word 'duty' or the word 'ought.' In fact we may define the meaning of the various ethical words in terms both of the different feelings they are ordinarily taken to express, and also the different responses which they are calculated to provoke.

We can now see why it is impossible to find a criterion for determining the validity of ethical judgements. It is not because they have an 'absolute' validity which is mysteriously independent of ordinary sense-experience, but because they have no objective validity whatsoever. If a sentence makes no statement at all, there is obviously no sense in asking whether what it says is true or false. And we have seen that sentences which simply express moral judgements do not say anything. They are pure expressions of feeling and as such do not come under the category of truth and falsehood. They are unverifiable for the same reason as a cry of pain or a word of command is unverifiable—because they do not express genuine propositions.

Thus, although our theory of ethics might fairly be said to be radically subjectivist, it differs in a very important respect from the orthodox subjectivist theory. For the orthodox subjectivist does not deny, as we do, that the sentences of a moralizer express genuine propositions. All he denies is that they express propositions of a unique non-empirical character. His own view is that they express propositions about the speaker's feelings. If this were so, ethical judgements clearly would be capable of being true or false.

They would be true if the speaker had the relevant feelings, and false if he had not. And this is a matter which is, in principle, empirically verifiable. Furthermore they could be significantly contradicted. For if I say, 'Tolerance is a virtue,' and someone answers, 'You don't approve of it,' he would, on the ordinary subjectivist theory, be contradicting me. On our theory, he would not be contradicting me, because, in saying that tolerance was a virtue, I should not be making any statement about my own feelings or about anything else. I should simply be evincing my feelings, which is not at all the same thing as saying that I have them.

The distinction between the expression of feeling and the assertion of feeling is complicated by the fact that the assertion that one has a certain feeling often accompanies the expression of that feeling, and is then, indeed, a factor in the expression of that feeling. Thus I may simultaneously express boredom and say that I am bored, and in that case my utterance of the words, 'I am bored,' is one of the circumstances which make it true to say that I am expressing or evincing boredom. But I can express boredom without actually saying that I am bored. I can express it by my tone and gestures, while making a statement about something wholly unconnected with it, or by an ejaculation, or without uttering any words at all. So that even if the assertion that one has a certain feeling always involves the expression of that feeling, the expression of a feeling assuredly does not always involve the assertion that one has it. And this is the important point to grasp in considering the distinction between our theory and the ordinary subjectivist theory. For whereas the subjectivist holds that ethical statements actually assert the existence of certain feelings, we hold that ethical statements are expressions and excitants of feeling which do not necessarily involve any assertions.

We have already remarked that the main objection to the ordinary subjectivist theory is that the validity of ethical judgements is not determined by the nature of their author's feelings. And this is an objection which our theory escapes. For it does not imply that the existence of any feelings is a necessary and sufficient condition of the validity of an ethical judgement. It implies, on the contrary, that ethical judgements have no validity.

There is, however, a celebrated argument against subjectivist theories which our theory does not escape. It has been pointed out by Moore that if ethical statements were simply statements about the speaker's feelings, it would be impossible to argue about questions of value.[1] To take a typical example: if a man said that thrift was a virtue, and another replied that it was a vice, they would not, on this theory, be disputing with one another. One would be saying that he approved of thrift, and the other that *he* didn't;

---

[1] G. E. Moore, 'The Nature of Moral Philosophy', in *Philosophical Studies* (Routledge and Kegan Paul: London, 1951), 310–39.

and there is no reason why both these statements should not be true. Now Moore held it to be obvious that we do dispute about questions of value, and accordingly concluded that the particular form of subjectivism which he was discussing was false.

It is plain that the conclusion that it is impossible to dispute about questions of value follows from our theory also. For as we hold that such sentences as 'Thrift is a virtue' and 'Thrift is a vice' do not express propositions at all, we clearly cannot hold that they express incompatible propositions. We must therefore admit that if Moore's argument really refutes the ordinary subjectivist theory, it also refutes ours. But, in fact, we deny that it does refute even the ordinary subjectivist theory. For we hold that one really never does dispute about questions of value.

This may seem, at first sight, to be a very paradoxical assertion. For we certainly do engage in disputes which are ordinarily regarded as disputes about questions of value. But, in all such cases, we find, if we consider the matter closely, that the dispute is not really about a question of value, but about a question of fact. When someone disagrees with us about the moral value of a certain action or type of action, we do admittedly resort to argument in order to win him over to our way of thinking. But we do not attempt to show by our arguments that he has the 'wrong' ethical feeling towards a situation whose nature he has correctly apprehended. What we attempt to show is that he is mistaken about the facts of the case. We argue that he has misconceived the agent's motive: or that he has misjudged the effects of the action, or its probable effects in view of the agent's knowledge; or that he has failed to take into account the special circumstances in which the agent was placed. Or else we employ more general arguments about the effects which actions of a certain type tend to produce, or the qualities which are usually manifested in their performance. We do this in the hope that we have only to get our opponent to agree with us about the nature of the empirical facts for him to adopt the same moral attitude towards them as we do. And as the people with whom we argue have generally received the same moral education as ourselves, and live in the same social order, our expectation is usually justified. But if our opponent happens to have undergone a different process of moral 'conditioning' from ourselves, so that, even when he acknowledges all the facts, he still disagrees with us about the moral value of the actions under discussion, then we abandon the attempt to convince him by argument. We say that it is impossible to argue with him because he has a distorted or undeveloped moral sense; which signifies merely that he employs a different set of values from our own. We feel that our own system of values is superior, and therefore speak in such derogatory terms of his. But we cannot bring forward any arguments to show that our system is superior. For our judgement that it is so is itself a judgement of value, and accordingly outside the scope of argument. It is because argument fails us when we come to deal with pure questions of value, as distinct from questions of fact, that we finally resort to mere abuse.

In short, we find that argument is possible on moral questions only if some system of values is presupposed. If our opponent concurs with us in expressing moral disapproval of all actions of a given type *t*, then we may get him to condemn a particular action A, by bringing forward arguments to show that A is of type *t*. For the question whether A does or does not belong to that type is a plain question of fact. Given that a man has certain moral principles, we argue that he must, in order to be consistent, react morally to certain things in a certain way. What we do not and cannot argue about is the validity of these moral principles. We merely praise or condemn them in the light of our own feelings.

If anyone doubts the accuracy of this account of moral disputes, let him try to construct even an imaginary argument on a question of value which does not reduce itself to an argument about a question of logic or about an empirical matter of fact. I am confident that he will not succeed in producing a single example. And if that is the case, he must allow that its involving the impossibility of purely ethical arguments is not, as Moore thought, a ground of objection to our theory, but rather a point in favour of it.

Having upheld our theory against the only criticism which appeared to threaten it, we may now use it to define the nature of all ethical enquiries. We find that ethical philosophy consists simply in saying that ethical concepts are pseudo-concepts and therefore unanalysable. The further task of describing the different feelings that the different ethical terms are used to express, and the different reactions that they customarily provoke, is a task for the psychologist. There cannot be such a thing as ethical science, if by ethical science one means the elaboration of a 'true' system of morals. For we have seen that, as ethical judgements are mere expressions of feeling, there can be no way of determining the validity of any ethical system, and, indeed, no sense in asking whether any such system is true. All that one may legitimately enquire in this connection is, What are the moral habits of a given person or group of people, and what causes them to have precisely those habits and feelings? And this enquiry falls wholly within the scope of the existing social sciences.

It appears, then, that ethics, as a branch of knowledge, is nothing more than a department of psychology and sociology. And in case anyone thinks that we are overlooking the existence of casuistry, we may remark that casuistry is not a science, but is a purely analytical investigation of the structure of a given moral system. In other words, it is an exercise in formal logic.

When one comes to pursue the psychological enquiries which constitute ethical science, one is immediately enabled to account for the Kantian and hedonistic theories of morals. For one finds that one of the chief causes of moral behaviour is fear, both conscious and unconscious, of a god's displeasure, and fear of the enmity of society. And this, indeed, is the reason why moral precepts present themselves to some people as 'categorical' commands. And one finds, also, that the moral code of a society is partly determined by the beliefs of that society concerning the conditions of its own happiness—or, in other words, that a society tends to encourage or discourage a given type of conduct by the use of moral sanctions according as it appears to promote or detract from the contentment of the society as a whole. And this is the reason why altruism is recommended in most moral codes and egotism condemned. It is from the observation of this connection between morality and happiness that hedonistic or eudæmonistic theories of morals ultimately spring, just as the moral theory of Kant is based on the fact, previously explained, that moral precepts have for some people the force of inexorable commands. As each of these theories ignores the fact which lies at the root of the other, both may be criticized as being one-sided; but this is not the main objection to either of them. Their essential defect is that they treat propositions which refer to the causes and attributes of our ethical feelings as if they were definitions of ethical concepts. And thus they fail to recognise that ethical concepts are pseudo-concepts and consequently indefinable.

[*Language, Truth and Logic* (Victor Gollancz: London, 1967), 106–13. First published in 1936.]

JEAN-PAUL SARTRE

40 Condemned to Be Free

Dostoevsky once wrote 'If God did not exist, everything would be permitted'; and that, for existentialism, is the starting point. Everything is indeed permitted if God does not exist, and man is in consequence forlorn, for he cannot find anything to depend upon either within or outside himself. He discovers forthwith, that he is without excuse. For if indeed existence precedes essence, one will never be able to explain one's action by reference to a given and specific human nature; in other words, there is no determinism—man is free, man *is* freedom. Nor, on the other hand, if God does not exist, are we provided with any values or commands that could legitimize our behavior. Thus we have neither behind us, nor before us in a luminous realm of values, any means of justification or excuse. We are left alone, without excuse. That is what I mean when I say that man is condemned to be free. Condemned, because he did not create himself, yet is nevertheless at liberty, and from the moment that he is thrown into this world he is responsible for everything he does. The existentialist does not believe in the power of passion. He will never regard a grand passion as a destructive torrent upon which a man is swept into certain actions as by fate, and which, therefore, is an excuse for them. He thinks that man is responsible for his passion. Neither will an existentialist think that a man can find help through some sign being vouchsafed upon earth for his orientation: for he thinks that the man himself interprets the sign as he chooses. He thinks that every man, without any support or help whatever, is condemned at every instant to invent man. As Ponge has written in a very fine article, 'Man is the future of man.' That is exactly true. Only, if one took this to mean that the future is laid up in Heaven, that God knows what it is, it would be false, for then it would no longer even be a future. If, however, it means that, whatever man may now appear to be, there is a future to be fashioned, a virgin future that awaits him—then it is a true saying. But in the present one is forsaken.

As an example by which you may the better understand this state of abandonment, I will refer to the case of a pupil of mine, who sought me out in the following circumstances. His father was quarrelling with his mother and was also inclined to be a 'collaborator'; his elder brother had been killed in the German offensive of 1940 and this young man, with a sentiment somewhat primitive but generous, burned to avenge him. His mother was living alone with him, deeply afflicted by the semi-treason of his father and by the death of her eldest son, and her one consolation was in this young man. But he, at this moment, had the choice between going to England to join the Free French Forces or of staying near his mother and helping her to live. He fully realized that this woman lived only for him and that his disappearance—or perhaps his death—would plunge her into despair. He also realized that, concretely and in fact, every action he performed on his mother's behalf would be sure of effect in the sense of aiding her to live, whereas anything he did in order to go and fight would be an ambiguous action which might vanish like water into sand and serve no purpose. For instance, to set out for England he would have to wait indefinitely in a Spanish camp on the way through Spain; or, on arriving in England or in Algiers he might be put into an office to fill up forms. Consequently, he found himself confronted by two very different modes of action; the one concrete, immediate, but directed towards only one individual; and the other an action addressed to an end infinitely greater, a national collectivity, but for that very reason ambiguous—and it might be frustrated on the way. At the same time, he was hesitating between two kinds of morality; on the one side the morality of sympathy, of personal devotion and, on the other side, a morality of wider scope but of more debatable validity. He had to choose between those two. What could help him to choose? Could the Christian doctrine? No. Christian doctrine says: Act with charity, love your neighbour, deny yourself for others, choose the way which is hardest, and so forth. But which is the harder road? To whom does one owe the more brotherly love, the patriot or the mother? Which is the more useful aim, the general one of fighting in and for the whole community, or the precise aim of helping one particular person to live? Who can give an answer to that *à priori*? No one. Nor is it given in any ethical scripture. The Kantian ethic says, Never regard another as a means, but always as an end. Very well; if I remain with my mother, I shall be regarding her as the end and not as a means: but by the same token I am in danger of treating as means those who are fighting on my behalf; and the converse is also true, that if I go to the aid of the combatants I shall be treating them as the end at the risk of treating my mother as a means.

If values are uncertain, if they are still too abstract to determine the particular, concrete case under consideration, nothing remains but to trust in our instincts. That is what this young man tried to do; and when I saw him he said, 'In the end, it is feeling that counts; the direction in which it is really pushing me is the one I ought to choose. If I feel that I love my mother enough to sacrifice everything else for her—my will to be avenged, all my longings for action and adventure—then I stay with her. If, on the contrary, I feel that my love for her is not enough, I go.' But how does one estimate the strength of a feeling? The value of his feeling for his mother was determined precisely by the fact that he was standing by her. I may say that I love a certain friend enough to sacrifice such or such a sum of money for him, but I cannot prove that unless I have done it. I may say, 'I love my mother enough to remain with her,' if actually I have remained with her. I can only estimate the strength of this affection if I have performed an action by which it is defined and ratified. But if I then appeal to this affection to justify my action, I find myself drawn into a vicious circle.

Moreover, as Gide has very well said, a sentiment which is play-acting and one which is vital are two things that are hardly distinguishable one from another. To decide that I love my mother by staying beside her, and to play a comedy the upshot of which is that I do so—these are nearly the same thing. In other words, feeling is formed by the deeds that one does; therefore I cannot consult it as a guide to action. And that is to say that I can neither seek within myself for an authentic impulse to action, nor can I expect, from some ethic, formulae that will enable me to act. You may say that the youth did, at least, go to a professor to ask for advice. But if you seek counsel—from a priest, for example—you have selected that priest; and at bottom you already knew, more or less, what he would advise. In other words, to choose an adviser is nevertheless to commit oneself by that choice. If you are a Christian, you will say, Consult a priest; but there are collaborationists, priests who are resisters and priests who wait for the tide to turn: which will you choose? Had this young man chosen a priest of the resistance, or one of the collaboration, he would have decided beforehand the kind of advice he was to receive. Similarly, in coming to me, he knew what advice I should give him, and I had but one reply to make. You are free, therefore choose—that is to say, invent. No rule of general morality can show you what you ought to do: no signs are vouchsafed in this world.

['Existentialism is a Humanism', in W. Kaufman (ed.), *Existentialism from Dostoevsky to Sartre* (New Arena Library: New York, 1975), 352–6. First published in 1946.]

THOMAS NAGEL

41   The Objective Basis of Morality

Suppose you work in a library, checking people's books as they leave, and a friend asks you to let him smuggle out a hard-to-find reference work that he wants to own.

You might hesitate to agree for various reasons. You might be afraid that he'll be caught, and that both you and he will then get into trouble. You might want the book to stay in the library so that you can consult it yourself.

But you may also think that what he proposes is wrong—that he shouldn't do it and you shouldn't help him. If you think that, what does it mean, and what, if anything, makes it true?

To say it's wrong is not just to say it's against the rules. There can be bad rules which prohibit what isn't wrong—like a law against criticizing the government. A rule can also be bad because it requires something that *is* wrong—like a law that requires racial segregation in hotels and restaurants. The ideas of wrong and right are different from the ideas of what is and is not against the rules. Otherwise they couldn't be used in the evaluation of rules as well as of actions.

If you think it would be wrong to help your friend steal the book, then you will feel uncomfortable about doing it: in some way you won't want to do it, even if you are also reluctant to refuse help to a friend. Where does the desire not to do it come from; what is its motive, the reason behind it?

There are various ways in which something can be wrong, but in this case, if you had to explain it, you'd probably say that it would be unfair to other users of the library who may be just as interested in the book as your friend is, but who consult it in the reference room, where anyone who needs it can find it. You may also feel that to let him take it would betray your employers, who are paying you precisely to keep this sort of thing from happening.

These thoughts have to do with effects on others—not necessarily effects on their feelings, since they may never find out about it, but some kind of damage nevertheless. In general, the thought that something is wrong depends on its impact not just on the person who does it but on other people. They wouldn't like it, and they'd object if they found out.

But suppose you try to explain all this to your friend, and he says, 'I know the head librarian wouldn't like it if he found out, and probably some of the other users of the library would be unhappy to find the book gone, but who cares? I want the book; why should I care about them?'

The argument that it would be wrong is supposed to give him a reason not to do it. But if someone just doesn't care about other people, what reason does he have to refrain from doing any of the things usually thought to be wrong, if he can get away with it: what reason does he have not to kill, steal, lie, or hurt others? If he can get what he wants by doing such things, why shouldn't he? And if there's no reason why he shouldn't, in what sense is it wrong?

Of course most people do care about others to some extent. But if someone doesn't care, most of us wouldn't conclude that he's exempt from morality. A person who kills someone just to steal his wallet, without caring about the victim, is not automatically excused. The fact that he doesn't care doesn't make it all right: he *should* care. But *why* should he care?

There have been many attempts to answer this question. One type of answer tries to identify something else that the person already cares about, and then connect morality to it.

For example, some people believe that even if you can get away with awful crimes on this earth, and are not punished by the law or your fellow men, such acts are forbidden by God, who will punish you after death (and reward you if you didn't do wrong when you were tempted to). So even when it seems to be in your interest to do such a thing, it really isn't. Some people have even believed that if there is no God to back up moral requirements with the threat of punishment and the promise of reward, morality is an illusion: 'If God does not exist, everything is permitted.'

This is a rather crude version of the religious foundation for morality. A more appealing version might be that the motive for obeying God's commands is not fear but love. He loves you, and you should love Him, and should wish to obey His commands in order not to offend Him.

But however we interpret the religious motivation, there are three objections to this type of answer. First, plenty of people who don't believe in God still make judgments of right and wrong, and think no one should kill another for his wallet even if he can be sure to get away with it. Second, if God exists, and forbids what's wrong, that still isn't what *makes* it wrong. Murder is wrong in itself, and that's *why* God forbids it (if He does). God couldn't make just any old thing wrong—like putting on your left sock before your right—simply by prohibiting it. If God would punish you for doing that it would be inadvisable to do it, but it wouldn't be wrong. Third, fear of punishment and hope of reward, and even love of God, seem not to be the right motives for morality. If you think it's wrong to kill, cheat, or steal, you should want to avoid doing such things because they are bad things to do to the victims, not just because you fear the consequences for yourself, or because you don't want to offend your Creator.

This third objection also applies to other explanations of the force of morality which appeal to the interests of the person who must act. For example, it may be said that you should treat others with consideration so that they'll do the same for you. This may be sound advice, but it is valid only so far as you think what you do will affect how others treat you. It's not a reason for doing the right thing if others won't find out about it, or against doing the wrong thing if you can get away with it (like being a hit and run driver).

There is no substitute for a direct concern for other people as the basis of morality. But morality is supposed to apply to everyone: and can we assume that everyone has such a concern for others? Obviously not: some people are very selfish, and even those who are not selfish may care only about the people they know, and not about everyone. So where will we find a reason that everyone has not to hurt other people, even those they don't know?

Well, there's one general argument against hurting other people which can be given to anybody who understands English (or any other language), and which seems to show that he has *some* reason to care about others, even if in the end his selfish motives are so strong that he persists in treating other people badly anyway. It's an argument that I'm sure you've heard, and it goes like this: 'How would you like it if someone did that to you?'

It's not easy to explain how this argument is supposed to work. Suppose you're about to steal someone else's umbrella as you leave a restaurant in a rainstorm, and a bystander says, 'How would you like it if someone did that to you?' Why is it supposed to make you hesitate, or feel guilty?

Obviously the direct answer to the question is supposed to be, 'I wouldn't like it at all!' But what's the next step? Suppose you were to say, 'I wouldn't like it if someone did that to me. But luckily no one *is* doing it to me. I'm doing it to someone else, and I don't mind that at all!'

This answer misses the point of the question. When you are asked how you would like it if someone did that to you, you are supposed to think about all the feelings you would have if someone stole your umbrella. And that includes more than just 'not liking it'—as you wouldn't 'like it' if you stubbed your toe on a rock. If someone stole your umbrella you'd *resent* it. You'd have feelings about the umbrella thief, not just about the loss of the umbrella. You'd think, 'Where does he get off, taking my umbrella that I bought with my hard-earned money and that I had the foresight to bring after reading the weather report? Why didn't he bring his own umbrella?' and so forth.

When our own interests are threatened by the inconsiderate behavior of others, most of us find it easy to appreciate that those others have a reason to be more considerate. When you are hurt, you probably feel that other people should care about it: you don't think it's no concern of theirs, and that they have no reason to avoid hurting you. That is the feeling that the 'How would you like it?' argument is supposed to arouse.

Because if you admit that you would *resent* it if someone else did to you what you are now doing to him, you are admitting that you think he would have a reason not to do it to you. And if you admit that, you have to consider what that reason is. It couldn't be just that it's *you* that he's hurting, of all the people in the world. There's no special reason for him not to steal *your* umbrella, as opposed to anyone else's. There's nothing so special about you. Whatever the reason is, it's a reason he would have against hurting anyone else in the same way. And it's a reason anyone else would have too, in a similar situation, against hurting you or anyone else.

But if it's a reason anyone would have not to hurt anyone else in this way, then it's a reason *you* have not to hurt someone else in this way (since *anyone* means *everyone*). Therefore it's a reason not to steal the other person's umbrella now.

This is a matter of simple consistency. Once you admit that another person would have a reason not to harm you in similar circumstances, and once you admit that the reason he would have is very general and doesn't apply only to you, or to him, then to be consistent you have to admit that the same reason applies to you now. You shouldn't steal the umbrella, and you ought to feel guilty if you do.

Someone could escape from this argument if, when he was asked, 'How would you like it if someone did that to you?' he answered, 'I wouldn't resent it at all. I wouldn't *like* it if someone stole my umbrella in a rainstorm, but I wouldn't think there was any reason for him to consider my feelings about it.' But how many people could honestly give that answer? I think most people, unless they're crazy, would think that their own interests and harms matter, not only to themselves, but in a way that gives other people a reason to care about them too. We all think that when we suffer it is not just bad *for us*, but *bad, period*.

The basis of morality is a belief that good and harm to particular people (or animals) is good or bad not just from their point of view, but from a more general point of view, which every thinking person can understand. That means that each person has a reason to consider not only his own interests but the interests of others in deciding what to do. And it isn't enough if he is considerate only of some others—his family and friends, those he specially cares about. Of course he will care more about certain people, and also about himself. But he has some reason to consider the effect of what he does on the good or harm of everyone. If he's like most of us, that is what he thinks others should do with regard to him, even if they aren't friends of his.

[*What Does it All Mean?* (Oxford University Press: New York, 1987), 59–67.]

42   The Argument from 'Queerness'

There are no objective values. This is a bald statement of the thesis of this chapter, but before arguing for it I shall try to clarify and restrict it in ways that may meet some objections and prevent some misunderstanding.

The statement of this thesis is liable to provoke one of three very different reactions. Some will think it not merely false but pernicious; they will see it as a threat to morality and to everything else that is worthwhile, and they will find the presenting of such a thesis in what purports to be a book on ethics paradoxical or even outrageous. Others will regard it as a trivial truth, almost too obvious to be worth mentioning, and certainly too plain to be worth much argument. Others again will say that it is meaningless or empty, that no real issue is raised by the question whether values are or are not part of the fabric of the world. But, precisely because there can be these three different reactions, much more needs to be said.

The claim that values are not objective, are not part of the fabric of the world, is meant to include not only moral goodness, which might be most naturally equated with moral value, but also other things that could be more loosely called moral values or disvalues—rightness and wrongness, duty, obligation, an action's being rotten and contemptible, and so on. [. . .]

We may make this issue clearer by referring to Kant's distinction between hypothetical and categorical imperatives. [. . .] A categorical imperative would express a reason for acting which was unconditional in the sense of not being contingent upon any present desire of the agent to whose satisfaction the recommended action would contribute as a means—or more directly: 'You ought to dance', if the implied reason is just that you want to dance or like dancing, is still a hypothetical imperative. Now Kant himself held that moral judgements are categorical imperatives, or perhaps are all applications of one categorical imperative, and it can plausibly be maintained at least that many moral judgements contain a categorically imperative element. So far as ethics is concerned, my thesis that there are no objective values is specifically the denial that any such categorically imperative element is objectively valid. The objective values which I am denying would be action-directing absolutely, not contingently (in the way indicated) upon the agent's desires and inclinations.

Another way of trying to clarify this issue is to refer to moral reasoning or moral arguments. In practice, of course, such reasoning is seldom fully explicit: but let us suppose that we could make explicit the reasoning that supports some evaluative conclusion, where this conclusion has some action-guiding force that is not contingent upon desires or purposes or chosen ends. Then what I am saying is that somewhere in the input to this argument—perhaps in one or more of the premisses, perhaps in some part of the form of the argument—there will be something which cannot be objectively validated—some premiss which is not capable of being simply true, or some form of argument which is not valid as a matter of general logic, whose authority or cogency is not objective, but is constituted by our choosing or deciding to think in a certain way. [. . .]

Traditionally [the denial of objective values] has been supported by arguments of two main kinds, which I shall call the argument from relativity and the argument from queerness. [. . .]

The argument from relativity has as its premiss the well-known variation in moral codes from one society to another and from one period to another, and also the differences in moral beliefs between different groups and classes within a complex community. Such variation is in itself merely a truth of descriptive morality, a fact of anthropology which entails neither first order nor second order ethical views. Yet it may indirectly support second order subjectivism: radical differences between first order moral judgements make it difficult to treat those judgements as apprehensions of objective truths. But it is not the mere occurrence of disagreements that tells against the objectivity of values. Disagreement on questions in history or biology or cosmology does not show that there are no objective issues in these fields for investigators to disagree about. But such scientific disagreement results from speculative inferences or explanatory hypotheses based on inadequate evidence, and it is hardly plausible to interpret moral disagreement in the same way. Disagreement about moral codes seems to reflect people's adherence to and participation in different ways of life. The causal connection seems to be mainly that way round: it is that people approve of monogamy because they participate in a monogamous way of life rather than that they participate in a monogamous way of life because they approve of monogamy. Of course, the standards may be an idealization of the way of life from which they arise: the monogamy in which people participate may be less complete, less rigid, than that of which it leads them to approve. This is not to say that moral judgements are purely conventional. Of course there have been and are moral heretics and moral reformers, people who have turned against the established rules and practices of their own communities for moral reasons, and often for moral reasons that we would endorse. But this can usually be understood as the extension, in ways which, though new and unconventional, seemed to them to be required for consistency, of rules to which they already adhered as arising out of an existing way of life. In short, the argument from relativity has some force simply because the actual variations in the moral codes are more readily explained by the hypothesis that they reflect ways of life than by the hypothesis that they express perceptions, most of them seriously inadequate and badly distorted, of objective values.

But there is a well-known counter to this argument from relativity, namely to say that the items for which objective validity is in the first place to be claimed are not specific moral rules or codes but very general basic principles which are recognized at least implicitly to some extent in all society—such principles as provide the foundations of what Sidgwick has called different methods of ethics: the principle of universalizability, perhaps, or the rule that one ought to conform to the specific rules of any way of life in which one takes part, from which one profits, and on which one relies, or some utilitarian principle of doing what tends, or seems likely, to promote the general happiness. It is easy to show that such general principles, married with differing concrete circumstances, different existing social patterns or different preferences, will beget different specific moral rules; and there is some plausibility in the claim that the specific rules thus generated will vary from community to community or from group to group in close agreement with the actual variations in accepted codes.

The argument from relativity can be only partly countered in this way. To take this line the moral objectivist has to say that it is only in these principles that the objective moral character attaches immediately to its descriptively specified ground or subject: other moral judgements are objectively valid or true, but only derivatively and contingently—if things had been otherwise, quite different sorts of actions would have been right. And despite the prominence in recent philosophical ethics of universalization, utilitarian principles, and the like, these are very far from constituting the whole of what is actually affirmed as basic in ordinary moral thought. [. . .] That is, people judge that some things are good or right, and others are bad or wrong, not because—or at any rate not only because—they exemplify some general principle for which widespread implicit acceptance could be claimed, but because something about those things arouses certain responses immediately in them, though they would arouse radically and irresolvably different responses in others. 'Moral sense' or 'intuition' is an initially more plausible description of what supplies many of our basic moral judgements than 'reason'. With regard to all these starting points of moral thinking the argument from relativity remains in full force.

Even more important, however, and certainly more generally applicable, is the argument from queerness. This has two parts, one metaphysical, the other epistemological. If there were objective values, then they would be entities or qualities or relations of a very strange sort, utterly different from anything else in the universe. Correspondingly, if we were aware of them, it would have to be by some special faculty of moral perception or intuition, utterly different from our ordinary ways of knowing everything else.

[. . .] Intuitionism has long been out of favour, and it is indeed easy to point out its implausibilities. What is not so often stressed, but is more important, is that the central thesis of intuitionism is one to which any objectivist view of values is in the end committed: intuitionism merely makes unpalatably plain what other forms of objectivism wrap up. Of course the suggestion that moral judgements are made or moral problems solved by just sitting down and having an ethical intuition is a travesty of actual moral thinking. But, however complex the real process, it will re-quire (if it is to yield authoritatively prescriptive conclusions) some input of this distinctive sort, either premises or forms of argument or both. When we ask the awkward question, how we can be aware of this authoritative prescriptivity, of the truth of these distinctively ethical premises or of the cogency of this distinctively ethical pattern of reasoning, none of our ordinary accounts of sensory perception or introspection or the framing and confirming of explanatory hypotheses or inference or logical construc-tion or conceptual analysis, or any combination of these, will provide a satisfactory answer; 'a special sort of intuition' is a lame answer, but it is the one to which the clear-headed objectivist is compelled to resort.

Indeed, the best move for the moral objectivist is not to evade this issue, but to look for companions in guilt. For example, Richard Price argues that it is not moral knowledge alone that such an empiricism as those of Locke and Hume is unable to account for, but also our knowledge and even our ideas of essence, number, identity, diversity, solidity, inertia, substance, the necessary existence and infinite extension of time and space, necessity and possibility in general, power, and causation. If the understanding, which Price defines as the faculty within us that discerns truth, is also a source of new simple ideas of so many other sorts, may it not also be a power of immediately perceiving right and wrong, which yet are real characters of actions?

This is an important counter to the argument from queerness. The only adequate reply to it would be to show how, on empiricist foundations, we can construct an account of the ideas and beliefs and knowledge that we have of all these matters. I cannot even begin to do that here, though I have undertaken some parts of the task elsewhere. I can only state my belief that satisfactory accounts of most of these can be given in empirical terms. If some supposed metaphysical necessities or essences resist such treatment, then they too should be included, along with objective values, among the targets of the argument from queerness.

This queerness does not consist simply in the fact that ethical statements are 'unverifiable'. Although logical positivism with its verifiability theory of descriptive meaning gave an impetus to non-cognitive accounts of ethics, it is not only logical positivists but also empiricists of a much more liberal sort who should find objective values hard to accommodate. Indeed, I would not only reject the verifiability principle but also deny the conclusion commonly drawn from it, that moral judgements lack descriptive meaning. The assertion that there are objective values or intrinsically prescriptive entities or features of some kind, which ordinary moral judgements presuppose, is, I hold, not meaningless but false.

Plato's Forms give a dramatic picture of what objective values would have to be. The Form of the Good is such that knowledge of it provides the knower with both a direction and an overriding motive; something's being good both tells the person who knows this to pursue it and makes him pursue it. An objective good would be sought by anyone who was acquainted with it, not because of any contingent fact that this person, or every person, is so constituted that he desires this end, but just because the end has to-be-pursuedness somehow built into it. Similarly, if there were objective principles of right and wrong, any wrong (possible) course of action would have not-to-be-doneness somehow built into it. Or we should have something like Clarke's necessary relations of fitness between situations and actions, so that a situation would have a demand for such-and-such an action somehow built into it.

The need for an argument of this sort can be brought out by reflection on Hume's argument that 'reason'—in which at this stage he includes all sorts of knowing as well as reasoning—can never be an 'influencing motive of the will'. Someone might object that Hume has argued unfairly from the lack of influencing power (not contingent upon desires) in ordinary objects of knowledge and ordinary reasoning, and might maintain that values differ from natural objects precisely in their power, when known, automatically to influence the will. To this Hume could, and would need to, reply that this objection involves the postulating of value-entities or value-features of quite a different order from anything else with which we are acquainted, and of a corresponding faculty with which to detect them. That is, he would have to supplement his explicit argument with what I have called the argument from queerness.

Another way of bringing out this queerness is to ask, about anything that is supposed to have some objective moral quality, how this is linked with its natural features. What is the connection between the natural fact that an action is a piece of deliberate cruelty—say, causing pain just for fun—and the moral fact that it is wrong? It cannot be an entailment, a logical or semantic necessity. Yet it is not merely that the two features occur together. The wrongness must somehow be 'consequential' or 'supervenient'; it is wrong because it is a piece of deliberate cruelty. But just what *in the world* is signified by this 'because'? And how do we know the relation that it signifies, if this is something more than such actions being socially condemned, and condemned by us too, perhaps through our having absorbed attitudes from our social environment? It is not even sufficient to postulate a faculty which 'sees' the wrongness: something must be postulated which can see at once the natural features that constitute the cruelty, and the wrongness, and the mysterious consequential link between the two. Alternatively, the intuition required might be the perception that wrongness is a higher order property belonging to certain natural properties; but what is this belonging of properties to other properties, and how can we discern it? How much simpler and more comprehensible the situation would be if we could replace the moral quality with some sort of subjective response which could be causally related to the detection of the natural features on which the supposed quality is said to be consequential.

[*Ethics: Inventing Right and Wrong* (Penguin: Harmondsworth, 1977), 15, 27–30, 35–41.]

COLIN McGINN

43 Evolution and the Basis of Morality

[Having presented] the evolutionary reason for why there could not be a gene for kin-unrelated altruism, namely that such a gene would be automatically selected against, [. . .] how can we explain the upsurge and continuance of morality in the human species? This is in fact a difficult question; from the point of view of evolution the deep and pervasive hold of morality on human conduct must seem anomalous. (It is otherwise with prudence, whatever the structural parallels with morality may be.) Dawkins himself asserts that we have the capacity, alone among animals, to 'rebel against our genes', but he offers no suggestion on how this is constitutionally possible for us, given that our constitution is answerable to the genes that built it.[1] Surely we would expect that morality will be cordially selected out, when once, by some evolutionary blunder, it has been let in. (To say that it is a matter of 'culture' merely labels the problem.) Part of the answer, no doubt, is that the human species is no longer in a state of nature; the pressures of brute natural selection are therefore cushioned. But this does not seem to go to the root of the matter if only because part of the explanation of our not being so is the prevalence of morality in human societies; and anyway, though this accounts in some measure for the stability of morality once established, it does not give a radical explanation of how the thing got started. It seems to me that cognitivism, unlike noncognitivism, has the resources for an answer to the problem. Cognitivism claims that the source of moral motives is reason, or a capacity to form an objective conception of the world. Furthermore, the requirements of morality are such as to be acknowledged (if not invariably acted upon) by any

[1] Richard Dawkins, *The Selfish Gene* (Granada Publishing Limited: London, 1978), 215.

rational being. Now we cannot help noticing that the cognitive capacity which confers moral sense on a being also has another function, indeed an evolutionary function. For rationality and the capacity to apprehend how the world works (what it is intrinsically like) are themselves tremendously advantageous characteristics for an individual, and hence a species, to possess: they are powerful aids to survival. That is presumably why the human species has developed the sort of brain it has. Now what I want to suggest is that morality is an inevitable corollary of evolutionarily useful intelligence: in becoming rational animals human beings, *eo ipso*, became creatures endowed with moral sense. It is important to this explanation that practical rationality be *inseparable* from susceptibility to moral requirements; for if it were possible to possess the one faculty without the other, then evolution could afford to dispense with morality while retaining reason. But I think that the Kantian thesis is right that rationality implies moral sense. If they are thus inseparable, then the price of eliminating morality from a species would be the elimination of (advanced) rationality from it; and, given the advantages of the latter, the price is too great. Morality, which jibs at the ruthless ways of natural selection, is the price the genes pay for intelligent survival machines. Presumably the price is not too high. This by-product theory[1] of the evolutionary origin of morality should be sharply contrasted with the noncognitivist account of its origin: for, on that account, it is hard to see why genetically determined altruistic desires should be necessary corollaries of characteristics whose evolutionary function, as predicted by gene selection theory, is confined to benefiting the individual and its kin. On the contrary, there seems no reason why such desires, if once they arose, would not be immediately vulnerable to the pressures for their extirpation outlined earlier. If we want to secure morality against the forces of natural selection, we need to associate it with possession of some characteristic whose evolutionary credentials are undisputed: I suggest that the cognitivist's associating it with reason meets this condition, while the noncognitivist's appetitive theory does not. [. . .]

The general thesis has been that morality is essentially such as to incline us in a direction contrary to that designed by the laws of natural selection; it cannot therefore be based upon, or derived from, such laws. What makes morality possible—namely, the cognitive character of moral reasons— involves no restriction of its scope, either to the family or to the group or to the species. On the contrary, the ground of a moral requirement—involving recognition of the reality of other creatures and their interests—recommends the extension of human moral concern beyond the bounds of our own species. In thus introducing morality into a world built according to principles of

---

[1] Chomsky in *Reflections on Language* (Fontana: London, 1976), 59, mentions the possibility of such an account of our advanced scientific and mathematical capacities.

ruthless competition, we signal our repudiation of the amoral tactics of gene selection. Animals unblessed with moral reason cannot do other than conform to the exigencies of natural selection; we can rise above them. Let us then employ our powers of reason, not in the immoral furtherance of interspecific exploitation, but to bring about its cessation.[1]

['Evolution, Animals, and the Basis of Morality', *Inquiry*, 22 (1979), 92–93, 98.]

VIRGINIA HELD

44 Reason, Gender, and Moral Theory

The history of philosophy, including the history of ethics, has been constructed from male points of view, and has been built on assumptions and concepts that are by no means gender-neutral. Feminists characteristically begin with different concerns and give different emphases to the issues we consider than do non-feminist approaches. [. . .]

Consider the ideals embodied in the phrase 'the man of reason.' As Genevieve Lloyd has told the story, what has been taken to characterize the man of reason may have changed from historical period to historical period, but in each, the character ideal of the man of reason has been constructed in conjunction with a rejection of whatever has been taken to be characteristic of the feminine. 'Rationality,' Lloyd writes, 'has been conceived as transcendence of the "feminine," and the "feminine" itself has been partly constituted by its occurrence within this structure.'[2]

This has of course fundamentally affected the history of philosophy and of ethics. The split between reason and emotion is one of the most familiar of philosophical conceptions. And the advocacy of reason 'controlling' unruly emotion, of rationality guiding responsible human action against the blindness of passion, has a long and highly influential history, almost as familiar to non-philosophers as to philosophers. We should certainly now be alert to the ways in which reason has been associated with male endeavor, emotion with female weakness, and the ways in which this is of course not an accidental association. [. . .]

The associations, between Reason, form, knowledge, and maleness, have persisted in various guises, and have permeated what has been thought to be moral knowledge as well as what has been thought to be scientific knowledge, and what has been thought to be the practice of morality. The associations between the philosophical concepts and gender cannot be

---

[1] I am grateful to Anita Avramides for comments on this work.
[2] Genevieve Lloyd, *The Man of Reason: 'Male' and 'Female' in Western Philosophy* (University of Minnesota Press: Minneapolis, 1984), 104.

merely dropped, and the concepts retained regardless of gender, because gender has been built into them in such a way that without it, they will have to be different concepts. As feminists repeatedly show, if the concept of 'human' were built on what we think about 'woman' rather than what we think about 'man,' it would be a very different concept. Ethics, thus, has not been a search for universal, or truly human guidance, but a gender-biased enterprise. [. . .]

In the area of moral theory in the modern era, the priority accorded to reason has taken two major forms. A) On the one hand has been the Kantian, or Kantian-inspired search for very general, abstract, deontological, universal moral principles by which rational beings should be guided. Kant's Categorical Imperative is a foremost example: it suggests that all moral problems can be handled by applying an impartial, pure, rational principle to particular cases. It requires that we try to see what the general features of the problem before us are, and that we apply an abstract principle, or rules derivable from it, to this problem. On this view, this procedure should be adequate for all moral decisions. We should thus be able to act as reason recommends, and resist yielding to emotional inclinations and desires in conflict with our rational wills.

B) On the other hand, the priority accorded to reason in the modern era has taken a Utilitarian form. The Utilitarian approach, reflected in rational choice theory, recognizes that persons have desires and interests, and suggests rules of rational choice for maximizing the satisfaction of these. While some philosophers in this tradition espouse egoism, especially of an intelligent and long-term kind, many do not. They begin, however, with assumptions that what are morally relevant are gains and losses of utility to theoretically isolatable individuals, and that the outcome at which morality should aim is the maximization of the utility of individuals. Rational calculation about such an outcome will, in this view, provide moral recommendations to guide all our choices. As with the Kantian approach, the Utilitarian approach relies on abstract general principles or rules to be applied to particular cases. And it holds that although emotion is, in fact, the source of our desires for certain objectives, the task of morality should be to instruct us on how to pursue those objectives most rationally. Emotional attitudes toward moral issues themselves interfere with rationality and should be disregarded. Among the questions Utilitarians can ask can be questions about which emotions to cultivate, and which desires to try to change, but these questions are to be handled in the terms of rational calculation, not of what our feelings suggest.

Although the conceptions of what the judgments of morality should be based on, and of how reason should guide moral decision, are different in Kantian and in Utilitarian approaches, both share a reliance on a highly abstract, universal principle as the appropriate source of moral guidance, and both share the view that moral problems are to be solved by the application of such an abstract principle to particular cases. Both share an admiration for the rules of reason to be appealed to in moral contexts, and both denigrate emotional responses to moral issues.

Many feminist philosophers have questioned whether the reliance on abstract rules, rather than the adoption of more context-respectful approaches, can possibly be adequate for dealing with moral problems, especially as women experience them.[1] Though Kantians may hold that complex rules can be elaborated for specific contexts, there is nevertheless an assumption in this approach that the more abstract the reasoning applied to a moral problem, the more satisfactory. And Utilitarians suppose that one highly abstract principle, The Principle of Utility, can be applied to every moral problem no matter what the context.

A genuinely universal or gender-neutral moral theory would be one which would take account of the experience and concerns of women as fully as it would take account of the experience and concerns of men. When we focus on the experience of women, however, we seem to be able to see a set of moral concerns becoming salient that differs from those of traditional or standard moral theory. Women's experience of moral problems seems to lead us to be especially concerned with actual relationships between embodied persons, and with what these relationships seem to require. Women are often inclined to attend to rather than to dismiss the particularities of the context in which a moral problem arises. And we often pay attention to feelings of empathy and caring to suggest what we ought to do rather than relying as fully as possible on abstract rules of reason. [. . .]

The work of psychologists such as Carol Gilligan and others has led to a clarification of what may be thought of as tendencies among women to approach moral issues differently. Rather than interpreting moral problems in terms of what could be handled by applying abstract rules of justice to particular cases, many of the women studied by Gilligan tended to be more concerned with preserving actual human relationships, and with expressing care for those for whom they felt responsible. Their moral reasoning was typically more embedded in a context of particular others than was the reasoning of a comparable group of men.[2] One should not equate tendencies women in fact display with feminist views, since the former may well be the result of the sexist, oppressive conditions in which

---

[1] For an approach to social and political as well as moral issues that attempts to be context-respectful, see Virginia Held, *Rights and Goods. Justifying Social Action* (University of Chicago Press: Chicago, 1989).

[2] See especially Carol Gilligan, *In a Different Voice. Psychological Theory and Women's Development* (Harvard University Press: Cambridge, Mass., 1988); and Eva Feder Kittay and Diana T. Meyers (eds.), *Women and Moral Theory* (Rowman and Allanheld: Totowa, NJ, 1987).

women's lives have been lived. But many feminists see our own conscious-ly considered experience as lending confirmation to the view that what has come to be called 'an ethic of care' needs to be developed. Some think it should supercede 'the ethic of justice' of traditional or standard moral theory. Others think it should be integrated with the ethic of justice and rules.

In any case, feminist philosophers are in the process of reevaluating the place of emotion in morality in at least two respects. First, many think morality requires the development of the moral emotions, in contrast to moral theories emphasizing the primacy of reason. As Annette Baier notes, the rationalism typical of traditional moral theory will be challenged when we pay attention to the role of parent. 'It might be important,' she writes, 'for father figures to have rational control over their violent urges to beat to death the children whose screams enrage them, but more than control of such nasty passions seems needed in the mother or primary parent, or parent-substitute, by most psychological theories. They need to love their children, not just to control their irritation,'[1] So the emphasis in many traditional theories on rational control over the emotions, 'rather than on cultivating desirable forms of emotion,'[2] is challenged by feminist ap-proaches to ethics.

Secondly, emotion will be respected rather than dismissed by many feminist moral philosophers in the process of gaining moral understanding. The experience and practice out of which feminist moral theory can be expected to be developed will include embodied feeling as well as thought. [. . .] Among the elements being reevaluated are feminine emotions. The 'care' of the alternative feminist approach to morality appreciates rather than rejects emotion. The caring relationships important to feminist mor-ality cannot be understood in terms of abstract rules or moral reasoning. And the 'weighing' so often needed between the conflicting claims of some relationships and others cannot be settled by deduction or rational calcula-tion. A feminist ethic will not just acknowledge emotion, as do Utilitarians, as giving us the objectives toward which moral rationality can direct us. It will embrace emotion as providing at least a partial basis for morality itself, and for moral understanding. [. . .]

Achieving and maintaining trusting, caring relationships is quite differ-ent from acting in accord with rational principles, or satisfying the indi-vidual desires of either self or other. Caring, empathy, feeling with others, being sensitive to each other's feelings, all may be better guides to what morality requires in actual contexts than may abstract rules of reason, or

---

[1] Annette Baier, 'The Need for More Than Justice', in Marsha Hanen and Kai Nielsen (eds.), *Science, Morality and Feminist Theory* (University of Calgary Press: Calgary, 1987), 55.
[2] Ibid.

rational calculation, or at least they may be necessary components of an adequate morality. [. . .]

['Feminist Transformations of Moral Theory', *Philosophy and Phenomenological Research*, 50 (supplement, Autumn 1990), 321–44.]

MICHAEL SMITH

45 Realism

Most of us take moral appraisal pretty much for granted. To the extent that we worry, we simply worry about *getting it right*. Philosophers too worry about getting the answers to moral questions right. However, traditionally, they have also been worried about the whole business of moral appraisal itself. The problem they have grappled with emerges when we focus on two distinctive features of moral practice; for, surprisingly, these features pull against each other, threatening to make the very idea of morality look altogether incoherent.

The first feature is implicit in our concern to get the answers to moral questions *right*, for this concern presupposes that there are correct answers to moral questions to be had, and thus that there exists a domain of distinctively *moral* facts. Moreover, we seem to think that these facts have a particular character, for the only relevant determinant of the rightness of an act would seem to be the circumstances in which that action takes place. Agents whose circumstances are identical face the same moral choice: if they perform the same act then either they both act rightly or they both act wrongly.

Something like this conception of moral facts seems to explain our preoccupation with moral argument. Since we are all in the same boat, so, it seems, we think that a conversation in which agents carefully muster and assess each other's reasons for and against their moral opinions is the best way to discover what the moral facts are. If the participants are open-minded and thinking clearly then we seem to think that such an argument should result in a *convergence* in moral opinion—a convergence upon the truth.

We may summarise this first feature of moral practice as follows: we seem to think that moral questions have correct answers, that these answers are made correct by objective moral facts, that these facts are determined by circumstances, and that, by arguing, we can discover what these facts are. The term 'objective' here simply signifies the possibility of a convergence in moral views of the kind just mentioned.

Consider now the second feature. Suppose we reflect and decide that we did the wrong thing in (say) refusing to give to famine relief. It seems we come to think we failed to do something for which there was a good reason.

And this has motivational implications. For now imagine the situation if we refuse again when next the opportunity arises. We will have refused to do what we think we have good reason to do, and this will occasion serious puzzlement. An explanation of some sort will need to be forthcoming (perhaps weakness of will or irrationality of some other kind). Why? Because, other things being equal, having a moral opinion seems to require having a corresponding reason, and therefore motivation, to act accordingly.

These two distinctive features of moral practice—the *objectivity* and the *practicality* of moral judgement—are widely thought to have both metaphysical and psychological implications. However, and unfortunately, these implications are the exact opposite of each other. In order to see why, we need to pause for a moment to reflect on the nature of human psychology.

According to the standard picture of human psychology—a picture we owe to David Hume—there are two main kinds of psychological state. On the one hand there are beliefs, states that purport to represent the way the world is. Since our beliefs purport to represent the world, they are subject to rational criticism: specifically, they are assessable in terms of truth and falsehood. And on the other hand there are also desires, states that represent how the world is to be. Desires are unlike beliefs in that they do not even purport to represent the way the world is. They are therefore not assessable in terms of truth and falsehood. Indeed, according to the standard picture, our desires are not subject to any sort of rational criticism at all. The fact that we have a certain desire is, with a proviso to be mentioned presently, simply a fact about ourselves to be acknowledged. In themselves, desires are all on a par, rationally neutral.

This is important, for it suggests that though facts about the world may rightly affect our beliefs, such facts should, again with a proviso to be mentioned presently, have no rational impact upon our desires. They may of course, have some *non*-rational impact. Seeing a spider, I may be overcome with a morbid fear and desire never to be near one. However this is not a change in my desires mandated by reason. It is a *non*-rational change in my desires.

Now for the proviso. Suppose, contrary to the example just given, I acquire an aversion to spiders because I come to believe, falsely, that they have an unpleasant odour. This is certainly an irrational aversion. However, this is not contrary to the spirit of the standard picture. For my aversion is *based on* a further desire and belief: my desire not to smell that unpleasant odour and my belief that that odour is given off by spiders. Since I can be rationally criticised for having the belief, as it is false, so I can be rationally criticised for having the aversion it helps to produce. The proviso is thus fairly minor: desires are subject to rational criticism, but only insofar as they are based on irrational beliefs. Desires that do not have this feature are not subject to rational criticism at all.

According to the standard picture, then, there are two kinds of psychological state—beliefs and desires—utterly distinct and different from each other. This picture is important because it provides us with a model for understanding human action. A human action is the product of these two forces: a desire representing the way the world is to be and a belief telling us how the world is, and thus how it has to be changed, so as to make it that way.

We said earlier that the objectivity and the practicality of moral judgement have both metaphysical and psychological implications. We can now say what they are. Consider first the objectivity of moral judgement: the idea that there are moral facts, determined by circumstances, and that, by arguing, we can discover what these objective moral facts are. This implies, metaphysically, that amongst the various facts there are in the world there aren't just facts about (say) the consequences of our actions on the well-being of sentient creatures, there are also distinctively *moral* facts: facts about the rightness and wrongness of our actions having these consequences. And, psychologically, the implication is thus that when we make a moral judgement we express our *beliefs* about the way these moral facts are. Our moral beliefs are representations of the way the world is *morally*.

Given the standard picture of human psychology, there is a further psychological implication. For whether or not people who have a certain moral belief desire to act accordingly must now be seen as a further and entirely separate question. They may happen to have a corresponding desire, they may not. However, either way, they cannot be rationally criticised.

But now consider the second feature, the practicality of moral judgement, the idea that to have a moral opinion simply *is*, contrary to what has just been said, to have a corresponding reason, and thus motivation, to act accordingly. Psychologically, since making a moral judgement entails having a certain desire, and no recognition of a fact about the world could rationally compel us to have one desire rather than another, this seems to imply that our judgement must really simply *be* an expression of that desire. And this psychological implication has a metaphysical counterpart. For, contrary to initial appearance, it seems that when we judge it right to give to famine relief (say), we *are not* responding to any moral fact. In judging it right to give to famine relief, we are really simply expressing our desire that people give to famine relief. It is as if we were yelling 'Hooray for giving to famine relief!'—no mention of a moral fact there, in fact, no factual claim at all.

We are now in a position to see why philosophers have been worried about the whole business of moral appraisal. The problem is that the *objectivity* and the *practicality* of moral judgement pull in quite opposite directions from each other. The objectivity of moral judgement suggests that there are moral facts, determined by circumstances, and that our moral judgements express our beliefs about what these facts are. But though this is presupposed by moral argument, it leaves it entirely mysterious how or why having a moral view has special links with what we are motivated to do. And the practicality of moral judgement suggests just the opposite, that our moral judgements express our desires. While this seems presupposed in the link between moral judgement and motivation, it leaves it entirely mysterious how or why moral judgements can be the subject of moral argument.

The very idea of morality may therefore be incoherent, for what is required to make sense of a moral judgement is a queer sort of fact about the universe: a fact whose recognition necessarily impacts upon our desires. But the standard picture of human psychology tells us that there are no such facts. Nothing could be everything a moral judgement purports to be—or so the standard picture tells us.

At long last we are in a position to see what this essay is about. For *moral realism* is simply the metaphysical view that there exist moral facts. The psychological counterpart to realism is cognitivism, the view that moral judgements express our beliefs about what these moral facts are. Moral realism thus contrasts with two alternative metaphysical views: *irrealism* and *moral nihilism*. According to the irrealists, there are no moral facts, but neither are moral facts required to make sense of moral practice. We can happily acknowledge that our moral judgements simply express our desires about how people behave. This is non-cognitivism, the psychological counterpart to irrealism. By contrast, according to the moral nihilists, the irrealists are right that there are no moral facts, but wrong about what is required to make sense of moral practice. Without moral facts moral practice is all a sham, much like religious practice without belief in God.

Which, then, should we believe: realism, irrealism or nihilism? I favour realism. Let me say why. We have assumed from the outset that judgements of right and wrong are judgements about our reasons for action. But though these judgements seem to concern a realm of facts about our reasons, what casts doubt on this is the standard picture of human psychology. For it tells us that, since judgements about our reasons have motivational implications, so they must really simply be expressions of our desires. It seems to me that here we see the real devil of the piece: the standard picture of human psychology's tacit conflation of *reasons* with *motives*. Seeing why this is so enables us to see why we may legitimately talk about our *beliefs* about the reasons we have, and why having such beliefs makes it rational to have corresponding desires; why such beliefs have motivational implications.

Imagine giving the baby a bath. As you do, it begins to scream uncontrollably. Nothing you do seems to help. As you watch, you are overcome with a desire to drown it in the bathwater. You are *motivated* to drown the baby. Does this entail that you have a *reason* to drown the baby? Commonsense tells us that, since this desire is not *worth* satisfying, it does not provide you with such a reason; that, in this case, you are motivated to do something you have *no* reason to do. But can the standard picture agree with commonsense on this score? No, it cannot. For your desire to drown the baby need be based on no false belief, and, as such, the standard picture tells us it is beyond rational criticism. There is no sense in which it is not worth satisfying—or so the standard picture tells us. But this is surely wrong.

The problem is that the standard picture gives no special privilege to what we would want if we were 'cool, calm and collected'. Yet commonsense tells us that not being cool, calm and collected may lead to all sorts of irrational emotional outbursts. Having those desires that we would have if we were cool, calm and collected thus seems to be an *independent* rational ideal. When cool, calm and collected, you would want that the baby isn't drowned, no matter how much it screams, and no matter how overcome you may be, in your uncool, uncalm and uncollected state, with a desire to drown it. This is why you have no reason to drown the baby. It seems to me that this insight is the key to reconciling the objectivity with the practicality of moral judgement.

Judgements of right and wrong express our beliefs about our reasons. But what sort of fact is a fact about our reasons? The preceding discussion suggests that they are not facts about what we *actually* desire, as the standard picture would have it, but are rather facts about what we *would* desire if we were in certain idealised conditions of reflection: if, say, we were well informed, cool, calm and collected.

According to this account, then, I have a reason to give to famine relief in my particular circumstances just in case, if I were in such idealised conditions of reflection, I would desire that, even when in my particular circumstances, I give to famine relief. Now this sort of fact may certainly be the object of a belief. And moreover having such a belief—a belief about our reasons—certainly seems to rationally require of us that we have corresponding desires.

In order to see this, suppose I believe I would desire to give to famine relief if I were cool, calm and collected but, being uncool, uncalm and uncollected, I don't desire to give to famine relief. Am I rationally criticizable for not having the desire? I surely am. After all, from my own point of view my beliefs and desires form a more coherent, and thus a rationally preferable, package if I do in fact desire what I believe I would desire if I were cool, calm and collected. This is because, since it is an independent rational ideal to have the desires I would have if I were cool, calm and collected so, from my own point of view, if I believe that I would have a certain desire under such conditions and yet fail to have it, my beliefs and desires fail to meet this ideal. To believe that I would desire to give to famine relief if I were cool, calm and collected and yet fail to desire to give to famine relief is thus to manifest a commonly recognizable species of rational failure.

If this is right then, contrary to the standard picture, a broader class of desires may be rationally criticized. The desires of those who fail to desire to do what they believe they have reason to do can be rationally criticized even though they may not be based on any false belief. And, if this is right, then the standard picture is wrong to suggest that a judgement with motivational implications must really be the expression of a desire. For a judgement about an agent's reasons has motivational implications—the rational agent is motivated accordingly—and yet it is the expression of a belief.

Have we said enough to solve the problem facing the moral realist? Not yet. Moral judgements aren't *just* judgements about the reasons we have. They are judgements about the reasons we have *where those reasons are determined entirely by our circumstances*. People in the same circumstances face the same moral choice: if they do the same then either they both act rightly (they both do what they have reason to do) or they both act wrongly (they both do what they have reason not to do). Does the account of reasons we have given support this?

Suppose our circumstances are identical. Is it right for each of us to give to famine relief? According to the story just told, it is right that I give to famine relief just in case I have a reason to do so, and I have such a reason just in case, if I were in idealised conditions of reflection—well informed, cool, calm and collected—I would desire to give to famine relief. And the same is true of you. If our circumstances are the same then, supposedly, we should both have such a reason or both lack such a reason. But do we?

The question is whether, if we were well informed, cool, calm and collected, we would all *converge* in the desires we have. Would we converge or would there always be the possibility of some non-rationally-explicable difference in our desires *even under such conditions*? The standard picture of human psychology now returns to center-stage. For it tells us that there is always the possibility of some non-rationally-explicable difference in our desires *even under such idealised conditions of reflection*. This is the residue of the standard picture's conception of desire as a psychological state that is beyond rational criticism.

If there is such a possibility then the realist's attempt to reconcile the objectivity and the practicality of moral judgement simply fails. For we are forced to accept that there is a *fundamental relativity* in the reasons we have. What we have reason to do is relative to what we would desire under idealised conditions of reflection, and this may differ from person to person. It is not wholly determined by our circumstances, as moral facts are supposed to be.

Many philosophers believe that there is always such a possibility; that our reasons are fundamentally relative. But this seems unwarranted to me. For it seems to me that moral practice is itself the forum in which we will *discover* whether there is a fundamental relativity in our reasons.

After all, in moral practice we attempt to change people's moral beliefs by engaging them in rational argument: i.e. by getting their beliefs to approximate those they would have under more idealised conditions of reflection. And sometimes we succeed. When we succeed, other things being equal, we succeed in changing their desires. How, then, can we say in advance that this procedure will never result in a massive *convergence* in moral beliefs? And, if it did result in a massive convergence in our moral beliefs—and thus in our desires—then why not say that this convergence would itself be best explained by the fact that the beliefs and desires that emerge have some *privileged* rational status? Something like such a convergence on certain mathematical judgements in mathematical practice lies behind our conviction that those claims enjoy a privileged rational status. So why not think that a like convergence in moral practice would show that those moral judgements and concerns enjoy the same privileged rational status? At this point, the standard picture's insistence that there is a fundamental relativity in our reasons begins to sound all too much like a hollow dogma.

The kind of moral realism described here endorses a conception of moral facts that is a far cry from the picture noted at the outset: moral facts as queer facts about the universe whose recognition necessarily impacts upon our desires. The realist has eschewed queer facts about the universe in favour of a more 'subjectivist' conception of moral facts. The realist's point, however, is that such a conception of moral facts may make them subjective only in the innocuous sense that they are facts about our reasons: i.e. facts about what we would *want* under certain idealised conditions of reflection. For wants are, admittedly, states enjoyed by subjects. But moral facts remain objective insofar as they are facts about what *we*, not just *you* or *I*, would want under such conditions. The existence of a moral fact—say, the rightness of giving to famine relief in certain circumstances—requires that, under idealised conditions of reflection, rational creatures would *converge* upon a desire to give to famine relief in such circumstances.

Of course, it must be said that moral argument has not yet produced the sort of convergence in our desires that would make the idea of a moral fact—a fact about the reasons we have entirely determined by our circumstances—look plausible. But neither has moral argument had much of a history in times in which we can engage in free reflection unhampered by a false biology (the Aristotelian tradition) or a false belief in God (the Judeo-Christian tradition). It remains to be seen whether sustained moral argument can elicit the requisite convergence in our moral beliefs, and corresponding desires, to make the idea of a moral fact look plausible. The kind of moral realism described here holds out the hope that it will. Only time will tell.

[Adapted from 'Realism', in P. Singer (ed.), *A Companion to Ethics* (Blackwell: Oxford, 1991), 399–410.]

PART II

The Content of Ethics: Judging Good Outcomes and Right Acts

Section A

Ultimate Good

The second part of this book is concerned not with the nature and origin of ethics, but rather with substantive issues within ethics; in other words, with normative ethics rather than with meta-ethics and other questions about ethics. Writings on the nature of the good life fall squarely within the domain of ethics, for they are based on conceptions of what is of intrinsic or ultimate value in a life. There are many things that we value, but few that we value for their own sake. Suppose that we value money, as most of us do. Why do we value it? Unless we are a Scrooge, we don't want to have money just in order to gloat over it. Do we want it in order to be able to buy a fine home or a luxury car? Perhaps, but why do we want those things? Because we believe that they will make us happy? But are material goods the way to happiness? And is happiness really the ultimate good? If not, what else could be?

These fundamental questions are part of the timeless human search for the best way to live. Today, there are two special reasons for examining ideas about what kind of life is really worth living. The first reason is the need to challenge the dominance of the assumption that the good life requires ever-rising standards of material affluence. This assumption is in opposition to the overwhelming majority of serious thinkers, past and present, from a wide variety of cultures. That does not show that the assumption is mistaken, but it gives us grounds to reflect and reconsider, especially since there is no evidence that—once we have provided for our basic needs—our increasing affluence makes us happier. The need for such reflection is greatly reinforced by the second reason for needing to revive discussion of this topic. We are running up against the limits of our planet's capacity to absorb the wastes produced by our affluent lifestyle. If we wish to avoid drastic change in the global climate, we may need to find a new ideal of the good life which is less reliant on a high level of material consumption.

The first six selections in this section provide a range of ideas from early thinkers. The Buddha describes the good life as a middle way between the pursuit of physical pleasure and the mortification of the body. As the ultimate goal, he takes 'the ceasing of woe', that is, a state beyond all passion, craving, and desire. Aristotle has a more positive ideal: for him, happiness is the end, and it is to be found in an active life that involves the pursuit of philosophical wisdom. This is the most intrinsically worthwhile life for a human being. Epicurus maintains that pleasure is the ultimate end; but those who know of him only because the word 'epicure' derives from his name will be surprised to find, in his letter to Menoeceus, a firm repudiation of those who live for the pleasures of eating and drinking. Instead, Epicurus advocates a simple life, in which we control our desires so as to maximize pleasure over the long term. The Stoics, rivals of the Epicureans in ancient Rome, went even further in subordinating desires to the commands of reason. Epictetus, who was born a slave, suggests that instead of desiring that reality be different, we should change our desires so that we want what actually happens. The Stoics think we should live according to reason, not desire. One wonders, though, how many Stoics were able to shrug off the loss of members of their families in the manner that Epictetus recommends.

I have included, among these ancient teachings about ultimate ideals, part of Jesus' Sermon on the Mount. It belongs here for two reasons. The first is that it shows the distinctive set of virtues that Jesus praised, thus setting an influential standard for how we ought to live in this life. The second is that this passage offers a different kind of justification for living in accordance with virtue. Jesus says nothing to link his list of virtues with a notion of an intrinsically good life, or with any other benefits in this world. Instead, his emphasis is on virtue as the only way of entering 'the kingdom of heaven'. This is in contrast to the Greek and Roman writers included in this section, who find living virtuously to be either its own reward or a path to the best life in this world. The dominance of Christian teaching in Western ethics may well have been responsible for the decline of the assumption that living well brings its own reward in this life. The bizarre extremes to which some early Christian saints took the idea of sacrificing present pleasures for the sake of the world to come are vividly described in the extract from W. E. H. Lecky's *History of European Morals from Augustus to Charlemagne*, one of the great works of late Victorian scholarship. Here we have a portrayal of what is, as Lecky calls it, an astonishing 'ideal of excellence' that held sway for about two centuries of European civilization.

With Voltaire's delightful 'Story of a Good Brahmin' we move into the modern era of discussion about the ends of life. Here the discussion tends to revolve around hedonism, the idea that pleasure or happiness is the ultimate good. While this view has by no means been universally accepted, the persistence of its attraction is shown by the fact that almost every alternative view defines itself in opposition to hedonism. Voltaire's story asks whether wisdom is to be valued—if we are happier when ignorant. Jeremy Bentham, the founding father of modern utilitarianism, is in no doubt that happiness is the criterion. Shall we agree with Bentham that, quantities of pleasure being equal, a simple game like push-pin is as good as poetry? Or will we side with Bentham's godson, John Stuart Mill, and hold that it is better to be Socrates dissatisfied than a satisfied fool? And is Mill's position really compatible with treating pleasure as the only good, as Mill maintained? Henry Sidgwick is characteristically more careful than either Bentham or Mill in trying to establish that 'desirable consciousness' (which is a very close relative of pleasure, if not necessarily limited only to that) is the only ultimate value.

Challenges to the hedonistic position have come from many directions. G. E. Moore, the Cambridge philosopher who had such a profound influence on the Bloomsbury set of writers and artists, rejects Sidgwick's insistence that only consciousness can be intrinsically good. He does give highest place, in his order of intrinsically valuable things, to conscious experiences, especially experiences of beauty and friendship. But he also thinks that beauty alone is intrinsically good, even when there is no possibility of anyone ever experiencing it. What is particularly interesting (and somewhat depressing) here is not only the disagreement between Sidgwick and Moore, but the fact that each insists that, given careful reflection, the view he espouses is *self-evidently* correct. Perhaps this is because, if such truths are not self-evident, there seems to be no way in which anyone can argue for them.

Discussions of ultimate value are not limited to works of philosophy or religion. In the conclusion of his autobiography, Gandhi harks back to an ancient Indian tradition, and sees the goal as truth and *ahimsa*, or harmlessness. The debate between the Controller and the Savage, from Aldous Huxley's *Brave New World*, is one of the classic literary confrontations between hedonism and an ideal of a life of struggle and conflict. Albert Camus's paradoxical portrait of Sisyphus as an existentialist hero takes this ideal of a life of struggle even further.

What, then, is the current state of the debate about ultimate value? In general terms, there are three main possibilities. One is, in broad terms, the view of the classical utilitarians: only some form of desirable consciousness can be intrinsically good. Robert Nozick argues that consciousness cannot have a monopoly on intrinsic value, because we want not only to have certain experiences, but to do certain things, to live our lives in contact with reality. The second possibility takes account of this kind of objection: it is based on the view that we are in no position to tell others what they are to regard as being desirable, and that we should therefore accept *whatever* anyone prefers as being, for that reason alone, of value. This view has given rise to a modern form of utilitarianism known as preference utilitarianism, because, instead of trying to maximize happiness, it seeks to bring about the fulfilment of preferences. In this section this view is put by William James. The third possibility is that we try to construct some objective list of intrinsic goods, a list that may include desirable forms of consciousness, but will go beyond it. One version of this third type of theory is the natural law tradition of ethics, represented here in a modern version by John Finnis, but with roots going back through Thomas Aquinas to Aristotle. Other writers might choose different lists of intrinsic values. In the final reading in this section, Derek Parfit considers the merits of each of these three possibilities and the different versions that they can take. When compared with the earlier writings in this section, his discussion shows how much more rigorous and precise the modern debate has become.

Then the Exalted One thus spake unto the company of Five Brethren:

'These two extremes, brethren, should not be followed by one who has gone forth as a wanderer:

Devotion to the pleasures of sense—a low and pagan practice, unworthy, unprofitable, the way of the world (on the one hand), and on the other hand devotion to self-mortification, which is painful, unworthy, unprofitable.

By avoiding these two extremes he who hath won the Truth (the Buddha) has gained knowledge of that *Middle Path* which giveth Vision, which giveth Knowledge, which causeth Calm, Insight, Enlightenment, and Nibbana.

And what, brethren, is that *Middle Path* which giveth Vision, which giveth Knowledge, which causeth Calm, Insight, Enlightenment, and Nibbana?

Verily it is this Ariyan Eightfold Path, that is to say:

RIGHT VIEW, RIGHT AIM, RIGHT SPEECH, RIGHT ACTION, RIGHT LIVING, RIGHT EFFORT, RIGHT MINDFULNESS, RIGHT CONTEMPLATION.

This, brethren, is that *Middle Path*, which giveth Vision, which giveth knowledge, which causeth Calm, Insight, Enlightenment, and Nibbana.

Now this, brethren, is the Ariyan Truth about *Suffering*:

Birth is Suffering, Decay is Suffering, Sickness is Suffering, Death is Suffering, likewise Sorrow and Grief, Woe, Lamentation and Despair. To be conjoined with things which we dislike, to be separated from things which we like—that also is Suffering. Not to get what one wants—that also is Suffering. In a word, this Body, this fivefold Mass which is based on *Grasping*, that is Suffering.

Now this, brethren, is the Ariyan Truth about *The Origin of Suffering*:

It is that *Craving* that leads downwards to birth, along with the Lure and the Lust that lingers longingly now here, now there: namely, the Craving for Sensation, the Craving to be born again, the Craving to have done with rebirth. Such, brethren, is the Ariyan Truth about *The Origin of Suffering*.

And this, brethren, is the Ariyan Truth about *The Ceasing of Suffering*:

Verily it is the utter passionless cessation of, the giving up, the forsaking, the release from, the absence of longing for, this *Craving*.

Now this, brethren, is the Ariyan Truth about *The Way leading to the Ceasing of Suffering*. Verily it is this Ariyan Eightfold Path, that is:

RIGHT VIEW, RIGHT AIM, RIGHT SPEECH, RIGHT ACTION, RIGHT LIVING, RIGHT EFFORT, RIGHT MINDFULNESS, RIGHT CONTEMPLATION.

* * * * * *

And the Exalted One said:

'Now what, brethren, is RIGHT VIEW?

The knowledge about Ill, the Arising of Ill, the Ceasing of Ill, and the Way leading to the Ceasing of Ill,—that, brethren, is called Right View.

And what, brethren, is RIGHT AIM?

The being set on Renunciation, on Non-resentment, on Harmlessness,—that, brethren, is called Right Aim.

And what, brethren, is RIGHT SPEECH?

Abstinence from lying speech, from backbiting and abusive speech, and from idle babble,—that, brethren, is called Right Speech.

And what, brethren, is RIGHT ACTION?

Abstinence from taking life, from taking what is not given, from wrong-doing in sexual passions,—that, brethren, is called Right Action.

And what, brethren, is RIGHT LIVING?

Herein, brethren, the Ariyan disciple, by giving up wrong living, gets his livelihood by right living,—that, brethren, is called Right Living.

And what, brethren, is RIGHT EFFORT?

Herein, brethren, a brother generates the will to inhibit the arising of evil immoral conditions that have not yet arisen: he makes an effort, he sets energy afoot, he applies his mind and struggles. Likewise (he does the same) to reject evil immoral conditions that have already arisen. Likewise (he does the same) to cause the arising of good conditions that have not yet arisen. Likewise he does the same to establish, to prevent the corruption, to cause the increase, the practice, the fulfilment of good conditions that have already arisen. This, brethren, is called Right Effort.

And what, brethren, is RIGHT MINDFULNESS?

Herein, brethren, a brother dwells regarding body as a compound, he dwells ardent, self-possessed, recollected, by controlling the covetousness and dejection that are in the world. So also with regard to Feelings, with regard to Perception, with regard to the Activities . . . with regard to Thought. This, brethren, is called RIGHT MINDFULNESS.

And what, brethren, is RIGHT CONTEMPLATION?

Herein, brethren, a brother, remote from sensual appetites, remote from evil conditions, enters upon and abides in the First Musing, which is accompanied by directed thought and sustained thought (on an object). It is born of solitude, full of zest and happiness.

Then, by the sinking down of thought directed and sustained, he enters on and abides in the Second Musing, which is an inner calming, a raising up of the will. In it there is no directed thought, no sustained thought. It is born of contemplation, full of zest and happiness.

Then again, brethren, by the fading away of the zest, he becomes balanced (indifferent) and remains mindful and self-possessed, and while still in the body he experiences the happiness of which the Ariyans aver 'the balanced thoughtful man dwells happily.' Thus he enters on the Third Musing and abides therein.

Then again, brethren, rejecting pleasure and pain, by the coming to an end of the joy and sorrow which he had before, he enters on and remains in the Fourth Musing, which is free from pain and free from pleasure, but is a state of perfect purity of balance and equanimity. This is called Right Contemplation.

This, brethren, is called the Ariyan Truth of the Way leading to the Ceasing of Woe.'

[*Some Sayings of the Buddha*, trans. F. L. Woodward (Oxford University Press: New York, 1973), 7–11. Originally 6th century.]

ARISTOTLE

47   The End for Human Nature

Now that we have spoken of the virtues, the forms of friendship, and the varieties of pleasure, what remains is to discuss in outline the nature of happiness, since this is what we state the end of human nature to be. Our discussion will be the more concise if we first sum up what we have said already. We said, then, that it is not a disposition; for if it were it might belong to someone who was asleep throughout his life, living the life of a plant, or, again, to someone who was suffering the greatest misfortunes. If these implications are unacceptable, and we must rather class happiness as an activity, as we have said before, and if some activities are necessary, and desirable for the sake of something else, while others are so in themselves, evidently happiness must be placed among those desirable in themselves, not among those desirable for the sake of something else; for happiness does not lack anything, but is self-sufficient. Now those activities are desirable in themselves from which nothing is sought beyond the activity. And of this nature virtuous actions are thought to be; for to do noble and good deeds is a thing desirable for its own sake.

Pleasant amusements also are thought to be of this nature: we choose them not for the sake of other things; for we are injured rather than benefited by them, since we are led to neglect our bodies and our property. But most of the people who are deemed happy take refuge in such pastimes, which is the reason why those who are ready-witted at them are highly esteemed at the courts of tyrants; they make themselves pleasant companions in the tyrants' favourite pursuits, and that is the sort of man they want. Now these things are thought to be of the nature of happiness because people in despotic positions spend their leisure in them, but perhaps such people prove nothing; for virtue and reason, from which good activities flow, do not depend on despotic position; nor, if these people, who have never tasted pure and generous pleasure, take refuge in the bodily pleasures, should these for that reason be thought more desirable; for boys, too, think the things that are valued among themselves are the best. It is to be expected, then, that, as different things seem valuable to boys and to men, so they should to bad men and to good. Now, as we have often maintained, those things are both valuable and pleasant which are such to the good man; and to each man the activity in accordance with his own disposition is most desirable, and therefore to the good man that which is in accordance with virtue. Happiness, therefore, does not lie in amusement; it would, indeed, be strange if the end were amusement, and one were to take trouble and suffer hardship all one's life in order to amuse oneself. For, in a word, everything that we choose we choose for the sake of something else—except happiness, which is an end. Now to exert oneself and work for the sake of amusement seems silly and utterly childish. But to amuse oneself in order that one may exert oneself, as Anacharsis[1] puts it, seems right; for amusement is a sort of relaxation, and we need relaxation because we cannot work continuously. Relaxation, then, is not an end; for it is taken for the sake of activity.

The happy life is thought to be virtuous; now a virtuous life requires exertion, and does not consist in amusement. And we say that serious things are better than laughable things and those connected with amusement, and that the activity of the better of any two things—whether it be two elements of our being or two men—is the more serious; but the activity of the better is *ipso facto* superior and more of the nature of happiness. And any chance person—even a slave—can enjoy the bodily pleasures no less than the best man; but no one assigns to a slave a share in happiness— unless he assigns to him also a share in human life. For happiness does not lie in such occupations, but, as we have said before, in virtuous activities.

If happiness is activity in accordance with virtue, it is reasonable that it should be in accordance with the highest virtue; and this will be that of the best thing in us. Whether it be reason or something else that is this element which is thought to be our natural ruler and guide and to take thought of things noble and divine, whether it be itself also divine or only the most divine element in us, the activity of this in accordance with its proper virtue will be perfect happiness. That this activity is contemplative we have already said.

Now this would seem to be in agreement both with what we said before and with the truth. For, firstly, this activity is the best (since not only is

---

[1] A Scythian prince who was believed to have travelled in Greece, and to have been the author of many aphorisms.

reason the best thing in us, but the objects of reason are the best of knowable objects); and, secondly, it is the most continuous, since we can contemplate truth more continuously than we can *do* anything. And we think happiness ought to have pleasure mingled with it, but the activity of philosophic wisdom is admittedly the pleasantest of virtuous activities; at all events the pursuit of it is thought to offer pleasures marvellous for their purity and their enduringness, and it is to be expected that those who know will pass their time more pleasantly than those who inquire. And the self-sufficiency that is spoken of must belong most to the contemplative activity. For while a philosopher, as well as a just man or one possessing any other virtue, needs the necessaries of life, when they are sufficiently equipped with things of that sort the just man needs people towards whom and with whom he shall act justly, and the temperate man, the brave man, and each of the others is in the same case, but the philosopher, even when by himself, can contemplate truth, and the better the wiser he is; he can perhaps do so better if he has fellow workers, but still he is the most self-sufficient. And this activity alone would seem to be loved for its own sake; for nothing arises from it apart from the contemplating, while from practical activities we gain more or less apart from the action. And happiness is thought to depend on leisure; for we are busy that we may have leisure, and make war that we may live in peace. Now the activity of the practical virtues is exhibited in political or military affairs, but the actions concerned with these seem to be unleisurely. Warlike actions are completely so (for no one chooses to be at war, or provokes war, for the sake of being at war; anyone would seem absolutely murderous if he were to make enemies of his friends in order to bring about battle and slaughter); but the action of the statesman also is unleisurely, and aims—beyond the political action itself—at despotic power and honours, or at all events happiness, for him and his fellow citizens—a happiness different from political action, and evidently sought as being different. So if among virtuous actions political and military actions are distinguished by nobility and greatness, and these are unleisurely and aim at an end and are not desirable for their own sake, but the activity of reason, which is contemplative, seems both to be superior in serious worth and to aim at no end beyond itself, and to have its pleasure proper to itself (and this augments the activity), and the self-sufficiency, leisureliness, unweariedness (so far as this is possible for man), and all the other attributes ascribed to the supremely happy man are evidently those connected with this activity, it follows that this will be the complete happiness of man, if it be allowed a complete term of life (for none of the attributes of happiness is incomplete).

But such a life would be too high for man; for it is not in so far as he is man that he will live so, but in so far as something divine is present in him; and by so much as this is superior to our composite nature is its activity superior to that which is the exercise of the other kind of virtue. If reason is divine, then, in comparison with man, the life according to it is divine in comparison with human life. But we must not follow those who advise us, being men, to think of human things, and, being mortal, of mortal things, but must, so far as we can, make ourselves immortal, and strain every nerve to live in accordance with the best thing in us; for even if it be small in bulk, much more does it in power and worth surpass everything. This would seem, too, to be each man himself, since it is the authoritative and better part of him. It would be strange, then, if he were to choose not the life of his self but that of something else. And what we said before will apply now: that which is proper to each thing is by nature best and most pleasant for each thing; for man, therefore, the life according to reason is best and pleasantest, since reason more than anything else *is* man. This life therefore is also the happiest.

[*The Nicomachean Ethics*, trans. W. D. Ross (Oxford University Press: London, 1959), 261–6. Written in *c*.340 BC.]

EPICURUS

48 The Pursuit of Pleasure

Let no one when young delay to study philosophy, nor when he is old grow weary of his study. For no one can come too early or too late to secure the health of his soul. And the man who says that the age of philosophy has either not yet come or has gone by is like the man who says that the age for happiness is not yet come to him, or has passed away. Wherefore both when young and old a man must study philosophy, that as he grows old he may be young in blessings through the grateful recollection of what has been, and that in youth he may be old as well, since he will know no fear of what is to come. We must then meditate on the things that make our happiness, seeing that when that is with us we have all, but when it is absent we do all to win it.

The things which I used unceasingly to commend to you, these do and practice, considering them to be the first principles of the good life. [. . .]

Become accustomed to the belief that death is nothing to us. For all good and evil consists in sensation, but death is deprivation of sensation. And therefore a right understanding that death is nothing to us makes the mortality of life enjoyable, not because it adds to it an infinite span of time, but because it takes away the craving for immortality. For there is nothing terrible in life for the man who has truly comprehended that there is nothing terrible in not living. So that the man speaks but idly who says that he fears death not because it will be painful when it comes, but because it is painful in anticipation. For that which gives no trouble when it comes is but an empty pain in anticipation. So death, the most terrifying of ills, is nothing to us, since so long as we exist, death is not with us; but when death comes, then we do not exist. It does not then concern either the living or the dead, since for the former it is not, and the latter are no more.

But the many at one moment shun death as the greatest of evils, at another yearn for it as a respite from the evils in life. But the wise man neither seeks to escape life nor fears the cessation of life, for neither does life offend him nor does the absence of life seem to be any evil. And just as with food he does not seek simply the larger share and nothing else, but rather the most pleasant, so he seeks to enjoy not the longest period of time, but the most pleasant.

And he who counsels the young man to live well, but the old man to make a good end, is foolish, not merely because of the desirability of life, but also because it is the same training which teaches to live well and to die well. Yet much worse still is the man who says it is good not to be born, but 'once born make haste to pass the gates of Death.' For if he says this from conviction why does he not pass away out of life? For it is open to him to do so, if he had firmly made up his mind to this. But if he speaks in jest, his words are idle among men who cannot receive them.

We must then bear in mind that the future is neither ours, nor yet wholly not ours, so that we may not altogether expect it as sure to come, nor abandon hope of it, as if it will certainly not come.

We must consider that of desires some are natural, others vain, and of the natural some are necessary and others merely natural; and of the necessary some are necessary for happiness, others for the repose of the body, and others for very life. The right understanding of these facts enables us to refer all choice and avoidance to the health of the body and the soul's freedom from disturbance, since this is the aim of the life of blessedness. For it is to obtain this end that we always act, namely, to avoid pain and fear. And when this is once secured for us, all the tempest of the soul is dispersed, since the living creature has not to wander as though in search of something that is missing, and to look for some other thing by which he can fulfil the good of the soul and the good of the body. For it is then that we have need of pleasure, when we feel pain owing to the absence of pleasure; but when we do not feel pain, we no longer need pleasure. And for this cause we call pleasure the beginning and end of the blessed life. For we recognize pleasure as the first good innate in us, and from pleasure we begin every act of choice and avoidance, and to pleasure we return again, using the feeling as the standard by which we judge every good.

And since pleasure is the first good and natural to us, for this very reason we do not choose every pleasure, but sometimes we pass over many pleasures, when greater discomfort accrues to us as the result of them: and similarly we think many pains better than pleasures, since a greater pleasure comes to us when we have endured pains for a long time. Every pleasure then because of its natural kinship to us is good, yet not every pleasure is to be chosen: even as every pain also is an evil, yet not all are always of a nature to be avoided. Yet by a scale of comparison and by the consideration of advantages and disadvantages we must form our judgement on all these matters. For the good on certain occasions we treat as bad, and conversely the bad as good.

And again independence of desire we think a great good—not that we may at all times enjoy but a few things, but that, if we do not possess many, we may enjoy the few in the genuine persuasion that those have the sweetest pleasure in luxury who least need it, and that all that is natural is easy to be obtained, but that which is superfluous is hard. And so plain savours bring us a pleasure equal to a luxurious diet, when all the pain due to want is removed; and bread and water produce the highest pleasure, when one who needs them puts them to his lips. To grow accustomed therefore to simple and not luxurious diet gives us health to the full, and makes a man alert for the needful employments of life, and when after long intervals we approach luxuries disposes us better towards them, and fits us to be fearless of fortune.

When, therefore, we maintain that pleasure is the end, we do not mean the pleasures of profligates and those that consist in sensuality, as is supposed by some who are either ignorant or disagree with us or do not understand, but freedom from pain in the body and from trouble in the mind. For it is not continuous drinkings and revellings, nor the satisfaction of lusts, nor the enjoyment of fish and other luxuries of the wealthy table, which produce a pleasant life, but sober reasoning, searching out the motives for all choice and avoidance, and banishing mere opinions, to which are due the greatest disturbance of the spirit.

['Epicurus to Menoeceus' in *Epicurus: Extant Remains*, trans. C. Bailey (Clarendon Press: Oxford, 1926), 84–91. Written in *c*. 300 BC.]

EPICTETUS

49   **A Stoic View of Life**

8. Do not seek to have everything that happens happen as you wish, but wish for everything to happen as it actually does happen, and your life will be serene.

9. Disease is an impediment to the body, but not to the moral purpose, unless that consents. Lameness is an impediment to the leg, but not to the

moral purpose. And say this to yourself at each thing that befalls you; for you will find the thing to be an impediment to something else, but not to yourself.

10. In the case of everything that befalls you, remember to turn to yourself and see what faculty you have to deal with it. If you see a handsome lad or woman, you will find continence the faculty to employ here; if hard labour is laid upon you, you will find endurance; if reviling, you will find patience to bear evil. And if you habituate yourself in this fashion, your external impressions will not run away with you.

11. Never say about anything, 'I have lost it,' but only 'I have given it back.' Is your child dead? It has been given back. Is your wife dead? She has been given back. 'I have had my farm taken away.' Very well, this too has been given back. 'Yet it was a rascal who took it away.' But what concern is it of yours by whose instrumentality the Giver called for its return? So long as He gives it to you, take care of it as of a thing that is not your own, as travellers treat their inn.

12. If you wish to make progress, dismiss all reasoning of this sort: 'If I neglect my affairs, I shall have nothing to live on.' 'If I do not punish my slave-boy he will turn out bad.' For it is better to die of hunger, but in a state of freedom from grief and fear, than to live in plenty, but troubled in mind. And it is better for your slave-boy to be bad than for you to be unhappy. Begin, therefore, with the little things. Your paltry oil gets spilled, your miserable wine stolen; say to yourself, 'This is the price paid for a calm spirit, this the price for peace of mind.' Nothing is got without a price. And when you call your slave-boy, bear in mind that it is possible he may not heed you, and again, that even if he does heed, he may not do what you want done. But he is not in so happy a condition that your peace of mind depends upon him.

13. If you wish to make progress, then be content to appear senseless and foolish in externals, do not make it your wish to give the appearance of knowing anything; and if some people think you to be an important personage, distrust yourself. For be assured that it is no easy matter to keep your moral purpose in a state of conformity with nature, and, at the same time, to keep externals; but the man who devotes his attention to one of these two things must inevitably neglect the other.

14. If you make it your will that your children and your wife and your friends should live for ever, you are silly; for you are making it your will that things not under your control should be under your control, and that what is not your own should be your own. In the same way, too, if you make it your will that your slave-boy be free from faults, you are a fool; for you are making it your will that vice be not vice, but something else. If, however, it is your will not to fail in what you desire, this is in your power. Wherefore, exercise yourself in that which is in your power. Each man's

master is the person who has the authority over what the man wishes or does not wish, so as to secure it, or take it away. Whoever, therefore, wants to be free, let him neither wish for anything, nor avoid anything, that is under the control of others; or else he is necessarily a slave.

15. Remember that you ought to behave in life as you would at a banquet. As something is being passed around it comes to you; stretch out your hand and take a portion of it politely. It passes on; do not detain it. Or it has not come to you yet; do not project your desire to meet it, but wait until it comes in front of you. So act toward children, so toward a wife, so toward office, so toward wealth; and then some day you will be worthy of the banquets of the gods. But if you do not take these things even when they are set before you, but despise them, then you will not only share the banquet of the gods, but share also their rule. For it was by so doing that Diogenes and Heracleitus, and men like them, were deservedly divine and deservedly so called. [. . .]

48. This is the position and character of a layman: He never looks for either help or harm from himself, but only from externals. This is the position and character of the philosopher: He looks for all his help or harm from himself.

Signs of one who is making progress are: He censures no one, praises no one, blames no one, finds fault with no one, says nothing about himself as though he were somebody or knew something. When he is hampered or prevented, he blames himself. And if anyone compliments him, he smiles to himself at the person complimenting; while if anyone censures him, he makes no defence. He goes about like an invalid, being careful not to disturb, before it has grown firm, any part which is getting well. He has put away from himself his every desire, and has transferred his aversion to those things only, of what is under our control, which are contrary to nature. He exercises no pronounced choice in regard to anything. If he gives the appearance of being foolish or ignorant he does not care. In a word, he keeps guard against himself as though he were his own enemy lying in wait.

49. When a person gives himself airs because he can understand and interpret the books of Chrysippus, say to yourself, 'If Chrysippus had not written obscurely, this man would have nothing about which to give himself airs.'

But what is it I want? To learn nature and to follow her. I seek, therefore, someone to interpret her; and having heard that Chrysippus does so, I go to him. But I do not understand what he has written; I seek, therefore, the person who interprets Chrysippus. And down to this point there is nothing to justify pride. But when I find the interpreter, what remains is to put his precepts into practice; this is the only thing to be proud about. If, however, I admire the mere act of interpretation, what have I done but turned into a grammarian instead of a philosopher? The only difference, indeed, is that I interpret Chrysippus instead of Homer. Far from being proud, therefore, when somebody says to me, 'Read me Chrysippus,' I blush the rather, when I am unable to show him such deeds as match and harmonize with his words.

50. Whatever principles are set before you, stand fast by these like laws, feeling that it would be impiety for you to transgress them. But pay no attention to what somebody says about you, for this is, at length, not under your control.

51. How long will you still wait to think yourself worthy of the best things, and in nothing to transgress against the distinctions set up by the reason? You have received the philosophical principles which you ought to accept, and you have accepted them. What sort of a teacher, then, do you still wait for, that you should put off reforming yourself until he arrives? You are no longer a lad, but already a full-grown man. If you are now neglectful and easy-going, and always making one delay after another, and fixing first one day and then another, after which you will pay attention to yourself, then without realizing it you will make no progress, but, living and dying, will continue to be a layman throughout. Make up your mind, therefore, before it is too late, that the fitting thing for you to do is to live as a mature man who is making progress, and let everything which seems to you to be best be for you a law that must not be transgressed. And if you meet anything that is laborious, or sweet, or held in high repute, or in no repute, remember that *now* is the contest, and here before you are the Olympic games, and that it is impossible to delay any longer, and that it depends on a single day and a single action, whether progress is lost or saved. This is the way Socrates became what he was, by paying attention to nothing but his reason in everything that he encountered. And even if you are not yet a Socrates, still you ought to live as one who wishes to be a Socrates.

[Epictetus, *The Discourses*, ii, trans. W. A. Oldfather (Cambridge, Mass.: Harvard University Press, 1928), 491–7, 531–5. Written in *c.* 100 AD.]

50   The Sermon on the Mount

And seeing the multitudes, he went up into a mountain: and when he was set, his disciples came unto him:

2. And he opened his mouth, and taught them, saying,

3. Blessed *are* the poor in spirit: for theirs is the kingdom of heaven.

4. Blessed *are* they that mourn: for they shall be comforted.

5. Blessed *are* the meek: for they shall inherit the earth.

6. Blessed *are* they which do hunger and thirst after righteousness: for they shall be filled.

7. Blessed *are* the merciful: for they shall obtain mercy.

8. Blessed *are* the pure in heart: for they shall see God.

9. Blessed *are* the peacemakers: for they shall be called the children of God.

10. Blessed *are* they which are persecuted for righteousness' sake: for their's is the kingdom of heaven.

11. Blessed are ye, when *men* shall revile you, and persecute *you*, and shall say all manner of evil against you falsely, for my sake.

12. Rejoice, and be exceeding glad: for great *is* your reward in heaven: for so persecuted they the prophets which were before you.

13. Ye are the salt of the earth: but if the salt have lost his savour, wherewith shall it be salted? it is thenceforth good for nothing, but to be cast out, and to be trodden under foot of men.

14. Ye are the light of the world. A city that is set on an hill cannot be hid.

15. Neither do men light a candle, and put it under a bushel, but on a candlestick; and it giveth light unto all that are in the house.

16. Let your light so shine before men, that they may see your good works, and glorify your Father, which is in heaven.

17. Think not that I am come to destroy the law, or the prophets: I am not come to destroy, but to fulfil.

18. For verily I say unto you, Till heaven and earth pass, one jot or one tittle shall in no wise pass from the law, till all be fulfilled.

19. Whosoever therefore shall break one of these least commandments, and shall teach men so, he shall be called the least in the kingdom of heaven: but whosoever shall do and teach *them*, the same shall be called great in the kingdom of heaven.

20. For I say unto you, That except your righteousness shall exceed *the righteousness* of the scribes and Pharisees, ye shall in no case enter into the kingdom of heaven.

[The Gospel According to St Matthew 5: 1–20. Written in *c.* 85 AD.]

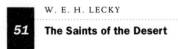

W. E. H. LECKY

51 The Saints of the Desert

Pilgrims wandered among the deserts, collecting accounts of the miracles and the austerities of the saints, which filled Christendom with admiration; and the strange biographies which were thus formed, wild and grotesque as they are, enable us to realise very vividly the general features of the anchorite life which became the new ideal of the Christian world.

There is, perhaps, no phase in the moral history of mankind of a deeper or more painful interest than this ascetic epidemic. A hideous, sordid, and emaciated maniac, without knowledge, without patriotism, without natural affection, passing his life in a long routine of useless and atrocious self-torture, and quailing before the ghastly phantoms of his delirious brain, had become the ideal of the nations which had known the writings of Plato and Cicero and the lives of Socrates and Cato. For about two centuries, the hideous maceration of the body was regarded as the highest proof of excellence. St Jerome declares, with a thrill of admiration, how he had seen a monk, who for thirty years had lived exclusively on a small portion of barley bread and of muddy water; another, who lived in a hole and never ate more than five figs for his daily repast; a third, who cut his hair only on Easter Sunday, who never washed his clothes, who never changed his tunic till it fell to pieces, who starved himself till his eyes grew dim, and his skin 'like a pumice stone,' and whose merits, shown by these austerities, Homer himself would be unable to recount. For six months, it is said, St Macarius of Alexandria slept in a marsh, and exposed his body naked to the stings of venomous flies. He was accustomed to carry about with him eighty pounds of iron. His disciple, St Eusebius, carried one hundred and fifty pounds of iron, and lived for three years in a dried-up well. St Sabinus would only eat corn that had become rotten by remaining for a month in water. St Besarion spent forty days and nights in the middle of thorn-bushes, and for forty years never lay down when he slept, which last penance was also during fifteen years practised by St Pachomius. Some saints, like St Marcian, restricted themselves to one meal a day, so small that they continually suffered the pangs of hunger. Of one of them it is related that his daily food was six ounces of bread and a few herbs; that he was never seen to recline on a mat or bed, or even to place his limbs easily for sleep; but that sometimes, from excess of weariness, his eyes would close at his meals, and the food would drop from his mouth. Other saints, however, ate only every second day; while many, if we could believe the monkish historian, abstained for whole weeks from all nourishment. St Macarius of Alexandria is said during an entire week to have never lain down, or eaten anything but a few uncooked herbs on Sunday. Of another famous saint, named John, it is asserted that for three whole years he stood in prayer, leaning upon a rock; that during all that time he never sat or lay down, and that his only nourishment was the Sacrament, which was brought him on Sundays. Some of the hermits lived in deserted dens of wild beasts, others in dried-up wells, while others found a congenial resting-place among the tombs. Some disdained all clothes, and crawled abroad like the wild beasts, covered only by their matted hair. In Mesopotamia, and part of Syria, there existed a sect known by the name of 'Grazers,' who never lived under a roof, who ate neither flesh nor bread, but who spent their time for ever on the mountain side, and ate grass like cattle. The cleanliness of the body was regarded as a pollution of the soul, and the saints who were most admired had become one hideous mass of clotted filth. St Athanasius relates with enthusiasm how St Antony, the patriarch of monachism, had never, to extreme old age, been guilty of washing his feet. The less constant St Pœmen fell into this habit for the first time when a very old man, and, with a glimmering of common sense, defended himself against the astonished monks by saying that he had 'learnt to kill not his body, but his passions.' St Abraham the hermit, however, who lived for fifty years after his conversion, rigidly refused from that date to wash either his face or his feet. He was, it is said, a person of singular beauty, and his biographer somewhat strangely remarks that 'his face reflected the purity of his soul.' St Ammon had never seen himself naked. A famous virgin named Silvia, though she was sixty years old and though bodily sickness was a consequence of her habits, resolutely refused, on religious principles, to wash any part of her body except her fingers. St Euphraxia joined a convent of one hundred and thirty nuns, who never washed their feet, and who shuddered at the mention of a bath. An anchorite once imagined that he was mocked by an illusion of the devil, as he saw gliding before him through the desert a naked creature black with filth and years of exposure, and with white hair floating to the wind. It was a once beautiful woman, St Mary of Egypt, who had thus, during forty-seven years, been expiating her sins. The occasional decadence of the monks into habits of decency was a subject of much reproach. 'Our fathers,' said the abbot Alexander, looking mournfully back to the past, 'never washed their faces, but we frequent the public baths.' It was related of one monastery in the desert, that the monks suffered greatly from want of water to drink; but at the prayer of the abbot Theodosius a copious stream was produced. But soon some monks, tempted by the abundant supply, diverged from their old austerity, and persuaded the abbot to avail himself of the stream for the construction of a bath. The bath was made. Once, and once only, did the monks enjoy their ablutions, when the stream ceased to flow. Prayers, tears, and fastings were in vain. A whole year passed. At last the abbot destroyed the bath, which was the object of the Divine displeasure, and the waters flowed afresh. But of all the evidences of the loathsome excesses to which this spirit was carried, the life of St Simeon Stylites is probably the most remarkable. It would be difficult to conceive a more horrible or disgusting picture than is given of the penances by which that saint commenced his ascetic career. He had bound a rope around him so that it became imbedded in his flesh, which putrefied around it. 'A horrible stench, intolerable to the bystanders, exhaled from his body and worms dropped from him whenever he moved, and they filled his bed.' Sometimes he left the monastery and slept in a dry well, inhabited, it is said, by dæmons. He built successively three pillars, the last being sixty feet high and scarcely two cubits in circumference, and on this pillar, during thirty years, he remained exposed to every change of climate, ceaselessly and rapidly bending his body in prayer almost to the level of his feet. A spectator attempted to number these rapid motions, but desisted from weariness when he had counted 1,244. For a whole year, we are told, St Simeon stood upon one leg, the other being covered with hideous ulcers, while his biographer was commissioned to stand by his side, to pick up the worms that fell from his body, and to replace them in the sores, the saint saying to the worm, 'Eat what God has given you.' From every quarter pilgrims of every degree thronged to do him homage. A crowd of prelates followed him to the grave. A brilliant star is said to have shone miraculously over his pillar; the general voice of mankind pronounced him to be the highest model of a Christian saint; and several other anchorites imitated or emulated his penances.

There is, if I mistake not, no department of literature the importance of which is more inadequately realised than the lives of the saints. Even where they have no direct historical value, they have a moral value of the very highest order. They may not tell us with accuracy what men did at particular epochs; but they display with the utmost vividness what they thought and felt, their measure of probability, and their ideal of excellence. Decrees of councils, elaborate treatises of theologians, creeds, liturgies, and canons, are all but the husks of religious history. They reveal what was professed and argued before the world, but not that which was realised in the imagination or enshrined in the heart. The history of art, which in its ruder day reflected with delicate fidelity the fleeting images of an anthropomorphic age, is in this respect invaluable; but still more important is that vast Christian mythology, which grew up spontaneously from the intellectual condition of the time, included all its dearest hopes, wishes, ideals, and imaginings, and constituted, during many centuries, the popular literature of Christendom. In the case of the saints of the deserts, there can be no question that the picture—which is drawn chiefly by eye-witnesses—however grotesque may be some of its details, is in its leading features historically true. It is true that self-torture was for some centuries regarded as the chief measure of human excellence, that tens of thousands of the most devoted men fled to the desert to reduce themselves by maceration nearly to the condition of the brute, and that this odious superstition had acquired an almost absolute ascendancy in the ethics of the age. The examples of asceticism I have cited are but a few out of many hundreds, and volumes might be written, and have been written, detailing them.

[*History of European Morals*, 10th edn. (Longmans Green and Co.: London, 1892), ii. 107–13.]

On my travels I met an old Brahmin, a very wise man, of marked intellect and great learning. Furthermore, he was rich and, consequently, all the wiser, because, lacking nothing, he needed to deceive nobody. His household was very well managed by three handsome women who set themselves out to please him. When he was not amusing himself with his women, he passed the time in philosophizing. Near his house, which was beautifully decorated and had charming gardens attached, there lived a narrow-minded old Indian woman: she was a simpleton, and rather poor.

Said the Brahmin to me one day: 'I wish I had never been born!' On my asking why, he answered: 'I have been studying forty years, and that is forty years wasted. I teach others and myself am ignorant of everything. Such a state of affairs fills my soul with so much humiliation and disgust that my life is intolerable. I was born in Time, I live in Time, and yet I do not know what Time is. I am at a point between two eternities, as our wise men say, and I have no conception of eternity. I am composed of matter: I think, but I have never been able to learn what produces my thought. I do not know whether or no my understanding is a simple faculty inside me, such as those of walking and digesting, and whether or no I think with my head as I grip with my hands. Not only is the cause of my thought unknown to me; the cause of my actions is equally a mystery. I do not know why I exist, and yet every day people ask me questions on all these points. I have to reply, and as I have nothing really worth saying I talk a great deal, and am ashamed of myself afterward for having talked.

'It is worse still when I am asked if Brahma was born of Vishnu or if they are both eternal. God is my witness that I have not the remotest idea, and my ignorance shows itself in my replies. "Ah, Holy One," people say to me, "tell us why evil pervades the earth." I am in as great a difficulty as those who ask me this question. Sometimes I tell them that everything is as well as can be, but those who have been ruined and broken in the wars do not believe a word of it—and no more do I. I retire to my home stricken at my own curiosity and ignorance. I read our ancient books, and they double my darkness. I talk to my companions: some answer me that we must enjoy life and make game of mankind; others think they know a lot and lose themselves in a maze of wild ideas. Everything increases my anguish. I am ready sometimes to despair when I think that after all my seeking I do not know whence I came, whither I go, what I am nor what I shall become.'

The good man's condition really worried me. Nobody was more rational or more sincere than he. I perceived that his unhappiness increased in proportion as his understanding developed and his insight grew.

The same day I saw the old woman who lived near him. I asked her if she had ever been troubled by the thought that she was ignorant of the nature of her soul. She did not even understand my question. Never in all her life had she reflected for one single moment on one single point of all those which tormented the Brahmin. She believed with all her heart in the metamorphoses of Vishnu and, provided she could obtain a little Ganges water wherewith to wash herself, thought herself the happiest of women.

Struck with this mean creature's happiness, I returned to my wretched philosopher. 'Are you not ashamed,' said I, 'to be unhappy when at your very door there lives an old automaton who thinks about nothing, and yet lives contentedly?'

'You are right,' he replied. 'I have told myself a hundred times that I should be happy if I were as brainless as my neighbor, and yet I do not desire such happiness.'

My Brahmin's answer impressed me more than all the rest. I set to examining myself, and I saw that in truth I would not care to be happy at the price of being a simpleton.

I put the matter before some philosophers, and they were of my opinion. 'Nevertheless,' said I, 'there is a tremendous contradiction in this mode of thought, for, after all, the problem is—how to be happy. What does it matter whether one has brains or not? Further, those who are contented with their lot are certain of their contentment, whereas those who reason are not certain that they reason correctly. It is quite clear, therefore,' I continued, 'that we must choose not to have common sense, however little common sense may contribute to our discomfort.' Everyone agreed with me, but I found nobody, notwithstanding, who was willing to accept the bargain of becoming a simpleton in order to become contented. From which I conclude that if we consider the question of happiness we must consider still more the question of reason.

But on reflection it seems that to prefer reason to felicity is to be very senseless. How can this contradiction be explained? Like all the other contradictions. It is matter for much talk.

[*The Portable Voltaire*, ed. Ben Ray Redman (Viking Press: New York, 1963), 436–8. First published in 1759.]

JEREMY BENTHAM

53 Push-Pin and Poetry

Taken collectively, and considered in their connexion with the happiness of society, the arts and sciences may be arranged in two divisions; viz.—1.

Those of amusement and curiosity; 2. Those of utility, immediate and remote. These two branches of human knowledge require different methods of treatment on the part of governments.

By arts and sciences of amusement, I mean those which are ordinarily called the *fine arts;* such as music, poetry, painting, sculpture, architecture, ornamental gardening, &c. &c. Their complete enumeration must be excused: it would lead us too far from our present subject, were we to plunge into the metaphysical discussions necessary for its accomplishment. Amusements of all sorts would be comprised under this head. [. . .]

By arts and sciences of curiosity, I mean those which in truth are pleasing, but not in the same degree as the fine arts, and to which at the first glance we might be tempted to refuse this quality. It is not that these arts and sciences of curiosity do not yield as much pleasure to those who cultivate them as the fine arts; but the number of those who study them is more limited. Of this nature are the sciences of heraldry, of medals, of pure chronology—the knowledge of ancient and barbarous languages, which present only collections of strange words,—and the study of antiquities, inasmuch as they furnish no instruction applicable to morality, or any other branch of useful or agreeable knowledge.

The utility of all these arts and sciences,—I speak both of those of amusement and curiosity,—the value which they possess, is exactly in proportion to the pleasure they yield. Every other species of pre-eminence which may be attempted to be established among them is altogether fanciful. Prejudice apart, the game of push-pin is of equal value with the arts and sciences of music and poetry. If the game of push-pin furnish more pleasure, it is more valuable than either. Everybody can play at push-pin: poetry and music are relished only by a few. The game of push-pin is always innocent: it were well could the same be always asserted of poetry. Indeed, between poetry and truth there is a natural opposition: false morals, fictitious nature. The poet always stands in need of something false. When he pretends to lay his foundations in truth, the ornaments of his superstructure are fictions; his business consists in stimulating our passions, and exciting our prejudices. Truth, exactitude of every kind, is fatal to poetry. The poet must see everything through coloured media, and strive to make every one else to do the same. It is true, there have been noble spirits, to whom poetry and philosophy have been equally indebted; but these exceptions do not counteract the mischiefs which have resulted from this magic art. If poetry and music deserve to be preferred before a game of push-pin, it must be because they are calculated to gratify those individuals who are most difficult to be pleased.

[*The Rationale of Reward*, in *The Works of Jeremy Bentham*, ii, ed. John Bowring (Russell and Russell, Inc.: New York, 1962), 253–4. First published in 1825.]

54 Higher and Lower Pleasures

The creed which accepts as the foundation of morals, Utility, or the Greatest Happiness Principle, holds that actions are right in proportion as they tend to promote happiness, wrong as they tend to produce the reverse of happiness. By happiness is intended pleasure, and the absence of pain; by unhappiness, pain, and the privation of pleasure. To give a clear view of the moral standard set up by the theory, much more requires to be said; in particular, what things it includes in the ideas of pain and pleasure; and to what extent this is left an open question. But these supplementary explanations do not affect the theory of life on which this theory of morality is grounded—namely, that pleasure, and freedom from pain, are the only things desirable as ends; and that all desirable things (which are as numerous in the utilitarian as in any other scheme) are desirable either for the pleasure inherent in themselves, or as means to the promotion of pleasure and the prevention of pain.

Now, such a theory of life excites in many minds, and among them in some of the most estimable in feeling and purpose, inveterate dislike. To suppose that life has (as they express it) no higher end than pleasure—no better and nobler object of desire and pursuit—they designate as utterly mean and grovelling; as a doctrine worthy only of swine, to whom the followers of Epicurus were, at a very early period, contemptuously likened; and modern holders of the doctrine are occasionally made the subject of equally polite comparisons by its German, French, and English assailants.

When thus attacked, the Epicureans have always answered, that it is not they, but their accusers, who represent human nature in a degrading light; since the accusation supposes human beings to be capable of no pleasures except those of which swine are capable. If this supposition were true, the charge could not be gainsaid, but would then be no longer an imputation; for if the sources of pleasure were precisely the same to human beings and to swine, the rule of life which is good enough for the one would be good enough for the other. The comparison of the Epicurean life to that of beasts is felt as degrading, precisely because a beast's pleasures do not satisfy a human being's conceptions of happiness. Human beings have faculties more elevated than the animal appetites, and when once made conscious of them, do not regard anything as happiness which does not include their gratification. I do not, indeed, consider the Epicureans to have been by any means faultless in drawing out their scheme of consequences from the utilitarian principle. To do this in any sufficient manner, many Stoic, as well as Christian elements require to be included. But there is no known Epicurean theory of life which does not assign to the pleasures of the intellect, of the feelings and imagination, and of the moral sentiments, a much higher value as pleasures than to those of mere sensation. It must be admitted, however, that utilitarian writers in general have placed the superiority of mental over bodily pleasures chiefly in the greater permanency, safety, uncostliness, &c., of the former—that is, in their circumstantial advantages rather than in their intrinsic nature. And on all these points utilitarians have fully proved their case; but they might have taken the other, and, as it may be called, higher ground, with entire consistency. It is quite compatible with the principle of utility to recognise the fact, that some *kinds* of pleasure are more desirable and more valuable than others. It would be absurd that while, in estimating all other things, quality is considered as well as quantity, the estimation of pleasures should be supposed to depend on quantity alone.

If I am asked, what I mean by difference of quality in pleasures, or what makes one pleasure more valuable than another, merely as a pleasure, except its being greater in amount, there is but one possible answer. Of two pleasures, if there be one to which all or almost all who have experience of both give a decided preference, irrespective of any feeling of moral obligation to prefer it, that is the more desirable pleasure. If one of the two is, by those who are competently acquainted with both, placed so far above the other that they prefer it, even though knowing it to be attended with a greater amount of discontent, and would not resign it for any quantity of the other pleasure which their nature is capable of, we are justified in ascribing to the preferred enjoyment a superiority in quality, so far outweighing quantity as to render it, in comparison, of small account.

Now it is an unquestionable fact that those who are equally acquainted with, and equally capable of appreciating and enjoying, both, do give a most marked preference to the manner of existence which employs their higher faculties. Few human creatures would consent to be changed into any of the lower animals, for a promise of the fullest allowance of a beast's pleasures; no intelligent human being would consent to be a fool, no instructed person would be an ignoramus, no person of feeling and conscience would be selfish and base, even though they should be persuaded that the fool, the dunce, or the rascal is better satisfied with his lot than they are with theirs. They would not resign what they possess more than he, for the most complete satisfaction of all the desires which they have in common with him. If they ever fancy they would, it is only in cases of unhappiness so extreme, that to escape from it they would exchange their lot for almost any other, however undesirable in their own eyes. A being of higher faculties requires more to make him happy, is capable probably of more acute suffering, and is certainly accessible to it at more points, than one of an inferior type; but in spite of these liabilities, he can never really wish to sink into what he feels to be a lower grade of existence. We may give what explanation we please of this unwillingness; we may attribute it to pride, a name which is given indiscriminately to some of the most and to some of the least estimable feelings of which mankind are capable; we may refer it to the love of liberty and personal independence, an appeal to which was with the Stoics one of the most effective means for the inculcation of it; to the love of power, or to the love of excitement, both of which do really enter into and contribute to it: but its most appropriate appellation is a sense of dignity, which all human beings possess in one form or other, and in some, though by no means in exact, proportion to their higher faculties, and which is so essential a part of the happiness of those in whom it is strong, that nothing which conflicts with it could be, otherwise than momentarily, an object of desire to them. Whoever supposes that this preference takes place at a sacrifice of happiness—that the superior being, in anything like equal circumstances, is not happier than the inferior—confounds the two very different ideas, of happiness, and content. It is indisputable that the being whose capacities of enjoyment are low, has the greatest chance of having them fully satisfied; and a highly-endowed being will always feel that any happiness which he can look for, as the world is constituted, is imperfect. But he can learn to bear its imperfections, if they are at all bearable; and they will not make him envy the being who is indeed unconscious of the imperfections, but only because he feels not at all the good which those imperfections qualify. It is better to be a human being dissatisfied than a pig satisfied; better to be Socrates dissatisfied than a fool satisfied. And if the fool, or the pig, is of a different opinion, it is because they only know their own side of the question. The other party to the comparison knows both sides.

It may be objected, that many who are capable of the higher pleasures, occasionally, under the influence of temptation, postpone them to the lower. But this is quite compatible with a full appreciation of the intrinsic superiority of the higher. Men often, from infirmity of character, make their election for the nearer good, though they know it to be the less valuable; and this no less when the choice is between two bodily pleasures, than when it is between bodily and mental. They pursue sensual indulgences to the injury of health, though perfectly aware that health is the greater good. It may be further objected, that many who begin with youthful enthusiasm for everything noble, as they advance in years sink into indolence and selfishness. But I do not believe that those who undergo this very common change, voluntarily choose the lower description of pleasures in preference to the higher. I believe that before they devote themselves exclusively to the one, they have already become incapable of the other. Capacity for the nobler feelings is in most natures a very tender plant, easily killed, not only by hostile influences, but by mere want of sustenance; and in the majority of young persons it speedily dies away if the occupations to which their position in life has devoted them, and the society into which it has thrown them, are not favourable to keeping that higher capacity in exercise. Men lose their high aspirations as they lose their intellectual tastes, because they have not time or opportunity for indulging them; and they addict themselves to inferior pleasures, not because they deliberately prefer them, but because they are either the only ones to which they have access, or the only ones which they are any longer capable of enjoying. It may be questioned whether any one who has remained equally susceptible to both classes of pleasures, ever knowingly and calmly preferred the lower; though many, in all ages, have broken down in an ineffectual attempt to combine both.

From this verdict of the only competent judges, I apprehend there can be no appeal. On a question which is the best worth having of two pleasures, or which of two modes of existence is the most grateful to the feelings, apart from its moral attributes and from its consequences, the judgment of those who are qualified by knowledge of both, or, if they differ, that of the majority among them, must be admitted as final. And there needs be the less hesitation to accept this judgment respecting the quality of pleasures, since there is no other tribunal to be referred to even on the question of quantity. What means are there of determining which is the acutest of two pains, or the intensest of two pleasurable sensations, except the general suffrage of those who are familiar with both? Neither pains nor pleasures are homogeneous, and pain is always heterogeneous with pleasure. What is there to decide whether a particular pleasure is worth purchasing at the cost of a particular pain, except the feelings and judgment of the experienced? When, therefore, those feelings and judgment declare the pleasures derived from the higher faculties to be preferable *in kind*, apart from the question of intensity, to those of which the animal nature, disjoined from the higher faculties, is susceptible, they are entitled on this subject to the same regard.

I have dwelt on this point, as being a necessary part of a perfectly just conception of Utility or Happiness, considered as the directive rule of human conduct. But it is by no means an indispensable condition to the acceptance of the utilitarian standard; for that standard is not the agent's own greatest happiness, but the greatest amount of happiness altogether; and if it may possibly be doubted whether a noble character is always the happier for its nobleness, there can be no doubt that it makes other people happier, and that the world in general is immensely a gainer by it. Utilitarianism, therefore, could only attain its end by the general cultivation of nobleness of character, even if each individual were only benefited by the nobleness of others, and his own, so far as happiness is concerned, were a sheer deduction from the benefit. But the bare enunciation of such an absurdity as this last, renders refutation superfluous.

According to the Greatest Happiness Principle, as above explained, the ultimate end, with reference to and for the sake of which all other things are desirable (whether we are considering our own good or that of other people), is an existence exempt as far as possible from pain, and as rich as possible in enjoyments, both in point of quantity and quality; the test of quality, and the rule for measuring it against quantity, being the preference felt by those who, in their opportunities of experience, to which must be added their habits of self-consciousness and self-observation, are best furnished with the means of comparison. This, being, according to the utilitarian opinion, the end of human action, is necessarily also the standard of morality; which may accordingly be defined, the rules and precepts for human conduct, by the observance of which an existence such as has been described might be, to the greatest extent possible, secured to all mankind; and not to them only, but, so far as the nature of things admits, to the whole sentient creation.

['Utilitarianism', *Essays on Ethics, Religion and Society*, ed. J. M. Robson, F. E. L. Priestley, and D. P. Dryer (University of Toronto Press: Toronto, 1969), 210–14. First published in 1861.]

WILLIAM JAMES

55   **Good as the Satisfaction of Demands**

Imagine an absolutely material world, containing only physical and chemical facts, and existing from eternity without a God, without even an interested spectator: would there be any sense in saying of that world that one of its states is better than another? Or if there were two such worlds possible, would there be any rhyme or reason in calling one good and the other bad,—good or bad positively, I mean, and apart from the fact that one might relate itself better than the other to the philosopher's private interests? But we must leave these private interests out of the account, for the philosopher is a mental fact, and we are asking whether goods and evils and obligations exist in physical facts *per se*. Surely there is no *status* for good and evil to exist in, in a purely insentient world. How can one physical fact, considered simply as a physical fact, be 'better' than another? Betterness is not a physical relation. In its mere material capacity, a thing can no more be good or bad than it can be pleasant or painful. Good for what? Good for the production of another physical fact, do you say? But what in a purely physical universe demands the production of that other fact? Physical facts simply *are* or are *not*; and neither when present or absent, can they be supposed to make demands. If they do, they can only do so by having desires; and then they have ceased to be purely physical facts, and have become facts of conscious sensibility. Goodness, badness, and obligation must be *realized* somewhere in order really to exist; and the first step in ethical philosophy is to see that no merely inorganic 'nature of things' can realize them. Neither moral relations nor the moral law can swing *in vacuo*. Their only habitat can be a mind which feels them; and no world composed of merely physical facts can possibly be a world to which ethical propositions apply.

The moment one sentient being, however, is made a part of the universe, there is a chance for goods and evils really to exist. Moral relations now have their *status*, in that being's consciousness. So far as he feels anything to be good, he *makes* it good. It *is* good, for him; and being good for him, is absolutely good, for he is the sole creator of values in that universe, and outside of his opinion things have no moral character at all.

In such a universe as that it would of course be absurd to raise the question of whether the solitary thinker's judgments of good and ill are true or not. Truth supposes a standard outside of the thinker to which he must conform; but here the thinker is a sort of divinity, subject to no higher judge. Let us call the supposed universe which he inhabits a *moral solitude*. In such a moral solitude it is clear that there can be no outward obligation, and that the only trouble the god-like thinker is liable to have will be over the consistency of his own several ideals with one another. Some of these will no doubt be more pungent and appealing than the rest, their goodness will have a profounder, more penetrating taste; they will return to haunt him with more obstinate regrets if violated. So the thinker will have to order his life with them as its chief determinants, or else remain inwardly discordant and unhappy. Into whatever equilibrium he may settle, though, and however he may straighten out his system, it will be a right system; for beyond the facts of his own subjectivity there is nothing moral in the world.

If now we introduce a second thinker with his likes and dislikes into the universe, the ethical situation becomes much more complex, and several possibilities are immediately seen to obtain.

One of these is that the thinkers may ignore each other's attitude about good and evil altogether, and each continue to indulge his own preferences, indifferent to what the other may feel or do. In such a case we have a world with twice as much of the ethical quality in it as our moral solitude, only it is without ethical unity. The same object is good or bad there, according as you measure it by the view which this one or that one of the thinkers takes. Nor can you find any possible ground in such a world for saying that one thinker's opinion is more correct than the other's, or that either has the truer moral sense. Such a world, in short, is not a moral universe but a moral dualism. Not only is there no single point of view within it from which the values of things can be unequivocally judged, but there is not even a demand for such a point of view, since the two thinkers are supposed to be indifferent to each other's thoughts and acts. Multiply the thinkers into a pluralism, and we find realized for us in the ethical sphere something like that world which the antique sceptics conceived of,—in which individual minds are the measures of all things, and in which no one 'objective' truth, but only a multitude of 'subjective' opinions, can be found.

But this is the kind of world with which the philosopher, so long as he holds to the hope of a philosophy, will not put up. Among the various ideals represented, there must be, he thinks, some which have the more truth or authority; and to these the others *ought* to yield, so that system and subordination may reign. Here in the word 'ought' the notion of *obligation* comes emphatically into view, and the next thing in order must be to make its meaning clear.

Since the outcome of the discussion so far has been to show us that nothing can be good or right except so far as some consciousness feels it to be good or thinks it to be right, we perceive on the very threshold that the real superiority and authority which are postulated by the philosopher to reside in some of the opinions, and the really inferior character which he supposes must belong to others, cannot be explained by any abstract moral 'nature of things' existing antecedently to the concrete thinkers themselves with their ideals. Like the positive attributes good and bad, the comparative ones better and worse must be *realized* in order to be real. If one ideal judgment be objectively better than another, that betterness must be made flesh by being lodged concretely in some one's actual perception. It cannot float in the atmosphere, for it is not a sort of meteorological phenomenon, like the aurora borealis or the zodiacal light. Its *esse* is *percipi*, like the *esse* of the ideals themselves between which it obtains. The philosopher, therefore, who seeks to know which ideal ought to have supreme weight and which one ought to be subordinated, must trace the *ought* itself to the *de facto* constitution of some existing consciousness, behind which, as one of the data of the universe, he as a purely ethical philosopher is unable to go. This consciousness must make the one ideal right by feeling it to be right, the other wrong by feeling it to be wrong. But now what particular consciousness in the universe *can* enjoy this prerogative of obliging others to conform to a rule which it lays down?

If one of the thinkers were obviously divine, while all the rest were human, there would probably be no practical dispute about the matter. The divine thought would be the model, to which the others should conform. But still the theoretic question would remain, What is the ground of the obligation, even here?

In our first essays at answering this question, there is an inevitable tendency to slip into an assumption which ordinary men follow when they are disputing with one another about questions of good and bad. They imagine an abstract moral order in which the objective truth resides; and each tries to prove that this pre-existing order is more accurately reflected in his own ideas than in those of his adversary. It is because one disputant is backed by this overarching abstract order that we think the other should submit. Even so, when it is a question no longer of two finite thinkers, but of God and ourselves,—we follow our usual habit, and imagine a sort of *de jure* relation, which antedates and overarches the mere facts, and would make it right that we should conform our thoughts to God's thoughts, even though he made no claim to that effect, and though we preferred *de facto* to go on thinking for ourselves.

But the moment we take a steady look at the question, *we see not only that without a claim actually made by some concrete person there can be no obligation, but that there is some obligation wherever there is a claim.* Claim and obligation are, in fact, coextensive terms; they cover each other exactly. Our ordinary attitude of regarding ourselves as subject to an overarching system of moral relations, true 'in themselves,' is therefore either an out-and-out superstition, or else it must be treated as a merely provisional abstraction from that real Thinker in whose actual demand upon us to think as he does our obligation must be ultimately based. In a theistic-ethical philosophy that thinker in question is, of course, the Deity to whom the existence of the universe is due.

I know well how hard it is for those who are accustomed to what I have called the superstitious view, to realize that every *de facto* claim creates in so far forth an obligation. We inveterately think that something which we call the 'validity' of the claim is what gives to it its obligatory character, and that this validity is something outside of the claim's mere existence as a matter of fact. It rains down upon the claim, we think, from some sublime dimension of being, which the moral law inhabits, much as upon the steel of the compass-needle the influence of the Pole rains down from out of the starry heavens. But again, how can such an inorganic abstract character of imperativeness, additional to the imperativeness which is in the concrete claim itself, *exist?* Take any demand, however slight, which any creature, however weak, may make. Ought it not, for its own sole sake, to be satisfied? If not, prove why not. The only possible kind of proof you could adduce would be the exhibition of another creature who should make a demand that ran the other way. The only possible reason there can be why any phenomenon ought to exist is that such a phenomenon actually is desired. Any desire is imperative to the extent of its amount; it *makes* itself valid by the fact that it exists at all. Some desires, truly enough, are small desires; they are put forward by insignificant persons, and we customarily make light of the obligations which they bring. But the fact that such personal demands as these impose small obligations does not keep the largest obligations from being personal demands. [. . .]

We may now consider that what we distinguished as the metaphysical question in ethical philosophy is sufficiently answered, and that we have learned what the words 'good,' 'bad,' and 'obligation' severally mean. They mean no absolute natures, independent of personal support. They are objects of feeling and desire, which have no foothold or anchorage in Being, apart from the existence of actually living minds.

Wherever such minds exist, with judgments of good and ill, and demands upon one another, there is an ethical world in its essential features. Were all other things, gods and men and starry heavens, blotted out from this universe, and were there left but one rock with two loving souls upon it, that rock would have as thoroughly moral a constitution as any possible world which the eternities and immensities could harbor. It would be a tragic constitution, because the rock's inhabitants would die. But while they lived, there would be real good things and real bad things in the universe; there would be obligations, claims, and expectations; obediences, refusals, and disappointments; compunctions and longings for harmony to come again, and inward peace of conscience when it was restored; there would, in short, be a moral life, whose active energy would have no limit but the intensity of interest in each other with which the hero and heroine might be endowed.

We, on this terrestrial globe, so far as the visible facts go, are just like the inhabitants of such a rock. Whether a God exist, or whether no God exist, in yon blue heaven above us bent, we form at any rate an ethical republic here below. And the first reflection which this leads to is that ethics have as genuine and real a foothold in a universe where the highest consciousness is human, as in a universe where there is a God as well. 'The religion of humanity' affords a basis for ethics as well as theism does. [. . .]

The best, on the whole, of these marks and measures of goodness seems to be the capacity to bring happiness. But in order not to break down fatally, this test must be taken to cover innumerable acts and impulses that never *aim* at happiness; so that, after all, in seeking for a universal principle we inevitably are carried onward to the *most* universal principle,—that *the essence of good is simply to satisfy demand*. The demand may be for anything under the sun. There is really no more ground for supposing that all our demands can be accounted for by one universal underlying kind of motive than there is ground for supposing that all physical phenomena are cases of a single law. The elementary forces in ethics are probably as plural as those of physics are. The various ideals have no common character apart from the fact that they are ideals. No single abstract principle can be so used as to yield to the philosopher anything like a scientifically accurate and genuinely useful casuistic scale.

A look at another peculiarity of the ethical universe, as we find it, will still further show us the philosopher's perplexities. As a purely theoretic problem, namely, the casuistic question would hardly ever come up at all. If the ethical philosopher were only asking after the best *imaginable* system of goods he would indeed have an easy task; for all demands as such are *primâ facie* respectable, and the best simply imaginary world would be one in which *every* demand was gratified as soon as made. Such a world would, however, have to have a physical constitution entirely different from that of the one which we inhabit. It would need not only a space, but a time, 'of *n*-dimensions,' to include all the acts and experiences incompatible with one another here below, which would then go on in conjunction,—such as spending our money, yet growing rich; taking our holiday, yet getting ahead with our work; shooting and fishing, yet doing no hurt to the beasts; gaining no end of experience, yet keeping our youthful freshness of heart; and the like. There can be no question that such a system of things, however brought about, would be the absolutely ideal system; and that if a philosopher could create universes *à priori*, and provide all the mechanical conditions, that is the sort of universe which he should unhesitatingly create.

But this world of ours is made on an entirely different pattern, and the casuistic question here is most tragically practical. The actually possible in this world is vastly narrower than all that is demanded; and there is always a *pinch* between the ideal and the actual which can only be got through by leaving part of the ideal behind. There is hardly a good which we can imagine except as competing for the possession of the same bit of space and time with some other imagined good. Every end of desire that presents itself appears exclusive of some other end of desire. Shall a man drink and smoke, *or* keep his nerves in condition?—he cannot do both. Shall he follow his fancy for Amelia, *or* for Henrietta?—both cannot be the choice of his heart. Shall he have the dear old Republican party, *or* a spirit of unsophistication in public affairs?—he cannot have both, etc. So that the ethical philosopher's demand for the right scale of subordination in ideals is the fruit of an altogether practical need. Some part of the ideal must be butchered, and he needs to know which part. It is a tragic situation, and no mere speculative conundrum, with which he has to deal. [. . .]

But do we not already see a perfectly definite path of escape which is open to him just because he is a philosopher, and not the champion of one particular ideal? Since everything which is demanded is by that fact a good, must not the guiding principle for ethical philosophy (since all demands conjointly cannot be satisfied in this poor world) be simply to satisfy at all times *as many demands as we can?* That act must be the best act, accordingly, which makes for the *best whole*, in the sense of awakening the least sum of dissatisfactions. In the casuistic scale, therefore, those ideals must be written highest which *prevail at the least cost*, or by whose realization the least possible number of other ideals are destroyed. Since victory and defeat there must be, the victory to be philosophically prayed for is that of the more inclusive side,—of the side which even in the hour of triumph will to some degree do justice to the ideals in which the vanquished party's inter-ests lay. The course of history is nothing but the story of men's struggles from generation to generation to find the more and more inclusive order. *Invent some manner* of realizing your own ideals which will also satisfy the alien demands,—that and that only is the path of peace!

[*The Will to Believe and Other Essays in Popular Philosophy* (Longmans Green and Co.: New York, 1899), 189–205. First published in 1891.]

HENRY SIDGWICK

56 Desirable Consciousness

If then Ultimate Good can only be conceived as Desirable Consciousness—including the Consciousness of Virtue as a part but only as a part—are we to identify this notion with Happiness or Pleasure, and say with the Utilitarians that General Good is general happiness? Many would at this point of the discussion regard this conclusion as inevitable: to say that all other things called good are only means to the end of making conscious life better or more desirable, seems to them the same as saying that they are means to the end of happiness. But very important distinctions remain to be considered. According to the view taken in a previous chapter in affirming Ultimate Good to be Happiness or Pleasure, we imply (1) that nothing is desirable except desirable feelings, and (2) that the desirability of each feeling is only directly cognisable by the sentient individual at the time of feeling it, and that therefore this particular judgment of the sentient individual must be taken as final[1] on the question how far each element of feeling has the quality of Ultimate Good. Now no one, I conceive, would estimate in any other way the desirability of feeling considered merely as feeling: but it may be urged that our conscious experience includes besides Feelings, Cognitions and Volitions, and that the desirability of these must be taken into account, and is not to be estimated by the standard above stated. I think, however, that when we reflect on a cognition as a transient fact of an individual's psychical experience,—distinguishing it on the one hand from the feeling that normally accompanies it, and on the other hand from that relation of the knowing mind to the object known which is implied in the term 'true' or 'valid cognition'[2]—it is seen to be an element

---

[1] Final, that is, so far as the quality of the present feeling is concerned. I have pointed out that so far as any estimate of the desirability or pleasantness of a feeling involves comparison with feelings only represented in idea, it is liable to be erroneous through imperfections in the representation.

[2] The term 'cognition' without qualification more often implies what is signified by 'true' or 'valid': but for the present purpose it is necessary to eliminate this implication.

of consciousness quite neutral in respect of desirability: and the same may be said of Volitions, when we abstract from their concomitant feelings, and their relation to an objective norm or ideal, as well as from all their consequences. It is no doubt true that in ordinary thought certain states of consciousness—such as Cognition of Truth, Contemplation of Beauty, Volition to realise Freedom or Virtue—are sometimes judged to be preferable on other grounds than their pleasantness: but the general explanation of this seems to be that what in such cases we really prefer is not the present consciousness itself, but either effects on future consciousness more or less distinctly foreseen, or else something in the objective relations of the conscious being, not strictly included in his present consciousness.

The second of these alternatives may perhaps be made clearer by some illustrations. A man may prefer the mental state of apprehending truth to the state of half-reliance on generally accredited fictions, while recognising that the former state may be more painful than the latter, and independently of any effect which he expects either state to have upon his subsequent consciousness. Here, on my view, the real object of preference is not the consciousness of knowing truth, considered merely as consciousness,—the element of pleasure or satisfaction in this being more than outweighed by the concomitant pain,—but the relation between the mind and something else, which, as the very notion of 'truth' implies, is whatever it is independently of our cognition of it, and which I therefore call objective. This may become more clear if we imagine ourselves learning afterwards that what we took for truth is not really such: for in this case we should certainly feel that our preference had been mistaken; whereas if our choice had really been between two elements of transient consciousness, its reasonableness could not be affected by any subsequent discovery.

Similarly, a man may prefer freedom and penury to a life of luxurious servitude, not because the pleasant consciousness of being free outweighs in prospect all the comforts and securities that the other life would afford, but because he has a predominant aversion to that relation between his will and the will of another which we call slavery: or, again, a philosopher may choose what he conceives as 'inner freedom'—the consistent self-determination of the will—rather than the gratifications of appetite; though recognising that the latter are more desirable, considered merely as transient feelings. In either case, he will be led to regard his preference as mistaken, if he be afterwards persuaded that his conception of Freedom or self-determination was illusory; that we are all slaves of circumstances, destiny, etc.

So again, the preference of conformity to Virtue, or contemplation of Beauty, to a state of consciousness recognised as more pleasant seems to depend on a belief that one's conception of Virtue or Beauty corresponds to an ideal to some extent objective and valid for all minds. Apart from any consideration of future consequences, we should generally agree that a man who sacrificed happiness to an erroneous conception of Virtue or Beauty made a mistaken choice.

Still, it may be said that this is merely a question of definition: that we may take 'conscious life' in a wide sense, so as to include the objective relations of the conscious being implied in our notions of Virtue, Truth, Beauty, Freedom; and that from this point of view we may regard cognition of Truth, contemplation of Beauty, Free or Virtuous action, as in some measure preferable alternatives to Pleasure or Happiness—even though we admit that Happiness must be included as a part of Ultimate Good. In this case the principle of Rational Benevolence, which was stated as an indubitable intuition of the practical Reason, would not direct us to the pursuit of universal happiness alone, but of these 'ideal goods' as well, as ends ultimately desirable for mankind generally.

I think, however, that this view ought not to commend itself to the sober judgment of reflective persons. In order to show this, I must ask the reader to use the same twofold procedure that I before requested him to employ in considering the absolute and independent validity of common moral precepts. I appeal firstly to his intuitive judgment after due consideration of the question when fairly placed before it: and secondly to a comprehensive comparison of the ordinary judgments of mankind. As regards the first argument, to me at least it seems clear after reflection that these objective relations of the conscious subject, when distinguished from the consciousness accompanying and resulting from them, are not ultimately and intrinsically desirable; any more than material or other objects are, when considered apart from any relation to conscious existence. Admitting that we have actual experience of such preferences as have just been described, of which the ultimate object is something that is not merely consciousness: it still seems to me that when (to use Butler's phrase) we 'sit down in a cool hour,' we can only justify to ourselves the importance that we attach to any of these objects by considering its conduciveness, in one way or another, to the happiness of sentient beings.

The second argument, that refers to the common sense of mankind, obviously cannot be made completely cogent; since, as above stated, several cultivated persons do habitually judge that knowledge, art, etc.—not to speak of Virtue—are ends independently of the pleasure derived from them. But we may urge not only that all these elements of 'ideal good' are productive of pleasure in various ways; but also that they seem to obtain the commendation of Common Sense, roughly speaking, in proportion to the degree of this productiveness. This seems obviously true of Beauty; and will hardly be denied in respect of any kind of social ideal: it is paradoxical to maintain that any degree of Freedom, or any form of social order, would still be commonly regarded as desirable even if we were certain that it had no tendency to promote the general happiness. The case of Knowledge is rather more complex; but certainly Common Sense is most impressed with the value of knowledge, when its 'fruitfulness' has been demonstrated. It is, however, aware that experience has frequently shown how knowledge, long fruitless, may become unexpectedly fruitful, and how light may be shed on one part of the field of knowledge from another apparently remote: and even if any particular branch of scientific pursuit could be shown to be devoid of even this indirect utility, it would still deserve some respect on utilitarian grounds; both as furnishing to the inquirer the refined and innocent pleasures of curiosity, and because the intellectual disposition which it exhibits and sustains is likely on the whole to produce fruitful knowledge. Still in cases approximating to this last, Common Sense is somewhat disposed to complain of the misdirection of valuable effort; so that the meed of honour commonly paid to Science seems to be graduated, though perhaps unconsciously, by a tolerably exact utilitarian scale. Certainly the moment the legitimacy of any branch of scientific inquiry is seriously disputed, as in the recent case of vivisection, the controversy on both sides is generally conducted on an avowedly utilitarian basis.

The case of Virtue requires special consideration: since the encouragement in each other of virtuous impulses and dispositions is a main aim of men's ordinary moral discourse; so that even to raise the question whether this encouragement can go too far has a paradoxical air. Still, our experience includes rare and exceptional cases in which the concentration of effort on the cultivation of virtue has seemed to have effects adverse to general happiness, through being intensified to the point of moral fanaticism, and so involving a neglect of other conditions of happiness. If, then, we admit as actual or possible such 'infelicific' effects of the cultivation of Virtue, I think we shall also generally admit that, in the case supposed, conduciveness to general happiness should be the criterion for deciding how far the cultivation of Virtue should be carried.

At the same time it must be allowed that we find in Common Sense an aversion to admit Happiness (when explained to mean a sum of pleasures) to be the sole ultimate end and standard of right conduct. But this, I think, can be fully accounted for by the following considerations.

I. The term Pleasure is not commonly used so as to include clearly *all* kinds of consciousness which we desire to retain or reproduce: in ordinary usage it suggests too prominently the coarser and commoner kinds of such feelings; and it is difficult even for those who are trying to use it scientifically to free their minds altogether from the associations of ordinary usage, and to mean by Pleasure only Desirable Consciousness or Feeling of whatever kind. Again, our knowledge of human life continually suggests to us instances of pleasures which will inevitably involve as concomitant or consequent either a greater amount of pain or a loss of more important pleasures: and we naturally shrink from including even hypothetically in our conception of ultimate good these—in Bentham's phrase—'impure' pleasures; especially since we have, in many cases, moral or æsthetic instincts warning us against such pleasures. [. . .]

II. [M]any important pleasures can only be felt on condition of our experiencing desires for other things than pleasure. Thus the very acceptance of Pleasure as the ultimate end of conduct involves the practical rule that it is not always to be made the conscious end. Hence, even if we are considering merely the good of one human being taken alone, excluding from our view all effects of his conduct on others, still the reluctance of Common Sense to regard pleasure as the sole thing ultimately desirable may be justified by the consideration that human beings tend to be less happy if they are exclusively occupied with the desire of personal happiness. E.g. (as was before shown) we shall miss the valuable pleasures which attend the exercise of the benevolent affections if we do not experience genuinely disinterested impulses to procure happiness for others (which are, in fact, implied in the notion of 'benevolent affections').

III. But again, I hold that disinterested benevolence is not only thus generally in harmony with rational Self-love, but also in another sense and independently rational: that is, Reason shows me that if my happiness is desirable and a good, the equal happiness of any other person must be equally desirable. Now, when Happiness is spoken of as the sole ultimate good of man, the idea most commonly suggested is that each individual is to seek his own happiness at the expense (if necessary) or, at any rate, to the neglect of that of others: and this offends both our sympathetic and our rational regard for others' happiness. It is, in fact, rather the end of Egoistic than of Universalistic Hedonism, to which Common Sense feels an aversion. And certainly one's individual happiness is, in many respects, an unsatisfactory mark for one's supreme aim, apart from any direct collision into which the exclusive pursuit of it may bring us with rational or sympathetic Benevolence. It does not possess the characteristics which, as Aristotle says, we 'divine' to belong to Ultimate Good: being (so far, at least, as it can be empirically foreseen) so narrow and limited, of such necessarily brief duration, and so shifting and insecure while it lasts. But Universal Happiness, desirable consciousness or feeling for the innumerable multitude of sentient beings, present and to come, seems an End that satisfies our imagination by its vastness, and sustains our resolution by its comparative security.

It may, however, be said that if we require the individual to sacrifice his own happiness to the greater happiness of others on the ground that it is reasonable to do so, we really assign to the individual a different ultimate end from that which we lay down as the ultimate Good of the universe of sentient beings: since we direct him to take, as ultimate, Happiness for the Universe, but Conformity to Reason for himself. I admit the substantial truth of this statement, though I should avoid the language as tending to obscure the distinction before explained between 'obeying the dictates' and 'promoting the dictation' of reason. But granting the alleged difference, I do not see that it constitutes an argument against the view here maintained, since the individual is essentially and fundamentally different from the larger whole—the universe of sentient beings—of which he is conscious of being a part; just because he has a known relation to similar parts of the same whole, while the whole itself has no such relation. I accordingly see no inconsistency in holding that while it *would* be reasonable for the aggregate of sentient beings, if it could act collectively, to aim at its own happiness only as an ultimate end—and would be reasonable for any individual to do the same, if he were the only sentient being in the universe—it may yet be *actually* reasonable for an individual to sacrifice his own Good or happiness for the greater happiness of others.

At the same time I admit that, in the earlier age of ethical thought which Greek philosophy represents, men sometimes judged an act to be 'good' *for the agent*, even while recognising that its consequences would be on the whole painful to him,—as (*e.g.*) a heroic exchange of a life full of happiness for a painful death at the call of duty. I attribute this partly to a confusion of thought between what it is reasonable for an individual to desire, when he considers his own existence alone, and what he must recognise as reasonably to be desired, when he takes the point of view of a larger whole: partly, again, to a faith deeply rooted in the moral consciousness of mankind, that there cannot be really and ultimately any conflict between the two kinds of reasonableness. But when 'Reasonable Self-love' has been clearly distinguished from Conscience, as it is by Butler and his followers, we find it is naturally understood to mean desire for one's own Happiness: so that in fact the interpretation of 'one's own good,' which was almost peculiar in ancient thought to the Cyrenaic and Epicurean heresies, is adopted by some of the most orthodox of modern moralists. Indeed it often does not seem to have occurred to these latter that this notion can have any other interpretation. If, then, when any one hypothetically concentrates his attention on himself, Good is naturally and almost inevitably conceived to be Pleasure, we may reasonably conclude that the Good of any number of similar beings, whatever their mutual relations may be, cannot be essentially different in quality.

IV. But lastly, from the universal point of view no less than from that of the individual, it seems true that Happiness is likely to be better attained if the extent to which we set ourselves consciously to aim at it be carefully restricted. And this not only because action is likely to be more effective if our effort is temporarily concentrated on the realisation of more limited ends—though this is no doubt an important reason:—but also because the fullest development of happy life for each individual seems to require that he should have other external objects of interest besides the happiness of other conscious beings. And thus we may conclude that the pursuit of the ideal objects before mentioned, Virtue, Truth, Freedom, Beauty, etc., *for their own sakes*, is indirectly and secondarily, though not primarily and absolutely, rational; on account not only of the happiness that will result from their attainment, but also of that which springs from their disinterested pursuit. While yet if we ask for a final criterion of the comparative value of the different objects of men's enthusiastic pursuit, and of the limits within which each may legitimately engross the attention of mankind, we shall none the less conceive it to depend upon the degree in which they respectively conduce to Happiness.

[*The Methods of Ethics*, 7th edn. (Macmillan: London, 1907), 398–406.]

G. E. MOORE

57 Beauty and Friendship

'No one,' says Prof. Sidgwick, 'would consider it rational to aim at the production of beauty in external nature, apart from any possible contemplation of it by human beings.' Well, I may say at once, that I, for one, do consider this rational; and let us see if I cannot get any one to agree with me. Consider what this admission really means. It entitles us to put the following case. Let us imagine one world exceedingly beautiful. Imagine it as beautiful as you can; put into it whatever on this earth you most admire—mountains, rivers, the sea; trees, and sunsets, stars and moon. Imagine these all combined in the most exquisite proportions, so that no one thing jars against another, but each contributes to increase the beauty of the whole. And then imagine the ugliest world you can possibly conceive. Imagine it simply one heap of filth, containing everything that is most disgusting to us, for whatever reason, and the whole, as far as may be, without one redeeming feature. Such a pair of worlds we are entitled to compare: they fall within Prof. Sidgwick's meaning, and the comparison is highly relevant to it. The only thing we are not entitled to imagine is that any human being ever has or ever, by any possibility, *can*, live in either, can ever see and enjoy the beauty of the one or hate the foulness of the other. Well, even so, supposing them quite apart from any possible contemplation by human beings; still, is it irrational to hold that it is better that the beautiful world should exist, than the one which is ugly? Would it not be well, in any case, to do what we could to produce it rather than the other? Certainly I cannot help thinking that it would; and I hope that some may agree with me in this extreme instance. The instance is extreme. It is highly improbable, not to say, impossible, we should ever have such a choice before us. In any actual choice we should have to consider the possible effects of our action upon conscious beings, and among these possible effects there are always some, I think, which ought to be preferred to the existence of mere beauty. But this only means that in our present state, in which but a very small portion of the good is attainable, the pursuit of beauty for its own sake must always be postponed to the pursuit of some greater good, which is equally attainable. But it is enough for my purpose, if it be admitted that, *supposing* no greater good were at all attainable, then beauty must in itself be regarded as a greater good than ugliness; if it be admitted that, in that case, we should not be left without any reason for preferring one course of action to another, we should not be left without any duty whatever, but that it would then be our positive duty to make the world more beautiful, so far as we were able, since nothing better than beauty could then result from our efforts. If this be once admitted, if in any imaginable case you do admit that the existence of a more beautiful thing is better in itself than that of one more ugly, quite apart from its effects on any human feeling, then Prof. Sidgwick's principle has broken down. Then we shall have to include in our ultimate end something beyond the limits of human existence. I admit, of course, that our beautiful world would be better still, if there were human beings in it to contemplate and enjoy its beauty. But that admission makes nothing against my point. If it be once admitted that the beautiful world *in itself* is better than the ugly, then it follows, that however many beings may enjoy it, and however much better their enjoyment may be than it is itself, yet its mere existence adds *something* to the goodness of the whole: it is not only a means to our end, but also itself a part thereof. [. . .]

By far the most valuable things, which we know or can imagine, are certain states of consciousness, which may be roughly described as the pleasures of human intercourse and the enjoyment of beautiful objects. No one, probably, who has asked himself the question, has ever doubted that personal affection and the appreciation of what is beautiful in Art or Nature, are good in themselves; nor, if we consider strictly what things are worth having *purely for their own sakes*, does it appear probable that any one will think that anything else has *nearly* so great a value as the things which are included under these two heads. I have myself urged that the mere existence of what is beautiful does appear to have *some* intrinsic value; but I regard it as indubitable that Prof. Sidgwick was so far right, in the view there discussed, that such mere existence of what is beautiful has value, so small as to be negligible, in comparison with that which attaches to the *consciousness* of beauty. This simple truth may, indeed, be said to be universally recognised. What has *not* been recognised is that it is the ultimate and fundamental truth of Moral Philosophy. That it is only for the sake of these things—in order that as much of them as possible may at some time exist—that any one can be justified in performing any public or private duty; that they are the *raison d'être* of virtue; that it is they—these complex wholes *themselves*, and not any constituent or characteristic of them—that form the rational ultimate end of human action and the sole criterion of social progress: these appear to be truths which have been generally overlooked.

[*Principia Ethica* (Cambridge University Press: Cambridge, 1922), 83–5, 188–9. First published in 1903.]

M. K. GANDHI

58   Truth and Ahimsa

It is not without a wrench that I have to take leave of the reader. I set a high value on my experiments. I do not know whether I have been able to do justice to them. I can only say that I have spared no pains to give a faithful narrative. To describe truth, as it has appeared to me, and in the exact manner in which I have arrived at it, has been my ceaseless effort. The exercise has given me ineffable mental peace, because, it has been my fond hope that it might bring faith in Truth and Ahimsa[1] to waverers.

My uniform experience has convinced me that there is no other God than Truth. And if every page of these chapters does not proclaim to the reader that the only means for the realization of Truth is Ahimsa, I shall deem all my labour in writing these chapters to have been in vain. And, even though my efforts in this behalf may prove fruitless, let the readers know that the vehicle, not the great principle, is at fault. After all, however sincere my strivings after Ahimsa may have been, they have still been imperfect and inadequate. The little fleeting glimpses, therefore, that I have been able to have of Truth can hardly convey an idea of the indescribable lustre of Truth, a million times more intense than that of the sun we daily see with our eyes. In fact what I have caught is only the faintest glimmer of that mighty effulgence. But this much I can say with assurance, as a result of all my experiments, that a perfect vision of Truth can only follow a complete realization of Ahimsa.

To see the universal and all-pervading Spirit of Truth face to face one must be able to love the meanest of creation as oneself. And a man who aspires after that cannot afford to keep out of any field of life. That is why my devotion to Truth has drawn me into the field of politics; and I can say without the slightest hesitation, and yet in all humility, that those who say that religion has nothing to do with politics do not know what religion means.

---

[1] 'Ahimsa' is the Hindu principle of harmlessness, or non-violence, toward all sentient creatures. [Ed]

Identification with everything that lives is impossible without self-purification; without self-purification the observance of the law of Ahimsa must remain an empty dream; God can never be realized by one who is not pure of heart. Self-purification therefore must mean purification in all the walks of life. And purification being highly infectious, purification of oneself necessarily leads to the purification of one's surroundings.

But the path of self-purification is hard and steep. To attain to perfect purity one has to become absolutely passion-free in thought, speech and action; to rise above the opposing currents of love and hatred, attachment and repulsion. I know that I have not in me as yet that triple purity, in spite of constant ceaseless striving for it. That is why the world's praise fails to move me, indeed it very often stings me. To conquer the subtle passions seems to me to be harder far than the physical conquest of the world by the force of arms. Ever since my return to India I have had experiences of the dormant passions lying hidden within me. The knowledge of them has made me feel humiliated though not defeated. The experiences and experiments have sustained me and given me great joy. But I know that I have still before me a difficult path to traverse. I must reduce myself to zero. So long as a man does not of his own free will put himself last among his fellow creatures, there is no salvation for him. Ahimsa is the farthest limit of humility.

[*An Autobiography: The Story of My Experiments with Truth*, trans. M. Desai (Beacon Press: Boston, Mass., 1927), 503–5.]

ALDOUS HUXLEY

59 The Right to Be Unhappy

The room into which the three were ushered was the Controller's study.

'His fordship will be down in a moment.' The Gamma butler left them to themselves.

Helmholtz laughed aloud.

'It's more like a caffeine-solution party than a trial,' he said, and let himself fall into the most luxurious of the pneumatic armchairs. 'Cheer up, Bernard,' he added, catching sight of his friend's green unhappy face. But Bernard would not be cheered; without answering, without even looking at Helmholtz, he went and sat down on the most uncomfortable chair in the room, carefully chosen in the obscure hope of somehow deprecating the wrath of the higher powers.

The Savage meanwhile wandered restlessly round the room, peering with a vague superficial inquisitiveness at the books in the shelves, at the sound-track rolls and the reading-machine bobbins in their numbered pigeon-holes. On the table under the window lay a massive volume bound in limp black leather-surrogate, and stamped with large golden Ts. He picked it up and opened it. MY LIFE AND WORK, BY OUR FORD. The book had been published at Detroit by the Society for the Propagation of Fordian Knowledge. Idly he turned the pages, read a sentence here, a paragraph there, and had just come to the conclusion that the book didn't interest him, when the door opened, and the Resident World Controller for Western Europe walked briskly into the room.

Mustapha Mond shook hands with all three of them; but it was to the Savage that he addressed himself. 'So you don't much like civilization, Mr Savage,' he said.

The Savage looked at him. He had been prepared to lie, to bluster, to remain sullenly unresponsive; but, reassured by the good-humoured intelligence of the Controller's face, he decided to tell the truth, straightforwardly. 'No.' He shook his head.

Bernard started and looked horrified. What would the Controller think? To be labelled as the friend of a man who said that he didn't like civilization—said it openly and, of all people, to the Controller—it was terrible. 'But, John,' he began. A look from Mustapha Mond reduced him to an abject silence.

'Of course,' the Savage went on to admit, 'there are some very nice things. All that music in the air, for instance . . .'

'Sometimes a thousand twangling instruments will hum about my ears, and sometimes voices.'

The Savage's face lit up with a sudden pleasure. 'Have you read it too?' he asked. 'I thought nobody knew about that book here, in England.'

'Almost nobody. I'm one of the very few. It's prohibited, you see. But as I make the laws here, I can also break them. With impunity, Mr Marx,' he added, turning to Bernard. 'Which I'm afraid you *can't* do.'

Bernard sank into a yet more hopeless misery.

'But why is it prohibited?' asked the Savage. In the excitement of meeting a man who had read Shakespeare he had momentarily forgotten everything else.

The Controller shrugged his shoulders. 'Because it's old; that's the chief reason. We haven't any use for old things here.'

'Even when they're beautiful?'

'Particularly when they're beautiful. Beauty's attractive, and we don't want people to be attracted by old things. We want them to like the new ones.'

'But the new ones are so stupid and horrible. Those plays, where there's nothing but helicopters flying about and you *feel* the people kissing.' He made a grimace. 'Goats and monkeys!' Only in Othello's words could he find an adequate vehicle for his contempt and hatred.

'Nice tame animals, anyhow,' the Controller murmured parenthetically.

'Why don't you let them see *Othello* instead?'

'I've told you; it's old. Besides, they couldn't understand it.'

Yes, that was true. He remembered how Helmholtz had laughed at *Romeo and Juliet*. 'Well, then,' he said, after a pause, 'something new that's like *Othello*, and that they could understand.'

'That's what we've all been wanting to write,' said Helmholtz, breaking a long silence.

'And it's what you never will write,' said the Controller. 'Because, if it were really like *Othello* nobody could understand it, however new it might be. And if it were new, it couldn't possibly be like *Othello*.'

'Why not?'

'Yes, why not?' Helmholtz repeated. He too was forgetting the unpleasant realities of the situation. Green with anxiety and apprehension, only Bernard remembered them; the others ignored him. 'Why not?'

'Because our world is not the same as Othello's world. You can't make flivvers without steel—and you can't make tragedies without social instability. The world's stable now. People are happy; they get what they want, and they never want what they can't get. They're well off; they're safe; they're never ill; they're not afraid of death; they're blissfully ignorant of passion and old age; they're plagued with no mothers or fathers; they've got no wives, or children, or loves to feel strongly about; they're so conditioned that they practically can't help behaving as they ought to behave. And if anything should go wrong, there's *soma*. Which you go and chuck out of the window in the name of liberty, Mr Savage. *Liberty!*' He laughed. 'Expecting Deltas to know what liberty is! And now expecting them to understand *Othello*! My good boy!'

The Savage was silent for a little. 'All the same,' he insisted obstinately, '*Othello*'s good, *Othello*'s better than those feelies.'

'Of course it is,' the Controller agreed. 'But that's the price we have to pay for stability. You've got to choose between happiness and what people used to call high art. We've sacrificed the high art. We have the feelies and the scent organ instead.'

'But they don't mean anything.'

'They mean themselves; they mean a lot of agreeable sensations to the audience.'

'But they're . . . they're told by an idiot.'

The Controller laughed. 'You're not being very polite to your friend Mr Watson. One of our most distinguished Emotional Engineers . . .'

'But he's right,' said Helmholtz gloomily. 'Because it *is* idiotic. Writing when there's nothing to say . . .'

'Precisely. But that requires the most enormous ingenuity. You're making flivvers out of the absolute minimum of steel—works of art out of practically nothing but pure sensation.'

The Savage shook his head. 'It all seems to me quite horrible.'

'Of course it does. Actual happiness always looks pretty squalid in comparison with the over-compensations for misery. And, of course, stability isn't nearly so spectacular as instability. And being contented has none of the glamour of a good fight against misfortune, none of the picturesqueness of a struggle with temptation, or a fatal overthrow by passion or doubt. Happiness is never grand. [. . .]

'In a properly organized society like ours, nobody has any opportunities for being noble or heroic. Conditions have got to be thoroughly unstable before the occasion can arise. Where there are wars, where there are divided allegiances, where there are temptations to be resisted, objects of love to be fought for or defended—there, obviously, nobility and heroism have some sense. But there aren't any wars nowadays. The greatest care is taken to prevent you from loving anyone too much. There's no such thing as a divided allegiance; you're so conditioned that you can't help doing what you ought to do. And what you ought to do is on the whole so pleasant, so many of the natural impulses are allowed free play, that there really aren't any temptations to resist. And if ever, by some unlucky chance, anything unpleasant should somehow happen, why, there's always *soma* to give you a holiday from the facts. And there's always *soma* to calm your anger, to reconcile you to your enemies, to make you patient and long-suffering. In the past you could only accomplish these things by making a great effort and after years of hard moral training. Now, you swallow two or three half-gramme tablets, and there you are. Anybody can be virtuous now. You can carry at least half your morality about in a bottle. Christianity without tears—that's what *soma* is.'

'But the tears are necessary. Don't you remember what Othello said? "If after every tempest come such calms, may the winds blow till they have wakened death." There's a story one of the old Indians used to tell us, about the Girl of Mátsaki. The young men who wanted to marry her had to do a morning's hoeing in her garden. It seemed easy; but there were flies and mosquitoes, magic ones. Most of the young men simply couldn't stand the biting and stinging. But the one that could—he got the girl.'

'Charming! But in civilized countries,' said the Controller, 'you can have girls without hoeing for them; and there aren't any flies or mosquitoes to sting you. We got rid of them all centuries ago.'

The Savage nodded, frowning. 'You got rid of them. Yes, that's just like you. Getting rid of everything unpleasant instead of learning to put up with it. Whether 'tis nobler in the mind to suffer the slings and arrows of outrageous fortune, or to take arms against a sea of troubles and by opposing end them. . . . But you don't do either. Neither suffer nor oppose. You just abolish the slings and arrows. It's too easy.' [. . .]

'What you need', the Savage went on, 'is something *with* tears for a change. Nothing costs enough here. [. . .]

'Isn't there something in that?' he asked, looking up at Mustapha Mond. 'Quite apart from God—though of course God would be a reason for it. Isn't there something in living dangerously?'

'There's a great deal in it,' the Controller replied. 'Men and women must have their adrenals stimulated from time to time.'

'What?' questioned the Savage, uncomprehending.

'It's one of the conditions of perfect health. That's why we've made the V.P.S. treatments compulsory.'

'V.P.S.?'

'Violent Passion Surrogate. Regularly once a month. We flood the whole system with adrenalin. It's the complete physiological equivalent of fear and rage. All the tonic effects of murdering Desdemona and being murdered by Othello, without any of the inconveniences.'

'But I like the inconveniences.'

'We don't,' said the Controller. 'We prefer to do things comfortably.'

'But I don't want comfort. I want God, I want poetry, I want real danger, I want freedom, I want goodness. I want sin.'

'In fact,' said Mustapha Mond, 'you're claiming the right to be unhappy.'

'All right, then,' said the Savage defiantly, 'I'm claiming the right to be unhappy.'

'Not to mention the right to grow old and ugly and impotent; the right to have syphilis and cancer; the right to have too little to eat; the right to be lousy; the right to live in constant apprehension of what may happen tomorrow; the right to catch typhoid; the right to be tortured by unspeakable pains of every kind.'

There was a long silence.

'I claim them all,' said the Savage at last.

Mustapha Mond shrugged his shoulders. 'You're welcome,' he said.

[*Brave New World* (Penguin: Harmondsworth, 1971), 171–4, 185–7. First published in 1932.]

ALBERT CAMUS

60 The Myth of Sisyphus

There is but one truly serious philosophical problem, and that is suicide. Judging whether life is or is not worth living amounts to answering the fundamental question of philosophy. All the rest—whether or not the world has three dimensions, whether the mind has nine or twelve categories—comes afterwards. These are games; one must first answer. And if it is true, as Nietzsche claims, that a philosopher, to deserve our respect, must preach by example, you can appreciate the importance of that reply, for it will precede the definitive act. These are facts the heart can feel; yet they call for careful study before they become clear to the intellect.

If I ask myself how to judge that this question is more urgent than that, I reply that one judges by the actions it entails. I have never seen anyone die for the ontological argument. Galileo, who held a scientific truth of great importance, abjured it with the greatest ease as soon as it endangered his life. In a certain sense, he did right.[1] That truth was not worth the stake. Whether the earth or the sun revolves around the other is a matter of profound indifference. To tell the truth, it is a futile question. On the other hand, I see many people die because they judge that life is not worth living. I see others paradoxically getting killed for the ideas or illusions that give them a reason for living (what is called a reason for living is also an excellent reason for dying). I therefore conclude that the meaning of life is the most urgent of questions. How to answer it? [. . .]

The Gods had condemned Sisyphus to ceaselessly rolling a rock to the top of a mountain, whence the stone would fall back of its own weight. They had thought with some reason that there is no more dreadful punishment than futile and hopeless labor.

If one believes Homer, Sisyphus was the wisest and most prudent of mortals. According to another tradition, however, he was disposed to practice the profession of highwayman. I see no contradiction in this. Opinions differ as to the reasons why he became the futile laborer of the underworld. To begin with, he is accused of a certain levity in regard to the gods. He stole their secrets. Ægina, the daughter of Æsopus, was carried off by Jupiter. The father was shocked by that disappearance and complained to Sisyphus. He, who knew of the abduction, offered to tell about it on condition that Æsopus would give water to the citadel of Corinth. To the celestial thunderbolts he preferred the benediction of water. He was punished for this in the underworld. Homer tells us also that Sisyphus had put Death in chains. Pluto could not endure the sight of his deserted, silent empire. He dispatched the god of war, who liberated Death from the hands of her conqueror.

It is said also that Sisyphus, being near to death, rashly wanted to test his wife's love. He ordered her to cast his unburied body into the middle of the public square. Sisyphus woke up in the underworld. And there, annoyed by an obedience so contrary to human love, he obtained from Pluto permission to return to earth in order to chastise his wife. But when he had seen again the face of this world, enjoyed water and sun, warm stones and the sea, he no longer wanted to go back to the infernal darkness. Recalls,

---

[1] From the point of view of the relative value of truth. On the other hand, from the point of view of virile behavior, this scholar's fragility may well make us smile.

signs of anger, warnings were of no avail. Many years more he lived facing the curve of the gulf, the sparkling sea, and the smiles of earth. A decree of the gods was necessary. Mercury came and seized the impudent man by the collar and, snatching him from his joys, led him forcibly back to the under-world, where his rock was ready for him.

You have already grasped that Sisyphus is the absurd hero. He *is*, as much through his passions as through his torture. His scorn of the gods, his hatred of death, and his passion for life won him that unspeakable penalty in which the whole being is exerted toward accomplishing nothing. This is the price that must be paid for the passions of this earth. Nothing is told us about Sisyphus in the underworld. Myths are made for the imagination to breathe life into them. As for this myth, one sees merely the whole effort of a body straining to raise the huge stone, to roll it and push it up a slope a hundred times over; one sees the face screwed up, the cheek tight against the stone, the shoulder bracing the clay-covered mass, the foot wedging it, the fresh start with arms outstretched, the wholly human security of two earth-clotted hands. At the very end of his long effort measured by skyless space and time without depth, the purpose is achieved. Then Sisyphus watches the stone rush down in a few moments toward that lower world whence he will have to push it up again toward the summit. He goes back down to the plain.

It is during that return, that pause, that Sisyphus interests me. A face that toils so close to stones is already stone itself! I see that man going back down with a heavy yet measured step toward the torment of which he will never know the end. That hour like a breathing-space which returns as surely as his suffering, that is the hour of consciousness. At each of those moments when he leaves the heights and gradually sinks towards the lairs of the gods, he is superior to his fate. He is stronger than his rock.

If this myth is tragic, that is because its hero is conscious. Where would his torture be, indeed, if at every step the hope of succeeding upheld him? The workman of today works every day in his life at the same tasks, and this fate is no less absurd. But it is tragic only at the rare moments when it becomes conscious. Sisyphus, proletarian of the gods, powerless and rebel-lious, knows the whole extent of his wretched condition: it is what he thinks of during his descent. The lucidity that was to constitute his torture at the same time crowns his victory. There is no fate that cannot be surmounted by scorn.

If the descent is thus sometimes performed in sorrow, it can also take place in joy. This word is not too much. Again I fancy Sisyphus returning toward his rock, and the sorrow was in the beginning. When the images of earth cling too tightly to memory, when the call of happiness becomes too insistent, it happens that melancholy rises in man's heart: this is the rock's victory, this is the rock itself. The boundless grief is too heavy to bear. These are our nights of Gethsemane. But crushing truths perish from being acknowledged. Thus, Œdipus at the outset obeys fate without knowing it. But from the moment he knows, his tragedy begins. Yet at the same moment, blind and desperate, he realizes that the only bond linking him to the world is the cool hand of a girl. Then a tremendous remark rings out: 'Despite so many ordeals, my advanced age and the nobility of my soul make me conclude that all is well.' Sophocles' Œdipus, like Dostoevsky's Kirilov, thus gives the recipe for the absurd victory. Ancient wisdom confirms modern heroism.

One does not discover the absurd without being tempted to write a manual of happiness. 'What! by such narrow ways—?' There is but one world, however. Happiness and the absurd are two sons of the same earth. They are inseparable. It would be a mistake to say that happiness necessarily springs from the absurd discovery. It happens as well that the feeling of the absurd springs from happiness. 'I conclude that all is well,' says Œdipus, and that remark is sacred. It echoes in the wild and limited universe of man. It teaches that all is not, has not been, exhausted. It drives out of this world a god who had come into it with dissatisfaction and a preference for futile sufferings. It makes of fate a human matter, which must be settled among men.

All Sisyphus' silent joy is contained therein. His fate belongs to him. His rock is his thing. Likewise, the absurd man, when he contemplates his torment, silences all the idols. In the universe suddenly restored to its silence, the myriad wondering little voices of the earth rise up. Unconscious, secret calls, invitations from all the faces, they are the necessary reverse and price of victory. There is no sun without shadow, and it is essential to know the night. The absurd man says yes and his effort will henceforth be unceasing. If there is a personal fate, there is no higher destiny, or at least there is but one which he concludes is inevitable and despicable. For the rest, he knows himself to be the master of his days. At that subtle moment when man glances backward over his life, Sisyphus returning toward his rock, in that slight pivoting he contemplates that series of unrelated actions which becomes his fate, created by him, combined under his memory's eye and soon sealed by his death. Thus, convinced of the wholly human origin of all that is human, a blind man eager to see who knows that the night has no end, he is still on the go. The rock is still rolling.

I leave Sisyphus at the foot of the mountain! One always finds one's burden again. But Sisyphus teaches the higher fidelity that negates the gods and raises rocks. He too concludes that all is well. This universe henceforth without a master seems to him neither sterile nor futile. Each atom of that stone, each mineral flake of that night-filled mountain, in itself forms a world. The struggle itself toward the heights is enough to fill a man's heart. One must imagine Sisyphus happy.

[*The Myth of Sisyphus and Other Essays*, trans. Justin O' Brien (Alfred Knopf: New York, 1969), 3–4, 119–23. First published in 1945.]

ROBERT NOZICK

61   The Experience Machine

Suppose there were an experience machine that would give you any experience you desired. Superduper neuropsychologists could stimulate your brain so that you would think and feel you were writing a great novel, or making a friend, or reading an interesting book. All the time you would be floating in a tank, with electrodes attached to your brain. Should you plug into this machine for life, preprogramming your life's experiences? If you are worried about missing out on desirable experiences, we can suppose that business enterprises have researched thoroughly the lives of many others. You can pick and choose from their large library or smorgasbord of such experiences, selecting your life's experiences for, say, the next two years. After two years have passed, you will have ten minutes or ten hours out of the tank, to select the experiences of your *next* two years. Of course, while in the tank you won't know that you're there; you'll think it's all actually happening. Others can also plug in to have the experiences they want, so there's no need to stay unplugged to serve them. (Ignore problems such as who will service the machines if everyone plugs in.) Would you plug in? *What else can matter to us, other than how our lives feel from the inside?* Nor should you refrain because of the few moments of distress between the moment you've decided and the moment you're plugged. What's a few moments of distress compared to a lifetime of bliss (if that's what you choose), and why feel any distress at all if your decision *is* the best one?

What does matter to us in addition to our experiences? First, we want to *do* certain things, and not just have the experience of doing them. In the case of certain experiences, it is only because first we want to do the actions that we want the experiences of doing them or thinking we've done them. (But *why* do we want to do the activities rather than merely to experience them?) A second reason for not plugging in is that we want to *be* a certain way, to be a certain sort of person. Someone floating in a tank is an indeterminate blob. There is no answer to the question of what a person is like who has long been in the tank. Is he courageous, kind, intelligent, witty, loving? It's not merely that it's difficult to tell; there's no way he is. Plugging into the machine is a kind of suicide. It will seem to some, trapped by a picture, that nothing about what we are like can matter except as it gets reflected in our experiences. But should it be surprising that what *we are* is important to us? Why should we be concerned only with how our time is filled, but not with what we are?

Thirdly, plugging into an experience machine limits us to a man-made reality, to a world no deeper or more important than that which people can construct. There is no *actual* contact with any deeper reality, though the experience of it can be simulated. Many persons desire to leave themselves open to such contact and to a plumbing of deeper significance. This clarifies the intensity of the conflict over psychoactive drugs, which some view as mere local experience machines, and others view as avenues to a deeper reality; what some view as equivalent to surrender to the experience machine, others view as following one of the reasons *not* to surrender!

We learn that something matters to us in addition to experience by imagining an experience machine and then realizing that we would not use it. We can continue to imagine a sequence of machines each designed to fill lacks suggested for the earlier machines. For example, since the experience machine doesn't meet our desire to *be* a certain way, imagine a transformation machine which transforms us into whatever sort of person we'd like to be (compatible with our staying us). Surely one would not use the transformation machine to become as one would wish, and thereupon plug into the experience machine! So something matters in addition to one's experiences *and* what one is like. Nor is the reason merely that one's experiences are unconnected with what one is like. For the experience machine might be limited to provide only experiences possible to the sort of person plugged in. Is it that we want to make a difference in the world? Consider then the result machine, which produces in the world any result you would produce and injects your vector input into any joint activity. We shall not pursue here the fascinating details of these or other machines. What is most disturbing about them is their living of our lives for us. Is it misguided to search for *particular* additional functions beyond the competence of machines to do for us? Perhaps what we desire is to live (an active verb) ourselves, in contact with reality. (And this, machines cannot do *for* us.)

[*Anarchy, State and Utopia* (Basic Books: New York, 1974), 42–5.]

JOHN FINNIS

62   **The Basic Values**

What *are* the basic aspects of my well-being? Here each one of us, however extensive his knowledge of the interests of other people and other cultures, is alone with his own intelligent grasp of the indemonstrable (because self-evident) first principles of his own practical reasoning. From one's capacity to grasp intelligently the basic forms of good as 'to-be-pursued' one gets one's ability, in the descriptive disciplines of history and anthropology, to sympathetically (though not uncritically) see the point of actions, life-styles, characters, and cultures that one would not choose for oneself. And one's speculative knowledge of other people's interests and achievements does not leave unaffected one's practical understanding of the forms of good that lie open to one's choice. But there is no inference from fact to value. At this point in our discourse (or private meditation), inference and proof are left behind (or left until later), and the proper form of discourse is: '. . . is a good, in itself, don't you think?'.

Remember: by 'good', 'basic good', 'value', 'well-being', etc. I do *not* yet mean 'moral good', etc.

What, then, are the basic forms of good for us?

A. Life

A first basic value, corresponding to the drive for self-preservation, is the value of life. The term 'life' here signifies every aspect of the vitality (*vita*, life) which puts a human being in good shape for self-determination. Hence, life here includes bodily (including cerebral) health, and freedom from the pain that betokens organic malfunctioning or injury. And the recognition, pursuit, and realization of this basic human purpose (or internally related group of purposes) are as various as the crafty struggle and prayer of a man overboard seeking to stay afloat until his ship turns back for him; the team-work of surgeons and the whole network of supporting staff, ancillary services, medical schools, etc.; road safety laws and programmes; famine relief expeditions; farming and rearing and fishing; food marketing; the resuscitation of suicides; watching out as one steps off the kerb. [. . .]

B. Knowledge

The second basic value is knowledge, considered as desirable for its own sake, not merely instrumentally.

C. Play

The third basic aspect of human well-being is play. A certain sort of moralist analysing human goods may overlook this basic value, but an anthropologist will not fail to observe this large and irreducible element in human culture. More importantly, each one of us can see the point of engaging in performances which have no point beyond the performance itself, enjoyed for its own sake. The performance may be solitary or social, intellectual or physical, strenuous or relaxed, highly structured or relatively informal, conventional or *ad hoc* in its pattern . . . An element of play can enter into any human activity, even the drafting of enactments, but is always analytically distinguishable from its 'serious' context; and some activities, enterprises, and institutions are entirely or primarily pure play. Play, then, has and is its own value.

D. Aesthetic Experience

The fourth basic component in our flourishing is aesthetic experience. Many forms of play, such as dance or song or football, are the matrix or occasion of aesthetic experience. But beauty is not an indispensable element of play. Moreover, beautiful form can be found and enjoyed in nature. Aesthetic experience, unlike play, need not involve an action of one's own; what is sought after and valued for its own sake may simply be the beautiful form 'outside' one, and the 'inner' experience of appreciation of its beauty. But often enough the valued experience is found in the creation and/or active appreciation of some *work* of significant and satisfying form.

E. Sociability (Friendship)

Fifthly, there is the value of that sociability which in its weakest form is realized by a minimum of peace and harmony amongst men, and which ranges through the forms of human community to its strongest form in the flowering of full friendship. Some of the collaboration between one person and another is no more than instrumental to the realization by each of his own individual purposes. But friendship involves acting for the sake of one's friend's purposes, one's friend's well-being. To be in a relationship of friendship with at least one other person is a fundamental form of good, is it not? [. . .]

F. Practical Reasonableness

Sixthly, there is the basic good of being able to bring one's own intelligence to bear effectively (in practical reasoning that issues in action) on the problems of choosing one's actions and lifestyle and shaping one's own character. Negatively, this involves that one has a measure of effective freedom; positively, it involves that one seeks to bring an intelligent and reasonable order into one's own actions and habits and practical attitudes. This order in turn has (i) an internal aspect, as when one strives to bring one's emotions and dispositions into the harmony of an inner peace of mind that is not merely the product of drugs or indoctrination nor merely passive in its orientation; and (ii) an external aspect, as when one strives to make one's actions (which are external in that they change states of affairs in the world and often enough affect the relations between persons) authentic, that is to say, genuine realizations of one's own freely ordered evaluations, preferences, hopes, and self-determination. This value is thus complex, involving freedom and reason, integrity and authenticity. But it has a sufficient unity to be treated as one; and for a label I choose 'practical reasonableness'.

G. 'Religion'

Seventhly, and finally in this list, there is the value of what, since Cicero, we summarily and lamely call 'religion'. For, as there is the order of means to ends, and the pursuit of life, truth, play, and aesthetic experience in some individually selected order of priorities and pattern of specialization, and the order that can be brought into human relations through collaboration, community, and friendship, and the order that is to be brought into one's character and activity through inner integrity and outer authenticity, so, finally there arise such questions as: (a) How are all these orders, which have their immediate origin in human initiative and pass away in death, related to the lasting order of the whole cosmos and to the origin, if any, of that order? (b) Is it not perhaps the case that human freedom, in which one rises above the determinism of instinct and impulse to an intelligent grasp of worthwhile forms of good, and through which one shapes and masters one's environment but also one's own character, is itself somehow subordinate to something which makes that human freedom, human intelligence, and human mastery possible (not just 'originally' but from moment to moment) and which is free, intelligent, and sovereign in a way (and over a range) no human being can be?

Misgivings may be aroused by the notion that one of the basic human values is the establishment and maintenance of proper relationships between oneself (and the orders one can create and maintain) and the divine. For there are, always, those who doubt or deny that the universal order-of-things has any origin beyond the 'origins' known to the natural sciences, and who answer question (b) negatively. But is it reasonable to deny that it is, at any rate, peculiarly important to have thought reasonably and (where possible) correctly about these questions of the origins of cosmic order and of human freedom and reason—whatever the answer to those questions turns out to be, and even if the answers have to be agnostic or negative? And does not that importance in large part consist in this: that if there is a transcendent origin of the universal order-of-things and of human freedom and reason, then one's life and actions are in fundamental disorder if they are not brought, as best one can, into some sort of harmony with whatever can be known or surmised about that transcendent other and its lasting order? More important for us than the ubiquity of expressions of religious concerns, in all human cultures, is the question: Does not one's own sense of 'responsibility', in choosing what one is to be and do, amount to a concern that is not reducible to the concern to live, play, procreate, relate to others, and be intelligent? Does not even a Sartre, taking as his *point de départ* that God does not exist (and that therefore 'everything is permitted'), none the less appreciate that he is 'responsible'—obliged to act with freedom and authenticity, and to will the liberty of other persons equally with his own—in choosing what he is to be; and all this, because, *prior to* any choice of his, 'man' is and is-to-be free?[1] And is this not a recognition (however residual) of, and concern about, an order of things 'beyond' each and every man? And so, without wishing to beg any question, may we not for convenience call that concern, which is concern for a good consisting in an irreducibly distinct form of order, 'religious'? [. . .]

An Exhaustive List?

Now besides life, knowledge, play, aesthetic experience, friendship, practical reasonableness, and religion, there are countless objectives and forms of good. But I suggest that these other objectives and forms of good will be found, on analysis, to be ways or combinations of ways of pursuing (not always sensibly) and realizing (not always successfully) one of the seven basic forms of good, or some combination of them.

Moreover, there are countless aspects of human self-determination and self-realization besides the seven basic aspects which I have listed. But these other aspects, such as courage, generosity, moderation, gentleness, and so on, are not themselves basic values; rather, they are ways (not means, but modes) of pursuing the basic values, and fit (or are deemed by some individual, or group, or culture, to fit) a man for their pursuit.

In this way we can analytically unravel even very 'peculiar' conventions, norms, institutions, and orders of preference, such as the aristocratic code of honour that demanded direct attacks on life in duelling.

Again, though the pursuit of the basic values is made psychologically possible by the corresponding inclinations and urges of one's nature, still there are many inclinations and urges that do not correspond to or support any basic value: for example, the inclination to take more than one's share, or the urge to gratuitous cruelty. There is no need to consider whether these urges are more, or less, 'natural' (in terms of frequency, universality, intensity, etc.) than those urges which correspond to the basic values. For I am not trying to justify our recognition and pursuit of basic values by deducing from, or even by pointing to, any set of inclinations. The point, rather, is that selfishness, cruelty, and the like, simply do not stand to something self-evidently good as the urge to self-preservation stands to the

---

[1] J.-P. Sartre, *L'Existentialisme est un humanisme* (Les Éditions Nagel: Paris, 1946), 36, 83–4.

self-evident good of human life. Selfishness, cruelty, etc., stand in need of some explanation, in a way that curiosity, friendliness, etc., do not. (This is not to say that physiologists and psychologists should not investigate the physical and psychosomatic substructure of curiosity, friendliness, etc.) Often enough the explanation will be that the pursuit of a value (say, truth), or of a standard material means to sustaining a value (say, food), becomes locked into a pattern of exclusiveness or inversion—producing selfish indifference to the inclusive realization of that same value in the lives of others, and to the intrinsic value of sharing goods in friendship. Or again, cruelty may be found to be an inverted form of pursuit of the value of freedom and self-determination and authenticity: a man may make himself 'feel real' to himself by subjecting others to his utter mastery. In the absence of such explanations, and of psychosomatic disease, we find these urges as baffling as persistent illogicality, as opaque and pointless as, say, a demand for a plate of mud for no reason at all.

But are there just seven basic values, no more and no less? And what is meant by calling them basic?

There is no magic in the number seven, and others who have reflected on these matters have produced slightly different lists, usually slightly longer. There is no need for the reader to accept the present list, just as it stands, still less its nomenclature (which simply gestures towards categories of human purpose that are each, though unified, nevertheless multi-faceted). My brief discussion of the problem of whether procreation should be treated as an analytically distinct category of human good illustrates the scope that exists for modification of the details of the list. Still, it seems to me that those seven purposes are all of the basic purposes of human action, and that any other purpose which you or I might recognize and pursue will turn out to represent, or be constituted of, some aspect(s) of some or all of them.

All Equally Fundamental

More important than the precise number and description of these values is the sense in which each is basic. First, each is equally self-evidently a form of good. Secondly, none can be analytically reduced to being merely an aspect of any of the others, or to being merely instrumental in the pursuit of any of the others. Thirdly, each one, when we focus on it, can reasonably be regarded as the most important. Hence there is no objective hierarchy amongst them. [. . .]

Is Pleasure The Point of it all?

The experience of discovery ('Eureka!') or creative play or living through danger are pleasurable, satisfying, and valuable; but it is because we want to make the discovery or to create or to 'survive' that we want the experiences. What matters to us, in the final analysis, is knowledge, significantly patterned or testing performances (and performing them), beautiful form (and appreciating it), friendship (and being a friend), freedom, self-direction, integrity, and authenticity, and (if such there be) the transcendent origin, ground, and end of all things (and *being* in accord with it). If these give pleasure, this experience is one aspect of their reality as human goods, which are not participated in fully unless their goodness is experienced as such. But a participation in basic goods which is emotionally dry, subjectively unsatisfying, nevertheless is good and meaningful as far as it goes.

So it is that the practical principles which enjoin one to participate in those basic forms of good, through the practically intelligent decisions and free actions that constitute one the person one is and is to be, have been called in the Western philosophical tradition the first principles of natural law, because they lay down for us the outlines of everything one could reasonably want to do, to have, and to be.

[*Natural Law and Natural Rights* (Clarendon Press: Oxford, 1980), 87–97.]

DEREK PARFIT

63 What Makes Someone's Life Go Best

What would be best for someone, or would be most in this person's interests, or would make this person's life go, for him, as well as possible? Answers to this question I call *theories about self-interest*. There are three kinds of theory. On *Hedonistic Theories*, what would be best for someone is what would make his life happiest. On *Desire-Fulfilment Theories*, what would be best for someone is what, throughout his life, would best fulfil his desires. On *Objective List Theories*, certain things are good or bad for us, whether or not we want to have the good things, or to avoid the bad things.

Narrow Hedonists assume, falsely, that pleasure and pain are two distinctive kinds of experience. Compare the pleasures of satisfying an intense thirst or lust, listening to music, solving an intellectual problem, reading a tragedy, and knowing that one's child is happy. These various experiences do not contain any distinctive common quality.

What pains and pleasures have in common are their relations to our desires. On the use of 'pain' which has rational and moral significance, all pains are when experienced unwanted, and a pain is worse or greater the more it is unwanted. Similarly, all pleasures are when experienced wanted, and they are better or greater the more they are wanted. These are the claims of *Preference-Hedonism*. On this view, one of two experiences is more pleasant if it is preferred.

This theory need not follow the ordinary uses of the words 'pain' and 'pleasure'. Suppose that I could go to a party to enjoy the various pleasures of eating, drinking, laughing, dancing, and talking to my friends. I could instead stay at home and read *King Lear*. Knowing what both alternatives would be like, I prefer to read *King Lear*. It extends the ordinary use to say that this would give me more pleasure. But on Preference-Hedonism, if we add some further assumptions given below, reading *King Lear* would give me a better evening. Griffin cites a more extreme case. Near the end of his life Freud refused pain-killing drugs, preferring to think in torment than to be confusedly euphoric. Of these two mental states, euphoria is more pleasant. But on Preference-Hedonism thinking in torment was, for Freud, a better mental state. It is clearer here not to stretch the meaning of the word 'pleasant'. A Preference-Hedonist should merely claim that, since Freud preferred to think clearly though in torment, his life went better if it went as he preferred.[1]

Consider next Desire-Fulfilment Theories. The simplest is the *Unrestricted* Theory. This claims that what is best for someone is what would best fulfil *all* of his desires, throughout his life. Suppose that I meet a stranger who has what is believed to be a fatal disease. My sympathy is aroused, and I strongly want this stranger to be cured. Much later, when I have forgotten our meeting, the stranger is cured. On the Unrestricted Desire-Fulfilment Theory, this event is good for me, and makes my life go better. This is not plausible. We should reject this theory.

Another theory appeals only to someone's desires about his own life. I call this the *Success Theory*. This theory differs from Preference-Hedonism in only one way. The Success Theory appeals to all of our preferences about our own lives. A Preference-Hedonist appeals only to preferences about those present features of our lives that are introspectively discernible. Suppose that I strongly want not to be deceived by other people. On Preference-Hedonism it would be better for me if I believe that I am not being deceived. It would be irrelevant if my belief is false, since this makes no difference to my state of mind. On the Success Theory, it would be worse for me if my belief is false. I have a strong desire about my own life—that I should not be deceived in this way. It is bad for me if this desire is not fulfilled, even if I falsely believe that it is.

When this theory appeals only to desires that are about our own lives, it may be unclear what this excludes. Suppose that I want my life to be such that all of my desires, whatever their objects, are fulfilled. This may seem to make the Success Theory, when applied to me, coincide with the Unrestricted Desire-Fulfilment Theory. But a Success Theorist should claim that

[1] J. P. Griffin, 'Are There Incommensurable Values?', *Philosophy and Public Affairs*, 7/1 (Autumn, 1977).

this desire is not really about my own life. This is like the distinction between a real change in some object, and a so-called *Cambridge-change*. An object undergoes a Cambridge-change if there is any change in the true statements that can be made about this object. Suppose that I cut my cheek while shaving. This causes a real change in me. It also causes a change in Confucius. It becomes true, of Confucius, that he lived on a planet in which later one more cheek was cut. This is merely a Cambridge-change.

Suppose that I am an exile, and cannot communicate with my children. I want their lives to go well. I might claim that I want to live the life of someone whose children's lives go well. A Success Theorist should again claim that this is not really a desire about my own life. If unknown to me one of my children is killed by an avalanche, this is not bad for me, and does not make my life go worse.

A Success Theorist *would* count some similar desires. Suppose that I try to give my children a good start in life. I try to give them the right education, good habits, and psychological strength. Once again, I am now an exile, and will never be able to learn what happens to my children. Suppose that, unknown to me, my children's lives go badly. One finds that the education that I gave him makes him unemployable, another has a mental breakdown, another becomes a petty thief. If my children's lives fail in these ways, and these failures are in part the result of mistakes I made as their parent, these failures in my children's lives would be judged to be bad for me on the Success Theory. One of my strongest desires was to be a successful parent. What is now happening to my children, though it is unknown to me, shows that this desire is not fulfilled. My life failed in one of the ways in which I most wanted it to succeed. Though I do not know this fact, it is bad for me, and makes it true that I have had a worse life. This is like the case where I strongly want not to be deceived. Even if I never know, it is bad for me both if I am deceived and if I turn out to be an unsuccessful parent. These are not introspectively discernible differences in my conscious life. On Preference-Hedonism, these events are not bad for me. On the Success Theory, they are.

Because they are thought by some to need special treatment, I mention next the desires that people have about what happens after they are dead. For a Preference-Hedonist, once I am dead, nothing bad can happen to me. A Success Theorist should deny this. Return to the case where all my children have wretched lives, because of the mistakes I made as their parent. Suppose that my children's lives all go badly only after I am dead. My life turns out to have been a failure, in one of the ways I cared about most. A Success Theorist should claim that, here too, this makes it true that I had a worse life.

Some Success Theorists would reject this claim. Their theory ignores the desires of the dead. I believe this theory to be indefensible. Suppose that I was asked, 'Do you want it to be true that you were a successful parent even after you are dead?' I would answer 'Yes'. It is irrelevant to my desire whether it is fulfilled before or after I am dead. These Success Theorists count it as bad for me if my desire is not fulfilled, even if, because I am an exile, I never know this. How then can it matter whether, when my desire is not fulfilled, I am dead? All that my death does is to *ensure* that I will never know this. If we think it irrelevant that I never know about the non-fulfilment of my desire, we cannot defensibly claim that my death makes a difference.

I turn now to questions and objections which arise for both Preference-Hedonism and the Success Theory.

Should we appeal only to the desires and preferences that someone actually has? Return to my choice between going to a party or staying at home to read *King Lear*. Suppose that, knowing what both alternatives would be like, I choose to stay at home. And suppose that I never later regret this choice. On one theory, this shows that staying at home to read *King Lear* gave me a better evening. This is a mistake. It might be true that, if I had chosen to go to the party, I would never have regretted that choice. According to this theory, this would have shown that going to the party gave me a better evening. This theory thus implies that each alternative would have been better than the other. Since this theory implies such contradictions, it must be revised. The obvious revision is to appeal not only to my actual preferences, in the alternative I choose, but also to the preferences that I would have had if I had chosen otherwise.[1]

In this example, whichever alternative I choose, I would never regret this choice. If this is true, can we still claim that one of the alternatives would give me a better evening? On some theories, when in two alternatives I would have such contrary preferences, neither alternative is better or worse for me. This is not plausible when one of my contrary preferences would have been much stronger. Suppose that, if I choose to go to the party, I shall be only mildly glad that I made this choice, but that, if I choose to stay and read *King Lear*, I shall be extremely glad. If this is true, reading *King Lear* gives me a better evening.

Whether we appeal to Preference-Hedonism or the Success Theory, we should not appeal only to the desires or preferences that I actually have. We should also appeal to the desires and preferences that I would have had, in the various alternatives that were, at different times, open to me. One of these alternatives would be best for me if it is the one in which I would have the strongest desires and preferences fulfilled. This allows us to claim that some alternative life would have been better for me, even if throughout my actual life I am glad that I chose this life rather than this alternative. [. . .]

---

[1] See P. Bricker, 'Prudence', *The Journal of Philosophy*, 83/7 (July, 1980).

Turn now to the third kind of Theory that I mentioned: the Objective List Theory. According to this theory, certain things are good or bad for people, whether or not these people would want to have the good things, or to avoid the bad things. The good things might include moral goodness, rational activity, the development of one's abilities, having children and being a good parent, knowledge, and the awareness of true beauty. The bad things might include being betrayed, manipulated, slandered, deceived, being deprived of liberty or dignity, and enjoying either sadistic pleasure, or aesthetic pleasure in what is in fact ugly.[1]

An Objective List Theorist might claim that his theory coincides with the Global version of the Success Theory. On this theory, what would make my life go best depends on what I would prefer, now and in the various alternatives, if I knew all of the relevant facts about these alternatives. An Objective List Theorist might say that the most relevant facts are what his theory claims—what would in fact be good or bad for me. And he might claim that anyone who knew these facts would want what is truly good for him, and want to avoid what would be bad for him.

If this was true, though the Objective List Theory would coincide with the Success Theory, the two theories would remain distinct. A Success Theorist would reject this description of the coincidence. On his theory, nothing is good or bad for people, whatever their preferences are. Something is bad for someone only if, knowing the facts, he wants to avoid it. And the relevant facts do not include the alleged facts cited by the Objective List Theorist. On the Success Theory it is, for instance, bad for someone to be deceived if and because this is not what he wants. The Objective List Theorist makes the reverse claim. People want not to be deceived because this is bad for them.

As these remarks imply, there is one important difference between on the one hand Preference-Hedonism and the Success Theory, and on the other hand the Objective List Theory. The first two kinds of theory give an account of self-interest which is entirely factual, or which does not appeal to facts about value. The account appeals to what a person does and would prefer, given full knowledge of the purely non-evaluative facts about the alternatives. In contrast, the Objective List Theory appeals directly to facts about value.

In choosing between these theories, we must decide how much weight to give to imagined cases in which someone's fully informed preferences would be bizarre. If we can appeal to these cases, they cast doubt on both Preference-Hedonism and the Success Theory. Consider the man that Rawls imagined who wants to spend his life counting the numbers of blades of grass in different lawns. Suppose that this man knows that he

[1] H. Sidgwick, *The Methods of Ethics*, (Macmillan: London, 1907), 111–12.

could achieve great progress if instead he worked in some especially useful part of Applied Mathematics. Though he could achieve such significant results, he prefers to go on counting blades of grass. On the Success Theory, if we allow this theory to cover all imaginable cases, it could be better for this person if he counts his blades of grass rather than achieves great and beneficial results in Mathematics.

The counter-example might be more offensive. Suppose that what someone would most prefer, knowing the alternatives, is a life in which, without being detected, he causes as much pain as he can to other people. On the Success Theory, such a life would be what is best for this person.

We may be unable to accept these conclusions. Ought we therefore to abandon this theory? [. . .] Suppose we agree that, in some imagined cases, what someone would most want both now and later, fully knowing about the alternatives, would *not* be what would be best for him. If we accept this conclusion, it may seem that we must reject both Preference-Hedonism and the Success Theory. [. . .]

It might be claimed instead that we can dismiss the appeal to such imagined cases. It might be claimed that what people would in fact prefer, if they knew the relevant facts, would always be something that we could accept as what is really good for them. Is this a good reply? If we agree that in the imagined cases what someone would prefer might be something that is bad for him, in these cases we have abandoned our theory. If this is so, can we defend our theory by saying that, in the actual cases, it would not go astray? I believe that this is not an adequate defence. But I shall not pursue this question here.

This objection may apply with less force to Preference-Hedonism. On this theory, what can be good or bad for someone can only be discernible features of his conscious life. These are the features that, at the time, he either wants or does not want. I asked above whether it is bad for people to be deceived because they prefer not to be, or whether they prefer not to be deceived because this is bad for them. Consider the comparable question with respect to pain. Some have claimed that pain is intrinsically bad, and that this is why we dislike it. As I have suggested, I doubt this claim. After taking certain kinds of drug, people claim that the quality of their sensations has not altered, but they no longer dislike these sensations. We would regard such drugs as effective analgesics. This suggests that the badness of a pain consists in its being disliked, and that it is not disliked because it is bad. The disagreement between these views would need much more discussion. But, if the second view is better, it is more plausible to claim that whatever someone wants or does not want to experience—however bizarre we find his desires—should be counted as being for this person truly pleasant or painful, and as being for that reason good or bad for him. There may still be cases where it is plausible to claim that it would be bad for someone if he enjoys certain kinds of pleasure. This might be claimed, for instance, about sadistic pleasure. But there may be few such cases.

If instead we appeal to the Success Theory, we are not concerned only with the experienced quality of our conscious life. We are concerned with such things as whether we are achieving what we are trying to achieve, whether we are being deceived, and the like. When considering this theory, we can more often plausibly claim that, even if someone knew the facts, his preferences might go astray, and fail to correspond to what would be good or bad for him.

Which of these different theories should we accept? I shall not attempt an answer here. But I shall end by mentioning another theory, which might be claimed to combine what is most plausible in these conflicting theories. It is a striking fact that those who have addressed this question have disagreed so fundamentally. Many philosophers have been convinced Hedonists; many others have been as much convinced that Hedonism is a gross mistake.

Some Hedonists have reached their view as follows. They consider an opposing view, such as that which claims that what is good for someone is to have knowledge, to engage in rational activity, and to be aware of true beauty. These Hedonists ask, 'Would these states of mind be good, if they brought no enjoyment, and if the person in these states of mind had not the slightest desire that they continue?' Since they answer No, they conclude that the value of these states of mind must lie in their being liked, and in their arousing a desire that they continue.

This reasoning assumes that the value of a whole is just the sum of the value of its parts. If we remove the part to which the Hedonist appeals, what is left seems to have no value, hence Hedonism is the truth.

Suppose instead that we claim that the value of a whole may not be a mere sum of the value of its parts. We might then claim that what is best for people is a composite. It is not just their being in the conscious states that they want to be in. Nor is it just their having knowledge, engaging in rational activity, being aware of true beauty, and the like. What is good for someone is neither just what Hedonists claim, nor just what is claimed by Objective List Theorists. We might believe that if we had *either* of these, *without the other*, what we had would have little or no value. We might claim, for example, that what is good or bad for someone is to have knowledge, to be engaged in rational activity, to experience mutual love, and to be aware of beauty, while strongly wanting just these things. On this view, each side in this disagreement saw only half of the truth. Each put forward as sufficient something that was only necessary. Pleasure with many other kinds of object has no value. And, if they are entirely devoid of pleasure, there is no value in knowledge, rational activity, love, or the awareness of beauty. What is of value, or is good for someone, is to have both; to be engaged in these activities, and to be strongly wanting to be so engaged.

[*Reasons and Persons* (Oxford University Press: Oxford, 1984), 493–502.]

Section B

Deciding What Is Right

INTRODUCTION

The great divide within ethics is between those who judge an act right or wrong in accordance with whether it produces the best consequences, and those who judge right and wrong by some rule or principle. This section presents the major theories on both sides of this divide, and examples of important lines of objection to each theory.

Those who judge acts by their consequences are now known as consequentialists. They used to be known as utilitarians, but that term can be confusing, because it is also used to refer to one specific kind of consequentialist, namely, those who judge acts by the net amount of pleasure or happiness that they produce. Since pleasure or happiness is not the only possible intrinsic good, there can be consequentialists who are not utilitarians, in this sense of the term. Opponents of consequentialism support several different theories. Those included here are: natural law theory (with which, for convenience of presentation, I group theories based on respect for rights, even though rights-based theories may or may not be based on claims about natural law); a Kantian approach to ethics; and a social contract theory of ethics.

The subsection on natural law and natural rights begins with Thomas Aquinas, the medieval scholastic who made it his life's work to harmonize Aristotle's philosophy with Christian teachings. The result remains the semi-official philosophy of the Roman Catholic Church to this day, and most adherents of natural law ethics are Roman Catholics. Natural law is not, as is sometimes imagined, based on favouring what is 'natural' as opposed to what is 'artificial'. As John Stuart Mill points out, appeals to 'nature' as the basis of ethical judgement often lead us astray. The idea behind natural law ethics is that we have, within our own nature, a guide to what is good for us. If we follow our own nature, we will flourish. The problem is to know what it is that our nature guides us to do, because there is no objective or agreed way of deciding what our nature is. The kind of material presented in Part IB of this book would be one place to start, but in fact natural law theorists have never taken part in this kind of empirical investigation. If they did, they would no doubt find that human nature is compatible with a variety of arrangements, some very different from the standards upheld by the Catholic Church.

The system of natural law ethics developed over many centuries by Catholic theologians and philosophers is of great interest, quite apart from one's views about the Catholic religion, because it reveals more clearly than any other system of ethics the difficulties of adhering to an ethic based on rules that must not be violated. Blaise Pascal's *Provincial Letters*, written in 1656–7 in the form of imaginary letters home from a student of theology, is a devastating critique of the way in which the Jesuits of his day were interpreting rules—for example, against killing or against telling lies—in order to get around them. But in case anyone thinks that such Jesuitical moral arguments existed only in the seventeenth century, I have included two modern applications of natural law theory. One is a Vatican statement that struggles to distinguish euthanasia, which it rejects, from some common and humane, but clearly life-shortening, ways of treating dying patients, which it does not want to prohibit. The other, a short passage on the ethics of obtaining semen for sterility tests, comes from a textbook on medical ethics by a twentieth-century Jesuit, Gerald Kelly. I do not want to suggest that Jesuits are more prone to draw contrived distinctions than anyone else. On the contrary, my point is that when we take inviolable rules as the basis of ethics, we have to be very precise about the boundaries of the rules; and in drawing these boundaries, the rules will be interpreted so as to enable us to achieve the ends that we judge desirable. The only viable alternative is to abandon the ethic of absolute rules.

Included within the same subsection are some writings on rights. John Finnis defends absolute rights on the basis of a natural law ethic of the kind just discussed, and contrasts this with alternative ethical approaches. John Locke represents a very different kind of natural law tradition. He begins with rights that exist in a state of nature, and argues that they are retained by the citizens even when the state of nature is past. This view of rights has been a major influence on the development of the American constitution, and thereby on ethical thinking in America, where there is a greater tendency to couch arguments in terms of rights than in any other country. Robert Nozick examines the way in which rights can be part of an ethical theory that is structured differently from a consequentialist ethic. Jeremy Bentham takes the opposite point of view: in his examination of the Declaration of Rights issued by the French National Assembly in 1791, he denounces the lofty appeals that the French revolutionaries made to 'natural and imprescriptible rights' as 'terrorist language' and 'nonsense upon stilts'.

Kant presented his own form of non-consequentialist ethic in several works. The first extract here is a further passage from his major work on ethics, *The Foundations of the Metaphysics of Morals*, which we met earlier in Part IC. It gives some examples of the application of the categorical imperative, and of Kant's ethics of duty. The second extract, taken from a brief essay 'On a Supposed Right to Lie from Altruistic Motives', shows how firmly Kant rejects any consideration of consequences, even when a life is at stake.

The two essays that follow explore aspects of Kant's ethics in the light of its impact on the lives of two very different people. Rae Langton draws on little-known correspondence between Kant and a young woman to show how Kant fails to respond properly to a real moral problem—and how a rather different Kant, more open to considering the consequences of actions, could have given a much more adequate reply. Jonathan Bennett's essay is not only about its titular character, the fictional Huckleberry Finn, but also about the regrettably non-fictional Heinrich Himmler and the Calvinist theologian Jonathan Edwards. Bennett's essay is a warning against any ethics that is based on the (recognizably Kantian) idea that our actions must be governed by our sense of duty, not our human sympathies.

We turn now to consequentialism, beginning with Jeremy Bentham's confident assertion of the principle of utility from the opening chapter of his major work on ethics, *Introduction to the Theory of Morals and Legislation*. This is followed by a passage from William Godwin's *Political Justice*, a work based on utilitarian foundations. In this extract Godwin is applying the principle that we ought to act so as to bring about the greatest good to a case in which you must choose between saving a great man or his chambermaid, who happens to be your mother. Ever since *Political Justice* first appeared in 1793, Godwin's decision in this hypothetical case has been seized on by critics of utilitarianism as an illustration of the inhuman tendencies of this doctrine.

In the selections from *The Methods of Ethics*, Henry Sidgwick considers some difficult issues for utilitarians. At the outset, there are questions about the scope of the principle. Should we try to produce the greatest amount of happiness for human beings or for all sentient creatures? And is it only good to increase happiness by making existing beings happier, or is it also good to bring into existence beings who will be happy? On the first question, virtually every utilitarian has given the more inclusive answer, as Sidgwick does; but on the second (which Sigwick raises here for the first time) there is continuing disagreement, and a certain amount of bafflement at the difficulty of finding a convincing answer that does not do violence to most people's intuitions.

Next Sidgwick considers that it may, on utilitarian grounds, be right to act in a certain way, but not openly to advocate that people should act in that way. In other words, utilitarians (and other consequentialists) may be compelled, by their own principles, to do good in secret. To some critics of utilitarianism, this possibility has seemed so paradoxical that they regard it as a ground for rejecting utilitarianism; for Sidgwick, however, it is merely an implication of the fact that we do not live in 'an ideal community of enlightened Utilitarians'. In the reading that follows, the contemporary utilitarian J. J. C. Smart continues the discussion about the relationship between utilitarianism and conventional moral rules, this time introducing another much-used hypothetical example, the desert island promise.

R. M. Hare has done more than any other twentieth-century philosopher to provide a theoretical basis for a modern form of consequentialism. The article reprinted here provides a summary version of his position, developed over the past forty years in *The Language of Morals*, *Freedom and Reason* and *Moral Thinking*, as well as in numerous articles. If Hare's argument is sound, this work has achieved three remarkable results: it has vindicated consequentialism as an ethical theory; it has reconciled consequentialism and Kant's method of moral reasoning (not, of course, Kant's actual moral views); and it has resolved the problem raised in Part IC of this book, by demonstrating that reason has a substantial role to play in ethics.

The subsection on consequentialism concludes with some celebrated objections, old and new: the challenge put by Dostoevsky in *The Karamazov Brothers*; W. D. Ross's stand on the intuitions of 'the plain man' about the specific character of our duties; John Rawls's assertion that utilitarianism fails to respect the separateness of persons; and Bernard Williams's claim that utilitarianism does not have a place for the value of integrity. Susan Wolf's essay 'Moral Saints' is a more radical attack on both consequentialist and Kantian moral theories, raising fundamental questions about the role of such theories as ultimate guides to how we ought to live.

In the final subsection, on social contract ethics, we seem to have come full circle, since the idea of a contract was one of the earliest explanations for the origin of ethics. But the twentieth-century revival of interest in contract ethics is not due to any belief that ethics had its origin in a social contract, either explicit or tacit. Instead, this interest is due to the hope that the social contract model can help us to grasp the basic principles of a justifiable system of ethics, and that, because it starts from the need to reach agreement between separate individuals, it can provide an alternative to consequentialist theories which neglect the separateness of persons. To demonstrate that a particular set of ethical principles would be agreed to by independent agents bargaining from a position of initial equality would give those ethical principles special significance. Perhaps, though, independent agents in this situation would choose whatever principles would maximize their prospects of getting what they want. In that case, contract ethics would take us straight back to a form of consequentialism, but one limited in scope to bringing about the greatest good of the contracting parties. Hence it is no surprise that, as Mary Midgley shows in the final reading in this section, the contract model takes no account of important aspects of ethics.

i Natural Law, Natural Rights

a The Theory

THOMAS AQUINAS

64   **Of the Natural Law**

[T]he precepts of the natural law are to the practical reason what the first principles of demonstrations are to the speculative reason, because both are self-evident principles. Now a thing is said to be self-evident in two ways: first, in itself; secondly, in relation to us. Any proposition is said to be self-evident in itself if its predicate is contained in the notion of the subject, although to one who knows not the definition of the subject it happens that such a proposition is not self-evident. For instance, this proposition, 'Man is a rational being,' is, in its very nature, self-evident, since who says 'man' says 'a rational being'; and yet to one who knows not what a man is, this proposition is not self-evident. Hence it is that, as Boethius says, certain axioms or propositions are universally self-evident to all; and such are those propositions whose terms are known to all, as, 'Every whole is greater than its part,' and, 'Things equal to one and the same are equal to one another.' But some propositions are self-evident only to the wise who understand the meaning of the terms of such propositions; thus to one who understands that an angel is not a body, it is self-evident that an angel is not circumspectively in a place; but this is not evident to the unlearned, for they cannot grasp it.

Now a certain order is to be found in those things that are apprehended universally. For that which, before aught else, falls under apprehension, is 'being,' the notion of which is included in all things whatsoever a man apprehends. Wherefore the first indemonstrable principle is that *the same thing cannot be affirmed and denied at the same time*, which is based on the notion of 'being' and 'not-being'; and on this principle all others are based. Now as 'being' is the first thing that falls under the apprehension simply, so 'good' is the first thing that falls under the apprehension of the practical reason, which is directed to action, since every agent acts for an end under the aspect of good. Consequently the first principle in the practical reason is one founded on the notion of good, viz., that *good is that which all things seek after*. Hence this is the first precept of law, that *good is to be done and ensued, and evil is to be avoided*. All other precepts of the natural law are based upon this, so that whatever the practical reason naturally apprehends as man's good (or evil) belongs to the precepts of the natural law as something to be done or avoided.

Since, however, good has the nature of an end, and evil the nature of a contrary, hence it is that all those things to which man has a natural inclination are naturally apprehended by reason as being good and, consequently, as objects of pursuit, and their contraries as evil and objects of avoidance. Wherefore the order of the precepts of the natural law is according to the order of natural inclinations. Because in man there is first of all an inclination to good in accordance with the nature which he has in common with all substances, inasmuch as every substance seeks the preservation of its own being, according to its nature; and by reason of this inclination, whatever is a means of preserving human life and of warding off its obstacles belongs to the natural law. Secondly, there is in man an inclination to things that pertain to him more specially, according to that nature which he has in common with other animals; and in virtue of this inclination, those things are said to belong to the natural law 'which nature has taught to all animals,' such as sexual intercourse, education of offspring, and so forth. Thirdly, there is in man an inclination to good, according to the nature of his reason, which nature is proper to him: thus man has a natural inclination to know the truth about God and to live in society; and in this respect, whatever pertains to this inclination belongs to the natural law, for instance, to shun ignorance, to avoid offending those among whom one has to live, and other such things regarding the above inclination. [. . .]

[T]o the natural law belong those things to which a man is inclined naturally; [and among these it is a special property of man to be inclined to act according to reason. Now reason proceeds from what is common, or general, to what is proper, or special. But there is a difference in this regard between the speculative reason and practical reason. The speculative reason is concerned primarily with what is necessary, that is, with those things which cannot be other than they are; and therefore, in the case of speculative reason, both the common principles and the special conclusions are necessarily true. In the case of the practical reason, on the other hand, which is concerned with contingent matters, such as human actions, even though there be some necessary truth in the common principles, yet the more we descend to what is proper and peculiar, the more deviations we find. Therefore in speculative matters the same truth holds among all men both as to principles and as to conclusions, even though all men do not discern this truth in the conclusions but only in those principles which are called axiomatic notions. In active matters, on the other hand, all men do not hold to the same truth or practical rectitude in what is peculiar and proper, but only in what is common. And even among those who hold to the same line of rectitude in proper and peculiar matters, such rectitude is not equally known to all. It is clear, therefore, that as far as common principles are concerned in the case of speculative as well as of practical reason the same truth and the same rectitude exists among all and is equally known to all. In the case, however, of the proper or peculiar conclusions of speculative reason, the same truth obtains among all, even though it is not known equally to all. For it is true among all men that the three angles of a triangle are equal to two right angles, even though not all men know this. But in the case of the proper or peculiar conclusions of the practical reason there is neither the same truth and rectitude among all men, nor, where it does exist, is it equally known to all. Thus it is true and right among all men that action proceed in accordance with reason. From this principle there follows as a proper conclusion that deposits should be restored to the owner. This conclusion is indeed true in the majority of cases. But a case may possibly arise in which such restitution is harmful and consequently contrary to reason; so, for example, if things deposited were claimed so that they might be used against the fatherland. This uncertainty increases the more particular the cases become: as, for example, if it were laid down that the restitution should take place in a certain way, with certain *definite* precautions; for as the limiting particular conditions become more numerous, so do the possibilities decrease that render the principle normally applicable, with the result that neither the restitution nor the failure to do so can be rigorously presented as right.

It follows therefore that natural law in its first common principles is the same among all men, both as to validity and recognition (something is right for all and is so by all recognized). But as to certain proper or derived norms, which are, as it were, conclusions of these common principles, they are valid and are so recognized by all men only in the majority of cases. For in special cases they may prove defective both as to validity because of certain particular impediments (just as things of nature in the sphere of generation and corruption prove to be defective because of impediments) and also as to recognition. And this because some men have a reason that has been distorted by passion, or by evil habits, or by bad natural relations. Such was the case among the ancient Germans, who failed to recognize theft as contrary to justice, as Julius Caesar relates, even though it is an explicit violation of natural law.

[*Summa Theologica*, II / i, Question 94, Articles 2 and 4, in *The Political Ideas of St Thomas Aquinas*, ed. Dino Bignongiari (Hafner: New York, 1953), 44–50. Written in 1266–77.]

JOHN LOCKE

65 Our Rights in the State of Nature

The state of nature has a law of nature to govern it, which obliges every one, and reason, which is that law, teaches all mankind, who will but consult it, that being all equal and independent, no one ought to harm another in his life, health, liberty, or possessions: for men being all the workmanship of one omnipotent, and infinitely wise maker; all the servants of one sovereign master, sent into the world by his order, and about his business; they are his property, whose workmanship they are, made to last during his, not one another's pleasure: and being furnished with like faculties, sharing all in one community of nature, there cannot be supposed any such subordination among us, that may authorize us to destroy one another, as if we were made for one another's uses, as the inferior ranks of creatures are for ours. Every one, as he is bound to preserve himself, and not to quit his station wilfully, so by the like reason, when his own preservation comes not in competition, ought he as much as he can to preserve the rest of mankind, and not unless it be to do justice on an offender, take away, or impair the life, or what tends to the preservation of the life, the liberty, health, limb or goods of another.

7. And that all men may be restrained from invading others rights, and from doing hurt to one another, and the law of nature be observed, which willeth the peace and preservation of all mankind, the execution of the law of nature is, in that state, put into every man's hands, whereby every one has a right to punish the transgressors of that law to such a degree, as may hinder its violation. For the law of nature would, as all other laws that concern men in this world, be in vain, if there were nobody that in the state of nature had a power to execute that law, and thereby preserve the innocent and restrain offenders. And if any one in the state of nature may punish another for any evil he has done, every one may do so: for in that state of perfect equality where naturally there is no superiority or jurisdiction of one over another, what any may do in prosecution of that law, every one must needs have a right to do.

8. And thus, in the state of nature, one man comes by a power over another; but yet no absolute or arbitrary power, to use a criminal, when he has got him in his hands, according to the passionate heats, or boundless extravagancy of his own will; but only to retribute to him, so far as calm reason and conscience dictates, what is proportionate to his transgression, which is so much as may serve for reparation and restraint: for these two are the only reasons why one man may lawfully do harm to another, which is that we call punishment. In transgressing the law of nature, the offender declares himself to live by another rule than that of reason and common equity, which is that measure God has set to the actions of men for their mutual security, and so he becomes dangerous to mankind, the tie, which is to secure them from injury and violence, being slighted and broken by him, which being a trespass against the whole species, and the peace and safety of it, provided for by the law of nature, every man upon this score, by the right he hath to preserve mankind in general, may restrain, or where it is necessary, destroy things noxious to them, and so may bring such evil

on any one, who hath transgressed that law, as may make him repent the doing of it, and thereby deter him, and, by his example others, from doing the like mischief. And in this case, and upon this ground, every man hath a right to punish the offender, and be executioner of the law of nature. [. . .]

14. 'Tis often asked as a mighty objection, where are, or ever were there any men in such a state of nature? To which it may suffice as an answer at present, that since all princes and rulers of *independent* governments all through the world, are in a state of nature, 'tis plain the world never was, nor never will be, without numbers of men in that state. I have named all governors of *independent* communities, whether they are, or are not, in league with others: for 'tis not every compact that puts an end to the state of nature between men, but only this one of agreeing together mutually to enter into one community, and make one body politic; other promises, and compacts, men may make one with another, and yet still be in the state of nature. The promises and bargains for truck, etc. between the two men in the desert island, mentioned by Garcilasso de la Vega, in his history of Peru; or between a Swiss and an Indian, in the woods of America, are binding to them, though they are perfectly in a state of nature, in reference to one another: for truth and keeping of faith belongs to men as men, and not as members of society.

15. To those that say, there were never any men in the state of nature, I will not only oppose the authority of the judicious Hooker, *Eccl. Pol.* lib. i. *sect.* 10, where he says, 'the laws which have been hitherto mentioned, *i.e.* the laws of nature, do bind men absolutely, even as they are men, although they have never any settled fellowship, never any solemn agreement amongst themselves what to do, or not to do: but forasmuch as we are not by ourselves sufficient to furnish ourselves with competent store of things, needful for such a life as our nature doth desire, a life fit for the dignity of man; therefore to supply those defects and imperfections which are in us, as living singly and solely by ourselves, we are naturally induced to seek communion and fellowship with others: this was the cause of men uniting themselves at first in politic societies.' But I moreover affirm, that all men are naturally in that state, and remain so, till by their own consents they make themselves members of some politic society; and I doubt not in the sequel of this discourse, to make it very clear. [. . .]

25. Whether we consider natural reason, which tells us that men, being once born, have a right to their preservation, and consequently to meat and drink and such other things as Nature affords for their subsistence, or *revelation*, which gives us an account of those grants God made of the world to Adam, and to Noah and his sons, 'tis very clear that God, as King David says, *Psalm* CXV. 16, *has given the earth to the children of men*, given it to mankind in common. But, this being supposed, it seems to some a very

great difficulty how any one should ever come to have a property in anything. [. . .] I shall endeavour to shew how men might come to have a property in several parts of that which God gave to mankind in common, and that without any express compact of all the commoners.

26. God, who hath given the world to men in common, hath also given them reason to make use of it to the best advantage of life and convenience. The earth and all that is therein is given to men for the support and comfort of their being. And though all the fruits it naturally produces, and beasts it feeds, belong to mankind in common, as they are produced by the spontaneous hand of nature, and no body has originally a private dominion exclusive of the rest of mankind in any of them, as they are thus in their natural state, yet being given for the use of men, there must of necessity be a means to appropriate them some way or other before they can be of any use, or at all beneficial, to any particular man. The fruit or venison which nourishes the wild Indian, who knows no enclosure, and is still a tenant in common, must be his, and so his—i.e. a part of him, that another can no longer have any right to it before it can do him any good for the support of his life.

27. Though the earth and all inferior creatures be common to all men, yet every man has a *property* in his own *person*. This nobody has any right to but himself. The *labour* of his body and the *work* of his hands, we may say, are properly his. Whatsoever, then, he removes out of the state that nature hath provided and left it in, he hath mixed his labour with it, and joined to it something that is his own, and thereby makes it his property. It being by him removed from the common state nature placed it in, it hath by this labour something annexed to it that excludes the common right of other men. For this labour being the unquestionable property of the labourer, no man but he can have a right to what that is once joined to, at least where there is enough, and as good left in common for others.

28. He that is nourished by the acorns he picked up under an oak, or the apples he gathered from the trees in the wood, has certainly appropriated them to himself. Nobody can deny but the nourishment is his. I ask, then, when did they begin to be his? when he digested? or when he ate? or when he boiled? or when he brought them home? or when he picked them up? And 'tis plain, if the first gathering made them not his, nothing else could. That labour put a distinction between them and common. That added something to them more than Nature, the common mother of all, had done, and so they became his private right. And will any one say he had no right to those acorns or apples he thus appropriated because he had not the consent of all mankind to make them his? Was it a robbery thus to assume to himself what belonged to all in common? If such a consent as that was necessary, man had starved, notwithstanding the plenty God had given him. We see in commons, which remain so by compact, that 'tis the taking any part of what is common, and removing it out of the state Nature leaves

it in, which begins the property, without which the common is of no use. And the taking of this or that part does not depend on the express consent of all the commoners. Thus, the grass my horse has bit, the turfs my servant has cut, and the ore I have digged in any place, where I have a right to them in common with others, become my property without the assignation or consent of any body. The labour that was mine, removing them out of that common state they were in, hath fixed my property in them.

['Second Treatise on Civil Government', in *Social Contract*, ed. E. Barker (Oxford University Press: London, 1960), 7–9, 14–15, 23–6. First published in 1690.]

THE VATICAN

66 Declaration on Euthanasia

In order that the question of euthanasia can be properly dealt with, it is first necessary to define the words used.

Etymologically speaking, in ancient times *euthanasia* meant an *easy death* without severe suffering. Today one no longer thinks of this original meaning of the word, but rather of some intervention of medicine whereby the sufferings of sickness or of the final agony are reduced, sometimes also with the danger of suppressing life prematurely. Ultimately, the word *euthanasia* is used in a more particular sense to mean 'mercy killing', for the purpose of putting an end to extreme suffering, or saving abnormal babies, the mentally ill or the incurably sick from the prolongation, perhaps for many years, of a miserable life, which could impose too heavy a burden on their families or on society.

It is therefore necessary to state clearly in what sense the word is used in the present document.

By euthanasia is understood an action or an omission which of itself or by intention causes death, in order that all suffering may in this way be eliminated. Euthanasia's terms of reference, therefore, are to be found in the intention of the will and in the methods used.

It is necessary to state firmly once more that nothing and no one can in any way permit the killing of an innocent human being, whether a foetus or an embryo, an infant or an adult, an old person, or one suffering from an incurable disease, or a person who is dying. Furthermore, no one is permitted to ask for this act of killing, either for himself or herself or for another person entrusted to his or her care, nor can he or she consent to it, either explicitly or implicitly. Nor can any authority legitimately recommend or permit such an action. For it is a question of the violation of the divine law, an offence against the dignity of the human person, a crime against life, and an attack on humanity.

It may happen that, by reason of prolonged and barely tolerable pain, for deeply personal or other reasons, people may be led to believe that they can legitimately ask for death or obtain it for others. Although in these cases the guilt of the individual may be reduced or completely absent, nevertheless the error of judgment into which the conscience falls, perhaps in good faith, does not change the nature of this act of killing, which will always be in itself something to be rejected. The pleas of gravely ill people who sometimes ask for death are not to be understood as implying a true desire for euthanasia; in fact it is almost always a case of an anguished plea for help and love. What a sick person needs, besides medical care, is love, the human and supernatural warmth with which the sick person can and ought to be surrounded by all those close to him or her, parents and children, doctors and nurses.

The Meaning of Suffering for Christians and the Use of Painkillers

Death does not always come in dramatic circumstances after barely tolerable sufferings. Nor do we have to think only of extreme cases. Numerous testimonies which confirm one another lead one to the conclusion that nature itself has made provision to render more bearable at the moment of death separations that would be terribly painful to a person in full health. Hence it is that a prolonged illness, advanced old age, or a state of loneliness or neglect can bring about psychological conditions that facilitate the acceptance of death.

Nevertheless the fact remains that death, often preceded or accompanied by severe and prolonged suffering, is something which naturally causes people anguish.

Physical suffering is certainly an unavoidable element of the human condition; on the biological level, it constitutes a warning of which no one denies the usefulness; but, since it affects the human psychological makeup, it often exceeds its own biological usefulness and so can become so severe as to cause the desire to remove it at any cost. [. . .]

But the intensive use of painkillers is not without difficulties, because the phenomenon of habituation generally makes it necessary to increase their dosage in order to maintain their efficacy. At this point it is fitting to recall a declaration by Pius XII, which retains its full force; in answer to a group of doctors who had put the question: 'Is the suppression of pain and consciousness by the use of narcotics . . . permitted by religion and morality to the doctor and the patient (even at the approach of death and if one foresees that the use of narcotics will shorten life)?', the Pope said: 'If no other means exist, and if, in the given circumstances, this does not prevent the carrying out of other religious and moral duties: Yes'. In this case, of course, death is in no way intended or sought, even if the risk of it is reasonably taken; the intention is simply to relieve pain effectively, using for this purpose painkillers available to medicine. [. . .]

Due Proportion in the Use of Remedies

Today it is very important to protect, at the moment of death, both the dignity of the human person and the Christian concept of life, against a technological attitude that threatens to become an abuse. Thus, some people speak of a 'right to die', which is an expression that does not mean the right to procure death either by one's own hand of by means of someone else, as one pleases, but rather the right to die peacefully with human and Christian dignity. From this point of view, the use of therapeutic means can sometimes pose problems.

In numerous cases, the complexity of the situation can be such as to cause doubts about the way ethical principles should be applied. In the final analysis, it pertains to the conscience either of the sick person, or of those qualified to speak in the sick person's name, or of the doctors, to decide, in the light of moral obligations and of the various aspects of the case.

Everyone has the duty to care for his or her own health or to seek such care from others. Those whose task it is to care for the sick must do so conscientiously and administer the remedies that seem necessary or useful.

However, is it necessary in all circumstances to have recourse to all possible remedies?

In the past, moralists replied that one is never obliged to use 'extraordinary' means. This reply, which as a principle still holds good, is perhaps less clear today, by reason of the imprecision of the term and the rapid progress made in the treatment of sickness. Thus some people prefer to speak of 'proportionate' and 'disproportionate' means. In any case, it will be possible to make a correct judgment as to the means by studying the type of treatment to be used, its degree of complexity or risk, its cost and the possibilities of using it, and comparing these elements with the result that can be expected, taking into account the state of the sick person and his or her physical and moral resources.

In order to facilitate the application of these general principles, the following clarifications can be added:

—If there are no other sufficient remedies, it is permitted, with the patient's consent, to have recourse to the means provided by the most advanced medical techniques, even if these means are still at the experimental stage and are not without a certain risk. By accepting them, the patient can even show generosity in the service of humanity.

—It is also permitted, with the patient's consent, to interrupt these means, where the results fall short of expectations. But for such a decision to be made, account will have to be taken of the reasonable wishes of the patient and the patient's family, as also of the advice of the doctors who are specially competent in the matter. The latter may in particular judge that the investment in instruments and personnel is disproportionate to the results foreseen; they may also judge that the techniques applied impose on the patient strain or suffering out of proportion with the benefits which he or she may gain from such techniques.

—It is also permissible to make do with the normal means that medicine can offer. Therefore one cannot impose on anyone the obligation to have recourse to a technique which is already in use but which carries a risk or is burdensome. Such a refusal is not the equivalent of suicide; on the contrary, it should be considered as an acceptance of the human condition, or a wish to avoid the application of a medical procedure disproportionate to the results that can be expected, or a desire not to impose excessive expense on the family or the community.

—When inevitable death is imminent in spite of the means used, it is permitted in conscience to take the decision to refuse forms of treatment that would only secure a precarious and burdensome prolongation of life, so long as the normal care due to the sick person in similar cases is not interrupted. In such circumstances the doctor has no reason to reproach himself with failing to help the person in danger.

[Sacred Congregation for the Declaration of the Faith, *Declaration on Euthanasia* (Vatican City, 1980), 6–11.]

JOHN FINNIS

67 Absolute Human Rights

Are there then no limits to what may be done in pursuit of protection of human rights or of other aspects of the common good? Are there no fixed points in that pattern of life which one must hold in one's mind's eye in resolving problems of rights? Are there no 'absolute' rights, rights that are not to be limited or overridden for the sake of any conception of the good life in community, not even 'to prevent catastrophe'?[1]

The answer of utilitarians, of course, is clear: there are no absolute human rights, for there are no ways of treating a person of which it can be said, by a consistent utilitarian, 'Whatever the consequences, nobody must ever be treated in this way'. What is more striking, perhaps, is the fact that, whatever may be commonly professed in the modern world, no contemporary government or élite manifests in its practice any belief in absolute human rights. For every government that has the physical capacity to make

[1] R. M. Dworkin, *Taking Rights Seriously* (Duckworth: London, 1977) 91.

its threats credible says this to its potential enemies: 'If you attack us and threaten to defeat us, we will kill all the hostages we hold; that is to say, we will incinerate or dismember as many of your old men and women and children, and poison as many of your mothers and their unborn offspring, as it takes to persuade you to desist; we do not regard as decisive the fact that they are themselves no threat to us; nor do we propose to destroy them merely incidentally, as an unsought-after side-effect of efforts to stop your armed forces in their attack on us; no, we will destroy your non-combatants precisely because you value them, and in order to *persuade* you to desist.' Those who say this, and have been preparing elaborately for years to act upon their threat (and most of them acted upon it massively, between 1943 and 1945, to say no more), cannot be said to accept that anyone has, in virtue of his humanity, any absolute right. These people subscribe to Bills of Rights which, like the Universal Declaration and its successors, clearly treat the right not to be tortured as (unlike most of the other 'inalienable' rights there proclaimed) subject to no exceptions. But their military policy involves courses of action which in all but name are torture on an unprecedented scale, inflicted for the same motive as an old-fashioned torturer seeking to change his victim's mind or the minds of those next in line for the torture. Nor is this just a matter of govern-ments and soldiers; many of these governments are freely elected, and their policy (as distinct from the dangers of pursuing it) arouses scant contro-versy among their electorates. And who does not notice the accomplished smoothness with which the issue is avoided by many who write about rights?

In its classical representatives the tradition of theorizing about natural law has never maintained that what I have called the requirements of practical reasonableness, as distinct from the basic human values or basic principles of practical reasonableness, are clearly recognized by all or even most people—on the contrary.[1] So we too need not hesitate to say that, notwithstanding the substantial consensus to the contrary, there are absol-ute human rights. For the seventh of the requirements of practical reason-ableness that I identified is this: that it is always unreasonable to choose directly against any basic value, whether in oneself or in one's fellow human beings. And the basic values are not mere abstractions; they are aspects of the real well-being of flesh-and-blood individuals. Correlative to the exceptionless duties entailed by this requirement are, therefore, excep-tionless or absolute human claim-rights—most obviously, the right not to have one's life taken directly as a means to any further end; but also the right not to be positively lied to in any situation (e.g. teaching, preaching,

---

[1] See e.g. Aquinas, *Summa Theologica*, I, q. 113, a. 1; I-II, q. 9, a. 5 ad 3; q. 14, a. 1 ad 3; q. 94, a. 4c; q. 99, a 2 ad 2.

research publication, news broadcasting) in which factual communication (as distinct from fiction, jest, or poetry) is reasonably expected; and the related right not to be condemned on knowingly false charges; and the right not to be deprived, or required to deprive oneself, of one's procreative capacity; and the right to be taken into respectful consideration in any assessment of what the common good requires.

Because these are claim-rights strictly correlative to duties entailed by the requirements of practical reasonableness, the difficult task of giving precision to the specification of these rights has usually been undertaken in terms of a casuistry of duties. And because an unwavering recognition of the literally immeasurable value of human personality in each of its basic aspects (the solid core of the notion of human dignity) requires us to discount the apparently measurable evil of looming catastrophes which really do threaten the common good and the enjoyment by others of *their* rights, that casuistry is more complex, difficult, and controvertible in its details than can be indicated in the foregoing summary list of absolute rights. That casuistry may be framed in terms of 'direct' choices or intentions, as against 'indirect' effects, and of 'means' as against 'incidents'. But reasonable judgments in this casuistry are not made by applying a 'logic' of 'directness and indirectness' of 'means and ends' or 'intended and unintended', drawn from the use of those notions in other enquiries or contexts. Rather, such judgments are arrived at by a steady determination to respect human good in one's own existence and the equivalent humanity or human rights of others, when that human good and those human rights fall directly into one's care and disposal—rather than trade off that good and those rights against some vision of future 'net best consequences', consequences which overall, both logically and practically, one cannot know, cannot control or dispose of, and cannot evaluate.

[*Natural Law and Natural Rights* (Oxford University Press: Oxford, 1980), 223–6.]

ROBERT NOZICK

68 **The Rationality of Side Constraints**

A proponent of the ultraminimal state may seem to occupy an inconsistent position. Greatly concerned to protect rights against violation, he makes this the sole legitimate function of the state; and he protests that all other functions are illegitimate because they themselves involve the violation of rights. Since he accords paramount place to the protection and nonviolation of rights, how can he support the ultraminimal state, which would seem to leave some persons' rights unprotected or illprotected? How can he support this *in the name of* the nonviolation of rights?

Moral Constraints and Moral Goals

This question assumes that a moral concern can function only as a moral *goal*, as an end state for some activities to achieve as their result. It may, indeed, seem to be a necessary truth that 'right,' 'ought,' 'should,' and so on, are to be explained in terms of what is, or is intended to be, productive of the greatest good, with all goals built into the good. Thus it is often thought that what is wrong with utilitarianism (which *is* of this form) is its too narrow conception of good. Utilitarianism doesn't, it is said, properly take rights and their nonviolation into account; it instead leaves them a derivative status. Many of the counterexample cases to utilitarianism fit under this objection, for example, punishing an innocent man to save a neighborhood from a vengeful rampage. But a theory may include in a primary way the nonviolation of rights, yet include it in the wrong place and the wrong manner. For suppose some condition about minimizing the total (weighted) amount of violations of rights is built into the desirable end state to be achieved. We then would have something like a 'utilitarianism of rights'; violations of rights (to be *minimized*) merely would replace the total happiness as the relevant end state in the utilitarian structure. (Note that we do not hold the nonviolation of our rights as our sole greatest good or even rank it first lexicographically to exclude trade-offs, if there is some desirable society we would choose to inhabit even though in it some rights of ours sometimes are violated, rather than move to a desert island where we could survive alone.) This still would require us to violate someone's rights when doing so minimizes the total (weighted) amount of the violation of rights in the society. For example, violating someone's rights might deflect others from *their* intended action of gravely violating rights, or might remove their motive for doing so, or might divert their attention, and so on. A mob rampaging through a part of town killing and burning *will* violate the rights of those living there. Therefore, someone might try to justify his punishing another *he* knows to be innocent of a crime that enraged a mob, on the grounds that punishing this innocent person would help to avoid even greater violations of rights by others, and so would lead to a minimum weighted score for rights violations in the society.

In contrast to incorporating rights into the end state to be achieved, one might place them as side constraints upon the actions to be done: don't violate constraints C. The rights of others determine the constraints upon your actions. (A *goal-directed* view with constraints added would be: among those acts available to you that don't violate constraints C, act so as to maximize goal G. Here, the rights of others would constrain your goal-directed behavior. I do not mean to imply that the correct moral view includes mandatory goals that must be pursued, even within the constraints.) This view differs from one that tries to build the side constraints C *into* the goal G. The side-constraint view forbids you to violate these moral constraints in the pursuit of your goals; whereas the view whose objective is to minimize the violation of these rights allows you to violate the rights (the constraints) in order to lessen their total violation in the society.[1]

The claim that the proponent of the ultraminimal state is inconsistent, we now can see, assumes that he is a 'utilitarian of rights.' It assumes that his goal is, for example, to minimize the weighted amount of the violation of rights in the society, and that he should pursue this goal even through means that themselves violate people's rights. Instead, he may place the nonviolation of rights as a constraint upon action, rather than (or in addition to) building it into the end state to be realized. The position held by this proponent of the ultraminimal state will be consistent one if his conception of rights holds that your being *forced* to contribute to another's welfare violates your rights, whereas someone else's not providing you with things you need greatly, including things essential to the protection of your rights, does not *itself* violate your rights, even though it avoids making it more difficult for someone else to violate them. (That conception will be consistent provided it does not construe the monopoly element of the ultraminimal state as itself a violation of rights.) That it is a consistent position does not, of course, show that it is an acceptable one.

Why Side Constraints?

Isn't it *irrational* to accept a side constraint C, rather than a view that directs minimizing the violations of C? (The latter view treats C as a condition rather than a constraint.) If nonviolation of C is so important, shouldn't that be the goal? How can a concern for the nonviolation of C lead to the refusal to violate C even when this would prevent other more extensive violations of C? What is the rationale for placing the nonviolation of rights as a side constraint upon action instead of including it solely as a goal of one's actions?

Side constraints upon action reflect the underlying Kantian principle that individuals are ends and not merely means; they may not be sacrificed or used for the achieving of other ends without their consent. Individuals are inviolable. More should be said to illuminate this talk of ends and means. Consider a prime example of a means, a tool. There is no side constraint on how we may use a tool, other than the moral constraints on how we may use it upon others. There are procedures to be followed to preserve it for

---

[1] The question of whether these side constraints are absolute, or whether they may be violated in order to avoid catastrophic moral horror, and if the latter, what the resulting structure might look like, is one I hope largely to avoid.

future use ('don't leave it out in the rain'), and there are more and less efficient ways of using it. But there is no limit on what we may do to it to best achieve our goals. Now imagine that there was an overrideable constraint C on some tool's use. For example, the tool might have been lent to you only on the condition that C not be violated unless the gain from doing so was above a certain specified amount, or unless it was necessary to achieve a certain specified goal. Here the object is not *completely* your tool, for use according to your wish or whim. But it is a tool nevertheless, even with regard to the overrideable constraint. If we add constraints on its use that may not be overridden, then the object may not be used as a tool *in those ways. In those respects*, it is not a tool at all. Can one add enough constraints so that an object cannot be used as a tool at all, in *any* respect?

Can behavior toward a person be constrained so that he is not to be used for any end except as he chooses? This is an impossibly stringent condition if it requires everyone who provides us with a good to approve positively of every use to which we wish to put it. Even the requirement that he merely should not object to any use we plan would seriously curtail bilateral exchange, not to mention sequences of such exchanges. It is sufficient that the other party stands to gain enough from the exchange so that he is willing to go through with it, even though he objects to one or more of the uses to which you shall put the good. Under such conditions, the other party is not being used solely as a means, in that respect. Another party, however, who would not choose to interact with you if he knew of the uses to which you *intend* to put his actions or good, *is* being used as a means, even if he receives enough to choose (in his ignorance) to interact with you. ('All along, you were just *using* me' can be said by someone who chose to interact only because he was ignorant of another's goals and of the uses to which he himself would be put.) Is it morally incumbent upon someone to reveal his intended uses of an interaction if he has good reason to believe the other would refuse to interact if he knew? Is he *using* the other person, if he does not reveal this? And what of the cases where the other does not choose to be of use at all? In getting pleasure from seeing an attractive person go by, does one use the other solely as a means? Does someone so use an object of sexual fantasies? These and related questions raise very interesting issues for moral philosophy; but not, I think, for political philosophy.

Political philosophy is concerned only with *certain* ways that persons may not use others; primarily, physically aggressing against them. A specific side constraint upon action toward others expresses the fact that others may not be used in the specific ways the side constraint excludes. Side constraints express the inviolability of others, in the ways they specify. These modes of inviolability are expressed by the following injunction: 'Don't use people in specified ways.' An end-state view, on the other hand, would express the view that people are ends and not merely means (if it chooses to express this view at all), by a different injunction: 'Minimize the use in specified ways of persons as means.' Following this precept itself may involve using someone as a means in one of the ways specified. Had Kant held this view, he would have given the second formula of the categorical imperative as, 'So act as to minimize the use of humanity simply as a means,' rather than the one he actually used: 'Act in such a way that you always treat humanity, whether in your own person or in the person of any other, never simply as a means, but always at the same time as an end.'

Side constraints express the inviolability of other persons. But why may not one violate persons for the greater social good? Individually, we each sometimes choose to undergo some pain or sacrifice for a greater benefit or to avoid a greater harm: we go to the dentist to avoid worse suffering later; we do some unpleasant work for its results; some persons diet to improve their health or looks; some save money to support themselves when they are older. In each case, some cost is borne for the sake of the greater overall good. Why not, *similarly*, hold that some persons have to bear some costs that benefit other persons more, for the sake of the overall social good? But there is no *social entity* with a good that undergoes some sacrifice for its own good. There are only individual people, different individual people, with their own individual lives. Using one of these people for the benefit of others, uses him and benefits the others. Nothing more. What happens is that something is done to him for the sake of others. Talk of an overall social good covers this up. (Intentionally?) To use a person in this way does not sufficiently respect and take account of the fact that he is a separate person, that his is the only life he has. *He* does not get some overbalancing good from his sacrifice, and no one is entitled to force this upon him—least of all a state or government that claims his allegiance (as other individuals do not) and that therefore scrupulously must be *neutral* between its citizens.

[*Anarchy, State and Utopia* (Basic Books: New York, 1974), 27–33.]

GERALD KELLY

69 Moral Aspects of Sterility Tests

In an age in which so much time, expense, and medical skill are spent in perfecting and explaining techniques of contraception, it is comforting to know that a large amount of effort and research is also being expended to cure infertility. The cure, of course, includes not only the therapy, but also the diagnostic procedures necessary to determine the cause of the infertility. I shall consider the moral aspects of some diagnostic procedures. [. . .]

The main problem relative to testing male infertility concerns the methods of obtaining semen for analysis. Unfortunately, we do not have the same harmony here between accepted medical practice and sound morality that exists with regard to diagnosis of the woman. All too often, physicians take it for granted that masturbation or some form of unnatural coitus is a permissible method of obtaining semen. Pope Pius XII scored this error in his address to participants in the Second World Congress of Fertility and Sterility, May 19, 1956. His condemnation explicitly referred only to masturbation, but it applies equally to any other unnatural sex act. Moreover, he was not stating anything new; he was simply giving the long-standing teaching of Catholic moralists, a teaching which is concisely formulated in directives 29 and 38. which read as follows:

29. The unnatural use of the sex faculty (e.g. masturbation) is never permitted, even for a laudable purpose.

38. Sterility tests involving the procurement of the male specimen by masturbation or unnatural intercourse are morally objectionable.

[. . .] I shall discuss the methods of obtaining semen under three classifications:

1. Sterility tests are *certainly illicit* when they involve the procuring of semen in any of the following ways.

a) masturbation;

b) the use of an unperforated condom or of a vaginal sheath which is the equivalent of a condom;

c) withdrawal before orgasm, with ejaculation outside the vagina.

In each of these cases there is an unnatural sex act: that is, the psychophysical processes that lead to the sexual orgasm are used in such a way that the orgasm itself takes place outside of coitus. It is true that there is an appearance of coitus in the second and third cases; but it is only an appearance. Ejaculation into the vagina is the determining factor of true coitus. The practices, therefore, are morally objectionable because they violate the principle: *It is never lawful, even for a laudable purpose, to use the generative faculty in an unnatural way.*

2. Sterility tests are *probably licit* when they involve the procuring of semen in any of the following ways:

a) intercourse with a condom so perforated that it allows some semen to be deposited in the vagina of the wife and also retains some semen for examination;

b) removal of semen, immediately or very soon after normal coitus, from the genital tract of the wife;

c) direct removal of semen, by aspiration, from testicles or epididymes;

d) expression of seminal fluid by massage, from seminal vesicles.

An action is said to be 'probably licit' when it is neither certainly right nor certainly wrong. That is the present status of each of the testing methods mentioned under this heading. Theologians are still debating them; and up to the present time reasons have been offered for and against each of these methods. It may be that in the future—even the very near future—some of the debatable points will be settled. Until these moral issues are further clarified, however, physicians may follow this practical rule: *When a testing method is not clearly wrong, that is, when there is some soundly probable reason for approving it, it may be used.*

A brief explanation of the theological controversies over these various methods may be helpful. As far as I know, the first theologian to mention the use of the perforated condom in his written works was the late Fr. Arthur Vermeersch, SJ, of the Gregorian University, Rome.[1] Fr. Vermeersch considered this method of obtaining semen to be immoral. His reason was that it involves the direct will to deposit some of the ejaculate outside of the vagina—something which makes it a 'partial onanism.' Agreeing with Fr. Vermeersch is Fr. Francis J. Connell, CSSR of the Catholic University of America.[2]

Favoring the licitness of the use of the perforated condom is Fr. J. McCarthy, of Maynooth College, Ireland, one of the clearest and most capable of present-day theological writers.[3] Fr. McCarthy believes that it is a mistake to analyze only the part of the act which involves the retaining of semen within the condom. He says that if the *entire* act is analyzed, it is seen to be *substantially natural* because a fair percentage of the semen is ejaculated into the vagina; and he believes that the mutilating of the act by retaining a small portion of the ejaculate in the condom may be justified for a proportionate reason. Fr. John J. Clifford, SJ, of the Seminary of St Mary of the Lake, Mundelein, Illinois, also thought the perforated condom may be used for obtaining a seminal specimen.[4] [. . .]

Although Fr. Vermeersch was opposed to the use of the perforated condom, he was very openly cooperative with physicians in trying to find a morally unobjectionable manner of obtaining a seminal specimen. It was he who first suggested that removal of semen from testicles or epididymes by aspiration or from vesicles by massage might be permitted. His reason for approving these methods was that the semen is thus obtained without

---

[1] *De castitate* (Rome: Gregorian University, 1921), 403.
[2] 'The Catholic Doctor', *American Ecclesiastical Review* (Dec. 1944), 439–48. In citing articles in this chapter, I am giving the complete reference, and not merely the page on which the pertinent opinions are stated.
[3] 'A Lawful Method of Procuring Seminal Specimens for Sterility Tests', *Irish Ecclesiastical Record* (June 1948), 533–6. The article is now incorporated into a book, *Problems in Theology* i. *The Sacraments* (The Newman Press: Westminster, Md., 1956), 430–3.
[4] 'Sterility Tests and Their Morality', *American Ecclesiastical Review* (Nov. 1942), 358–67.

stimulating the orgasmic processes; hence, there is no abuse of the sex faculty. Against Fr. Vermeersch, Fr. Benedict Merkelbach, OP, of the Angelicum, the Dominican university in Rome, argued that man's sole right to use his semen is confined to the exercise of the conjugal act.[1] Prominent theologians have lined up on each side of this debate; and today, though the original contestants are both deceased, the debate still goes on.

[*Medico-Moral Problems* (The Catholic Hospital Association of the United States and Canada: St Louis, 1958), 218–23.]

b. Criticism

BLAISE PASCAL

70 **Provincial Letters**

After I had soothed the good Father, whose talk had been somewhat disturbed by my story of Jean d'Alba, he resumed. [. . .]

'You should know then that this marvellous principle is our great method of *directing the intention*, which is so important in our morality. You have seen some of its features in passing, in certain principles I mentioned. For when I explained how servants can perform certain awkward commissions with a good conscience, did you not notice that it was only by deflecting their intention from the evil of which they are the accessories and applying it to the profit they get out of it? That is what *directing the intention* means. [. . .] But I now want to show you this great method in all its lustre, on the subject of homicide, which it justifies in innumerable circumstances, so that you may judge from such effects all that it is capable of producing.'

'I see already,' I said, 'that this will make everything permissible, nothing will escape it.'

'You go from one extreme to another,' answered the Father, 'you must cure yourself of that fault. As evidence that we do not permit everything, note, for instance, that we never tolerate anyone having the formal intention of sinning just for the sake of sinning; and that if anyone insists on having no other end in evil-doing but evil itself, we break with him; that is diabolical; to that there is no exception whether of age, sex or rank. But when people are not in this unhappy state of mind, then we try and put into practice our method of *directing the intention*, which consists in setting up as the purpose of one's action some lawful object. Not that we fail to deter men as far as we can from forbidden things, but when we cannot prevent

[1] *Quaestiones de castitate et luxuria* (La Pensée Catholique: Liège, 1936), 60–2.

the action, at least we purify the intention; and thus we correct the viciousness of the means by the purity of the end.

'That is how our Fathers have found a way to permit the acts of violence commonly practised in the defence of honour. For it is only a question of deflecting one's intention from the desire for vengeance, which is criminal, and applying it to the desire to defend one's honour, which according to our Fathers is lawful. And so it is that they fulfil all their duties to God and to men. For they content the world by permitting such actions; and they satisfy the Gospel by purifying intentions. That is something the ancients never knew; that is something you owe to our Fathers. Now do you understand?'

'Very well,' I said. 'You grant men the crude substance of things and give God this spiritual movement of the intention; and by this equitable allocation you unite human and divine laws. But Father, to tell you the truth, I am a little wary of your promises, and I feel doubtful whether your authors go as far as you.' [. . .]

'Show me,' I said, 'with all your direction of intention that it is lawful to fight a duel.'

'Our great Hurtado de Mendoza,' said the Father, 'will give you immediate satisfaction, in this passage quoted by Diana, p. 5, tr. 14, R. 99: "If a gentleman who is challenged to a duel is known not to be devout, and the sins which he is seen constantly committing without any scruples make it obvious that any refusal to duel will be motivated not by any fear of God but by cowardice; and so that it is said of him that he has the heart of a chicken and not a man, *gallina et non vir*, to preserve his honour he may be at the spot assigned, not, it is true, with the express intention of fighting a duel, but merely with that of self-defence if his challenger comes there to attack him unjustly. And in itself his action will be quite indifferent, for what harm can there be in going to a field, walking about waiting for someone and defending oneself if attacked? And so he is not sinning in any way, since it is by no means accepting a duel if the intention is directed to other circumstances. For acceptance of the duel consists in the express intention of fighting, which this man does not have." '

'You have not kept your word, Father. That is not really permitting the duel. On the contrary he avoids saying that it is one, in order to make it lawful, so sure is he that it is forbidden.'

'Ah ha!' said the Father, 'you are beginning to get there; I am delighted. All the same I might say that in this he is permitting everything requested by those who fight duels. But since I must give you a fair answer, our Father Layman will do it for me, by permitting duelling in direct terms, provided that one's intention is directed towards accepting it solely in order to preserve one's honour and fortune. It is in book 3, pt. 3, ch. iii, nn. 2 and 3: "If a soldier in the army, or a gentleman at court, finds himself liable to lose honour or fortune by not accepting a duel, I cannot see that we can condemn anyone accepting one in self-defence." Petrus Hurtado says the same thing, as quoted by our famous Escobar in tr. I, ex. 7, nn. 96 and 98, where he adds these words of Hurtado: "That one may fight a duel even to defend one's property if there is no other way of preserving it, because everyone has the right to defend his property, even by the death of his enemies." '

These passages made me wonder at seeing piety inspire the King to use his power to forbid and abolish duelling in the State, while it makes the Jesuits devote their subtlety to permitting and authorizing it in the Church. But the good Father was so well launched that it would have been unfair to stop him, so he went on as follows:

'Finally Sanchez—just look at the sort of men I am quoting—goes further. For he does not merely permit people to accept, but even to challenge to a duel, if the intention is properly directed. And our Escobar follows him in this in the same place, n. 97.'

'Father,' I said, 'I give him up if this is so; but I will never believe he wrote it unless I see it.'

'Read it for yourself then,' said he.

And indeed I read these words in Sanchez's *Moral Theology*, book 2, ch. xxxix, n. 7: 'It is quite reasonable to say that someone may fight a duel to save his life, his honour or some considerable amount of property, when it is established that an attempt is being made to rob him of these by lawsuits and chicanery, and that this is the only way to preserve them. And Navarrus very rightly says that in such an event it is lawful to accept or challenge to a duel: *licet acceptare et offerre duellum*. And also that one may kill one's enemy by stealth. And even on such occasions one must not have recourse to a duel if one can kill one's man by stealth, and thus get out of it. For by this means one will at once avoid risking one's life in a fight and taking part in the sin which one's enemy would commit by duelling.'

'That is a pious ambush, Father,' I said; 'but, however pious, it remains an ambush, since it makes it lawful to kill one's enemy treacherously.'

'Did I ever say,' replied the Father, 'that one may kill anyone treacherously? Heaven preserve me! I tell you that one may kill by stealth, and from that you conclude that one may kill treacherously, as if it were the same thing. Find out from Escobar, tr. 6, ex. 4, n. 26, what killing treacherously means; then you can talk. "We call killing treacherously when one kills someone who is quite unsuspecting. And that is why anyone who kills his enemy is not said to kill him treacherously, even if it is from behind or in an ambush: *licet per insidias, aut a tergo percutiat*." And in the same treatise, n. 56: "Anyone who kills his enemy after being reconciled with him and promising to make no more attempts on his life is not absolutely said to kill him treacherously, unless they had enjoyed intimate friendship: *arctior amicitia*."

'You see from this that you do not even know what the terms signify, and yet you talk like a doctor of divinity.'

'I admit,' I said, 'that this is new to me; and from this definition I learn that perhaps no one has ever killed anyone else treacherously. For people seldom think of murdering anyone but their enemies; however that may be, according to Sanchez, one may have no qualms in killing, I will not say treacherously again, but merely from behind or in an ambush, some slanderer who is suing us?'

'Yes,' said the Father, 'but provided that the intention is properly directed; you keep forgetting the main thing. This is what Molina maintains too, vol. IV, tr. 3, disp. 12. And even, according to our learned Reginaldus, book 21, ch. V, n. 57: "One may also kill any false witnesses whom he calls against us." And finally, according to our great and celebrated Fathers Tannerus and Emmanuel Sa, one may likewise kill false witnesses and the judge too, if he is in collusion with them. Here are his words, tr. 3, disp. 4, q. 8, n. 83: "Sotus and Lessius say that it is not lawful to kill the false witnesses and the judge who are conspiring to bring about the death of an innocent man, but Emmanuel Sa and other authors are right to refuse approval to this view, at least as regards conscience." And he further confirms in the same place that one may kill both judge and witnesses.'

'Father,' I said, 'I now pretty well understand your principle of directing the intention, but I should also like to understand its consequences, and all the cases in which this method enables us to kill. Let us then go back over those you have told me, for fear of misunderstanding, since ambiguity here could be dangerous. One must kill only in the right conditions and following a good probable opinion. Then you assured me that if one directs one's intention properly, one may, according to your Fathers, in preservation of honour, or even property, accept a duel, sometimes challenge to one, kill a false accuser by stealth, and his witnesses with him, and even the corrupt judge who favours them; and you also told me that anyone who has been slapped may, without avenging himself, seek redress at the point of the sword. But, Father, you have not told me to what extent.'

'You can hardly go wrong,' said the Father; 'for you may go as far as killing him. That is well proved by our learned Henriquez, book 14, ch. X, n. 3, and some of our other Fathers quoted by Escobar, tr. 1, ex. 7, n. 48, as follows: "You may kill a person who has slapped you, even if he runs away, provided that you avoid doing so out of hatred or vengeance, thus giving no occasion for these excessive murders so harmful to the state. The reason is that one may run after one's honour, as one does after stolen goods. For although your honour is not in the hands of your enemy, like belongings he might have stolen, yet it may be recovered in the same way, by showing signs of dignity and authority, and thus acquiring public esteem. And is it not in fact true that anyone who has been slapped is reputed dishonoured until he has killed his enemy?" '

That seemed so horrible to me that I could hardly contain myself; but in order to learn the rest I let him continue thus:

'One may even, to forestall a slap, kill the person intending to give it, if there is no other way of avoiding it. That is common ground among our Fathers. For example, Azorius, *Moral Inst.*, pt. 3, p. 105 (he is another of the 24 Elders): "Is it lawful for a man of honour to kill someone who intends to slap him or hit him with a stick? Some say not, and their reason is that the life of our neighbour is more precious than our honour; and moreover that it is cruel to kill a man merely to avoid a slap. But others say that it is lawful; and I certainly find that probable, if there is no other means of avoiding it. Otherwise the honour of the innocent would be continually exposed to the malice of the insolent." ' [. . .]

'That is enough on that subject; now I want to talk to you about the facilities we have provided for the avoidance of sin in social intercourse and intrigues. One of the most embarrassing problems is how to avoid lying, especially when one would like people to believe something untrue. This is where our doctrine of equivocation is marvellously helpful, for it allows one "to use ambiguous terms, conveying a different meaning to the hearer from that in which one understands them oneself", as Sanchez says, *Moral Works*, pt. 2, bk. 3, ch. vi, n. 13.'

'I know that, Father,' I said.

'We have published it so widely,' he continued, 'that in the end everyone has heard of it. But I wonder if you know what to do when one cannot find any equivocal terms?'

'No, Father.'

'I thought as much,' he said; 'it is new: the doctrine of mental restrictions. Sanchez gives it in the same place: "One may swear," he says, "that one has not done something, though one really has done it, by inwardly understanding that one did not do it on a certain day, or before one was born, or by implying some other similar circumstance, but using words with no meaning capable of conveying this; this is very convenient on many occasions, and is always quite legitimate when necessary, or useful, to health, honour or property." '

'What, Father! Is this not a lie, and even perjury?'

'No,' said the Father; 'Sanchez proves it in the same place, and our Father Filiutius too, tr. 25, ch. xi, n. 331: "because", he says, "it is the intention which determines the quality of an action." And he adds, n. 328, another safer means of avoiding a lie; after saying aloud "I swear that I did not do that" you add under your breath "today" or after saying aloud "I swear" you say under your breath "that I say", and then go on aloud "that I did not do that." You see that that is telling the truth.'

'I admit that,' I said; 'but we might find that it is telling the truth under one's breath and a lie aloud; anyhow I am afraid that a lot of people would not have enough presence of mind to use such methods.'

'Our Fathers,' he said, 'teach in the same place, for the sake of those who are unable to find such restrictions, that it is sufficient to avoid lying simply to say "that they did not do" what they had done, provided "they have the general intention of giving their words the meaning that a clever man would give them."

'Tell me the truth. You have many times found yourself embarrassed because you did not know about this?'

'Sometimes,' I said.

'And will you not likewise admit that it would be often very convenient to be dispensed in conscience from keeping certain of one's promises?'

'It would, Father,' I said, 'be extremely convenient.'

'Listen then to Escobar in tr. 3, ex. 3, n. 48, where he gives this general rule: "Promises are not binding if one has no intention of being bound when making them. Now it hardly ever happens that one does have such an intention unless one confirms them by oath or contract; so that when one simply says: I will do that, one means that one will do it unless one changes one's mind. For no one wants to deprive himself of his liberty in this way." He gives other rules that you can look at yourself, and ends by saying: "that all this comes from Molina and our other authors: *omnia ex Molina et aliis.*" And so it is not open to question.'

'Oh Father!' I said, 'I never knew that direction of the intention had the power to nullify promises.'

'You see,' said the Father, 'that this makes social intercourse much easier. But what has given us most trouble is regulating relations between men and women; for our Fathers are more reserved on matters of chastity. Not that they omit to deal with some rather curious and broad-minded questions, mainly for married or engaged persons.'

Thereupon I learnt some of the most extraordinary and beastly questions imaginable. He gave me enough of them to fill several letters; but I do not want even to quote the references, because you show my letters to all sorts of people, and I would not like to give those who only look for entertainment the opportunity of reading such things.

[*Provincial Letters*, VII, IX, trans. A. J. Krailsheimer (Penguin: Harmondsworth, 1967), 102–4, 106–10, 140–2. First published in 1656–7.]

JEREMY BENTHAM

71 Natural Rights

'*The end in view of every political association is the preservation of the natural and imprescriptible rights of man. These rights are liberty, property, security, and resistance to oppression.*' [Declaration of Rights, French National Assembly, 1791]

Sentence 1. The end in view of every political association, is the preservation of the natural and imprescriptible rights of man.

More confusion—more nonsense,—and the nonsense, as usual, dangerous nonsense. The words can scarcely be said to have a meaning: but if they have, or rather if they had a meaning, these would be the propositions either asserted or implied:—

1. That there are such things as rights anterior to the establishment of governments: for natural, as applied to rights, if it mean anything, is meant to stand in opposition to *legal*—to such rights as are acknowledged to owe their existence to government, and are consequently posterior in their date to the establishment of government.

2. That these rights *can not* be abrogated by government: for *can not* is implied in the form of the word imprescriptible, and the sense it wears when so applied, is the cut-throat sense above explained.

3. That the governments that exist derive their origin from formal associations, or what are now called *conventions:* associations entered into by a partnership contract, with all the members for partners,—entered into at a day prefixed, for a predetermined purpose, the formation of a new government where there was none before (for as to formal meetings holden under the control of an existing government, they are evidently out of question here) in which it seems again to be implied in the way of inference, though a necessary and an unavoidable inference, that all governments (that is, self-called governments, knots of persons exercising the powers of government) that have had any other origin than an association of the above description, are illegal, that is, no governments at all; resistance to them, and subversion of them, lawful and commendable; and so on.

Such are the notions implied in this first part of the article. How stands the truth of things? That there are no such things as natural rights—no such things as rights anterior to the establishment of government—no such things as natural rights opposed to, in contradistinction to, legal: that the expression is merely figurative; that when used, in the moment you attempt to give it a literal meaning it leads to error, and to that sort of error that leads to mischief—to the extremity of mischief. [. . .]

In proportion to the want of happiness resulting from the want of rights, a reason exists for wishing that there were such things as rights. But reasons for wishing there were such things as rights, are not rights;—a reason for wishing that a certain right were established, is not that right—want is not supply—hunger is not bread.

That which has no existence cannot be destroyed—that which cannot be destroyed cannot require anything to preserve it from destruction. *Natural rights* is simple nonsense: natural and imprescriptible rights, rhetorical nonsense,—nonsense upon stilts. But this rhetorical nonsense ends in the old strain of mischievous nonsense: for immediately a list of these pretended natural rights is given, and those are so expressed as to present to view legal rights. And of these rights, whatever they are, there is not, it seems, any one of which any government *can*, upon any occasion whatever, abrogate the smallest particle.

So much for terrorist language. What is the language of reason and plain sense upon this same subject? That in proportion as it is *right* or *proper, i.e.* advantageous to the society in question, that this or that right—a right to this or that effect—should be established and maintained, in that same proportion it is *wrong* that it should be abrogated: but that as there is no *right*, which ought not to be maintained so long as it is upon the whole advantageous to the society that it should be maintained, so there is no right which, when the abolition of it is advantageous to society, should not be abolished. To know whether it would be more for the advantage of society that this or that right should be maintained or abolished, the time at which the question about maintaining or abolishing is proposed, must be given, and the circumstances under which it is proposed to maintain or abolish it; the right itself must be specifically described, not jumbled with an undistinguishable heap of others, under any such vague general terms as property, liberty, and the like.

[*Anarchical Fallacies; Being an Examination of the Declarations of Rights Issued during the French Revolution*, in *the Works of Jeremy Bentham*, ii, ed. John Bowring (Russell and Russell Inc.: New York, 1962), 500–1. First published in 1823.]

JOHN STUART MILL

72 **On Nature**

Nature, natural, and the group of words derived from them, or allied to them in etymology, have at all times filled a great place in the thoughts and taken a strong hold on the feelings of mankind. That they should have done so is not surprising, when we consider what the words, in their primitive and most obvious signification, represent; but it is unfortunate that a set of terms which play so great a part in moral and metaphysical speculation, should have acquired many meanings different from the primary one, yet sufficiently allied to it to admit of confusion. The words have thus become entangled in so many foreign associations, mostly of a very powerful and tenacious character, that they have come to excite, and to be the symbols of, feelings which their original meaning will by no means justify; and which have made them one of the most copious sources of false taste, false philosophy, false morality, and even bad law. [. . .]

[T]hough perhaps no one could now be found who [. . .] adopts the so-called Law of Nature as the foundation of ethics, and endeavours consistently to reason from it, the word and its cognates must still be counted among those which carry great weight in moral argumentation. That any mode of thinking, feeling, or acting, is 'according to nature' is usually accepted as a strong argument for its goodness. If it can be said with any plausibility that 'nature enjoins' anything, the propriety of obeying the injunction is by most people considered to be made out: and conversely, the imputation of being contrary to nature, is thought to bar the door against any pretension on the part of the thing so designated, to be tolerated or excused; and the word unnatural has not ceased to be one of the most vituperative epithets in the language. Those who deal in these expressions, may avoid making themselves responsible for any fundamental theorem respecting the standard of moral obligation, but they do not the less imply such a theorem, and one which must be the same in substance with that on which the more logical thinkers of a more laborious age grounded their systematic treatises on Natural Law. [. . .]

The word Nature has two principal meanings: it either denotes the entire system of things, with the aggregate of all their properties, or it denotes things as they would be, apart from human intervention.

In the first of these senses, the doctrine that man ought to follow nature is unmeaning; since man has no power to do anything else than follow nature; all his actions are done through, and in obedience to, some one or many of nature's physical or mental laws.

In the other sense of the term, the doctrine that man ought to follow nature, or in other words, ought to make the spontaneous course of things the model of his voluntary actions, is equally irrational and immoral.

Irrational, because all human action whatever, consists in altering, and all useful action in improving, the spontaneous course of nature:

Immoral, because the course of natural phenomena being replete with everything which when committed by human beings is most worthy of abhorrence, any one who endeavoured in his actions to imitate the natural course of things would be universally seen and acknowledged to be the wickedest of men.

The scheme of Nature regarded in its whole extent, cannot have had, for its sole or even principal object, the good of human or other sentient beings. What good it brings to them, is mostly the result of their own exertions. Whatsoever, in nature, gives indication of beneficent design, proves this beneficence to be armed only with limited power; and the duty of man is to co-operate with the beneficent powers, not by imitating but by perpetually striving to amend the course of nature—and bringing that part of it over which we can exercise control, more nearly into conformity with a high standard of justice and goodness.

['Nature' in *Essays on Ethics, Religion and Society*, ed. J. M. Robson (University of Toronto Press: Toronto, 1969), 375–7, 401–2. First published in 1874.]

ii Kant's Ethics of Duty

a. The Theory

IMMANUEL KANT

73   **The Categorical Imperative**

There is [. . .] only one categorical imperative. It is: Act only according to that maxim by which you can at the same time will that it should become a universal law.

Now if all imperatives of duty can be derived from this one imperative as a principle, we can at least show what we understand by the concept of duty and what it means, even though it remain undecided whether that which is called duty is an empty concept or not.

The universality of law according to which effects are produced constitutes what is properly called nature in the most general sense (as to form), i.e., the existence of things so far as it is determined by universal laws. [By analogy], then, the universal imperative of duty can be expressed as follows: Act as though the maxim of your action were by your will to become a universal law of nature.

We shall now enumerate some duties, adopting the usual division of them into duties to ourselves and to others and into perfect and imperfect duties.

1. A man who is reduced to despair by a series of evils feels a weariness with life but is still in possession of his reason sufficiently to ask whether it would not be contrary to his duty to himself to take his own life. Now he asks whether the maxim of his action could become a universal law of nature. His maxim, however, is: For love of myself, I make it my principle to shorten my life when by a longer duration it threatens more evil than satisfaction. But it is questionable whether this principle of self-love could become a universal law of nature. One immediately sees a contradiction in a system of nature, whose law would be to destroy life by the feeling whose special office is to impel the improvement of life. In this case it would not exist as nature; hence that maxim cannot obtain as a law of nature, and thus it wholly contradicts the supreme principle of all duty.

2. Another man finds himself forced by need to borrow money. He well knows that he will not be able to repay it, but he also sees that nothing will be loaned him if he does not firmly promise to repay it at a certain time. He desires to make such a promise, but he has enough conscience to ask himself whether it is not improper and opposed to duty to relieve his distress in such a way. Now, assuming he does decide to do so, the maxim of his action

would be as follows: When I believe myself to be in need of money, I will borrow money and promise to repay it, although I know I shall never do so. Now this principle of self-love or of his own benefit may very well be compatible with his whole future welfare, but the question is whether it is right. He changes the pretension of self-love into a universal law and then puts the question: How would it be if my maxim became a universal law? He immediately sees that it could never hold as a universal law of nature and be consistent with itself; rather it must necessarily contradict itself. For the universality of a law which says that anyone who believes himself to be in need could promise what he pleased with the intention of not fulfilling it would make the promise itself and the end to be accomplished by it impossible; no one would believe what was promised to him but would only laugh at any such assertion as vain pretense.

3. A third finds in himself a talent which could, by means of some cultivation, make him in many respects a useful man. But he finds himself in comfortable circumstances and prefers indulgence in pleasure to troubling himself with broadening and improving his fortunate natural gifts. Now, however, let him ask whether his maxim of neglecting his gifts, besides agreeing with his propensity to idle amusement, agrees also with what is called duty. He sees that a system of nature could indeed exist in accordance with such a law, even though man (like the inhabitants of the South Sea Islands) should let his talents rust and resolve to devote his life merely to idleness, indulgence, and propagation—in a word, to pleasure. But he cannot possibly will that this should become a universal law of nature or that it should be implanted in us by a natural instinct. For, as a rational being, he necessarily wills that all his faculties should be developed, inasmuch as they are given to him for all sorts of possible purposes.

4. A fourth man, for whom things are going well, sees that others (whom he could help) have to struggle with great hardships, and he asks, 'What concern of mine is it? Let each one be as happy as heaven wills, or as he can make himself; I will not take anything from him or even envy him; but to his welfare or to his assistance in time of need I have no desire to contribute.' If such a way of thinking were a universal law of nature, certainly the human race could exist, and without doubt even better than in a state where everyone talks of sympathy and good will or even exerts himself occasionally to practice them while, on the other hand, he cheats when he can and betrays or otherwise violates the rights of man. Now although it is possible that a universal law of nature according to that maxim could exist, it is nevertheless impossible to will that such a principle should hold everywhere as a law of nature. For a will which resolved this would conflict with itself, since instances can often arise in which he would need the love and sympathy of others, and in which he would have robbed himself, by such a law of nature springing from his own will, of all hope of the aid he desires.

The foregoing are a few of the many actual duties, or at least of duties we hold to be real, whose derivation from the one stated principle is clear. We must be able to will that a maxim of our action become a universal law; this is the canon of the moral estimation of our action generally. Some actions are of such a nature that their maxim cannot even be *thought* as a universal law of nature without contradiction, far from it being possible that one could will that it should be such. In others this internal impossibility is not found, though it is still impossible to *will* that their maxim should be raised to the universality of a law of nature, because such a will would contradict itself. We easily see that the former maxim conflicts with the stricter or narrower (imprescriptable) duty, the latter with broader (meritorious) duty. Thus all duties, so far as the kind of obligation (not the object of their action) is concerned, have been completely exhibited by these examples in their dependence on the one principle.

When we observe ourselves in any transgression of a duty, we find that we do not actually will that our maxim should become a universal law. That is impossible for us; rather, the contrary of this maxim should remain as a law generally, and we only take the liberty of making an exception to it for ourselves or for the sake of our inclination, and for this one occasion. Consequently, if we weighed everything from one and the same standpoint, namely, reason, we would come upon a contradiction in our own will, viz., that a certain principle is objectively necessary as a universal law and yet subjectively does not hold universally but rather admits exceptions. However, since we regard our action at one time from the point of view of a will wholly conformable to reason and then from that of a will affected by inclinations, there is actually no contradiction, but rather an opposition of inclination to the precept of reason (*antagonismus*). In this the universality of the principle (*universalitas*) is changed into mere generality (*generalitas*), whereby the practical principle of reason meets the maxim halfway. Although this cannot be justified in our own impartial judgment, it does show that we actually acknowledge the validity of the categorical imperative and allow ourselves (with all respect to it) only a few exceptions which seem to us to be unimportant and forced upon us.

We have thus at least established that if duty is a concept which is to have significance and actual legislation for our actions, it can be expressed only in categorical imperatives and not at all in hypothetical ones. For every application of it we have also clearly exhibited the content of the categorical imperative which must contain the principle of all duty (if there is such). This is itself very much. But we are not yet advanced far enough to prove a priori that that kind of imperative really exists, that there is a practical law which of itself commands absolutely and without any incentives, and that obedience to this law is duty.

With a view to attaining this, it is extremely important to remember that we must not let ourselves think that the reality of this principle can be derived from the particular constitution of human nature. For duty is practical unconditional necessity of action; it must, therefore, hold for all rational beings (to which alone an imperative can apply), and only for that reason can it be a law for all human wills. Whatever is derived from the particular natural situation of man as such, or from certain feelings and propensities, or, even, from a particular tendency of the human reason which might not hold necessarily for the will of every rational being (if such a tendency is possible), can give a maxim valid for us but not a law; that is, it can give a subjective principle by which we may act but not an objective principle by which we would be directed to act even if all our propensity, inclination, and natural tendency were opposed to it. This is so far the case that the sublimity and intrinsic worth of the command is the better shown in a duty the fewer subjective causes there are for it and the more they are against it; the latter do not weaken the constraint of the law or diminish its validity.

Here we see philosophy brought to what is, in fact, a precarious position, which should be made fast even though it is supported by nothing in either heaven or earth. Here philosophy must show its purity, as the absolute sustainer of its laws, and not as the herald of those which an implanted sense or who knows what tutelary nature whispers to it. Those may be better than no laws at all, but they can never afford fundamental principles, which reason alone dictates. These fundamental principles must originate entirely a priori and thereby obtain their commanding authority; they can expect nothing from the inclination of men but everything from the supremacy of the law and due respect for it. Otherwise they condemn man to self-contempt and inner abhorrence.

Thus everything empirical is not only wholly unworthy to be an ingredient in the principle of morality but is even highly prejudicial to the purity of moral practices themselves. For, in morals, the proper and inestimable worth of an absolutely good will consists precisely in the freedom of the principle of action from all influences from contingent grounds which only experience can furnish. We cannot too much or too often warn against the lax or even base manner of thought which seeks principles among empirical motives and laws, for human reason in its weariness is glad to rest on this pillow. In a dream of sweet illusions (in which it embraces not Juno but a cloud), it substitutes for morality a bastard patched up from limbs of very different parentage, which looks like anything one wishes to see in it, but not like virtue to anyone who has ever beheld her in her true form.[1]

---

[1] To behold virtue in her proper form is nothing else than to exhibit morality stripped of all admixture of sensuous things and of every spurious adornment of reward or self-love. How much she then eclipses everything which appears charming to the senses can easily be seen by everyone with the least effort of his reason, if it be not spoiled for all abstraction.

The question then is: Is it a necessary law for all rational beings that they should always judge their actions by such maxims that they themselves could will to serve as universal laws? If it is such a law, it must be connected (wholly a priori) with the concept of the will of a rational being as such. But in order to discover this connection, we must, however reluctantly, take a step into metaphysics, although into a region of it different from speculative philosophy, i.e., the metaphysics of morals. In a practical philosophy it is not a question of assuming grounds for what happens but of assuming laws of what ought to happen even though it may never happen, that is to say, objective, practical laws. Hence in practical philosophy we need not inquire into the reasons why something pleases or displeases, how the pleasure of mere feeling differs from taste, and whether this is distinct from a general satisfaction of reason. Nor need we ask on what the feeling of pleasure or displeasure rests, how desires and inclinations arise, and how, finally, maxims arise from desires and inclination under the co-operation of reason. For all these matters belong to an empirical psychology, which would be the second part of physics, if we consider it as philosophy of nature so far as it rests on empirical laws. But here it is a question of objectively practical laws and thus of the relation of a will to itself so far as it determines itself only by reason; for everything which has a relation to the empirical automatically falls away, because if reason of itself alone determines conduct, it must necessarily do so a priori. The possibility of reason's thus determining conduct must now be investigated.

The will is thought of as a faculty of determining itself to action in accordance with the conception of certain laws. Such a faculty can be found only in rational beings. That which serves the will as the objective ground of its self-determination is an end, and, if it is given by reason alone, it must hold alike for all rational beings. On the other hand, that which contains the ground of the possibility of the action, whose result is an end, is called the means. The subjective ground of desire is the incentive, while the objective ground of volition is the motive. Thus arises the distinction between subjective ends, which rest on incentives, and objective ends, which depend on motives valid for every rational being. Practical principles are formal when they disregard all subjective ends; they are material when they have subjective ends, and thus certain incentives, as their basis. The ends which a rational being arbitrarily proposes to himself as consequences of his action are material ends and are without exception only relative, for only their relation to a particularly constituted faculty of desire in the subject gives them their worth. And this worth cannot, therefore, afford any universal principles for all rational beings or valid and necessary principles for every volition. That is, they cannot give rise to any practical laws. All these relative ends, therefore, are grounds for hypothetical imperatives only.

But suppose that there were something the existence of which in itself had absolute worth, something which, as an end in itself, could be a ground of definite laws. In it and only in it could lie the ground of a possible categorical imperative, i.e., of a practical law.

Now, I say, man and, in general, every rational being exists as an end in himself and not merely as a means to be arbitrarily used by this or that will. In all his actions, whether they are directed to himself or to other rational beings, he must always be regarded at the same time as an end. All objects of inclinations have only a conditional worth, for if the inclinations and the needs founded on them did not exist, their object would be without worth. The inclinations themselves as the sources of needs, however, are so lacking in absolute worth that the universal wish of every rational being must be indeed to free themselves completely from them. Therefore, the worth of any objects to be obtained by our actions is at all times conditional. Beings whose existence does not depend on our will but on nature, if they are not rational beings, have only a relative worth as means and are therefore called "things"; on the other hand, rational beings are designated "persons," because their nature indicates that they are ends in themselves, i.e., things which may not be used merely as means. Such a being is thus an object of respect and, so far, restricts all [arbitrary] choice. Such beings are not merely subjective ends whose existence as a result of our action has a worth for us but are objective ends, i.e., beings whose existence in itself is an end. Such an end is one for which no other end can be substituted, to which these beings should serve merely as means. For, without them, nothing of absolute worth could be found, and if all worth is conditional and thus contingent, no supreme practical principle for reason could be found anywhere.

Thus if there is to be a supreme practical principle and a categorical imperative for the human will, it must be one that forms an objective principle of the will from the conception of that which is necessarily an end for everyone because it is an end in itself. Hence this objective principle can serve as a universal practical law. The ground of this principle is: rational nature exists as an end in itself. Man necessarily thinks of his own existence in this way; thus far it is a subjective principle of human actions. Also every other rational being thinks of his existence by means of the same rational ground which holds also for myself: thus it is at the same time an objective principle from which, as a supreme practical ground, it must be possible to derive all laws of the will. The practical imperative, therefore, is the following: Act so that you treat humanity, whether in your own person or in that of another, always as an end and never as a means only.

[*The Foundations of the Metaphysics of Morals* in *The Philosophy of Immanuel Kant*, iv, trans. L. W. Beck (University of Chicago Press: Chicago, 1949), 80–7. First published in 1785.]

On a Supposed Right to Lie from Altruistic Motives

In the journal *France* for 1797, Part VI, No. 1, page 123, in an article entitled 'On Political Reactions' by Benjamin Constant, there appears the following passage:

The moral principle, 'It is a duty to tell the truth,' would make any society impossible if it were taken singly and unconditionally. We have proof of this in the very direct consequences which a German philosopher has drawn from this principle. This philosopher goes so far as to assert that it would be a crime to lie to a murderer who asked whether our friend who is pursued by him had taken refuge in our house.

The French philosopher on page 124 refutes this principle in the following manner:

It is a duty to tell the truth. The concept of duty is inseparable from the concept of right. A duty is that which in one being corresponds to the rights of another. Where there are no rights, there are no duties. To tell the truth is thus a duty; but it is a duty only in respect to one who has a right to the truth. But no one has a right to a truth which injures others.

The πρῶτον ψεῦδος in this argument lies in the sentence: 'To tell the truth is a duty, but it is a duty only toward one who has a right to the truth.'

It must first be noted that the expression, 'to have a right to truth' is without meaning. One must rather say, 'Man has a right to his own truthfulness (*veracitas*),' i.e. to the subjective truth in his own person. For to have objectively a right to truth would mean that it is a question of one's will (as in questions of what belongs to individuals generally) whether a given sentence is to be true or false. This would certainly produce an extraordinary logic.

Now the first question is: Does a man, in cases where he cannot avoid answering 'Yes' or 'No,' have a right to be untruthful? The second question is: Is he not in fact bound to tell an untruth, when he is unjustly compelled to make a statement, in order to protect himself or another from a threatened misdeed?

Truthfulness in statements which cannot be avoided is the formal duty of an individual to everyone, however great may be the disadvantage accruing to himself or to another. If, by telling an untruth, I do not wrong him who unjustly compels me to make a statement, nevertheless by this falsification, which must be called a lie (though not in a legal sense), I commit a wrong against duty generally in a most essential point. That is, so far as in me lies I cause that declarations should in general find no credence, and hence that all rights based on contracts should be void and lose their force, and this is a wrong done to mankind generally.

Thus the definition of a lie as merely an intentional untruthful declaration to another person does not require the additional condition that it must harm another, as jurists think proper in their definition (*mendacium est falsiloquium in praeiudicium alterius*). For a lie always harms another; if not some other particular man, still it harms mankind generally, for it vitiates the source of law itself.

This benevolent lie, however, can become punishable under civil law through an accident (*casus*), and that which escapes liability to punishment only by accident can also be condemned as wrong even by external laws. For instance, if by telling a lie you have prevented murder, you have made yourself legally responsible for all the consequences; but if you have held rigorously to the truth, public justice can lay no hand on you, whatever the unforeseen consequences may be. After you have honestly answered the murderer's question as to whether his intended victim is at home, it may be that he has slipped out so that he does not come in the way of the murderer, and thus that the murder may not be committed. But if you had lied and said he was not at home when he had really gone out without your knowing it, and if the murderer had then met him as he went away and murdered him, you might justly be accused as the cause of his death. For if you had told the truth as far as you knew it, perhaps the murderer might have been apprehended by the neighbors while he searched the house and thus the deed might have been prevented. Therefore, whoever tells a lie, however well intentioned he might be, must answer for the consequences, however unforeseeable they were, and pay the penalty for them even in a civil tribunal. This is because truthfulness is a duty which must be regarded as the ground of all duties based on contract, and the laws of these duties would be rendered uncertain and useless if even the least exception to them were admitted.

To be truthful (honest) in all declarations, therefore, is a sacred and absolutely commanding decree of reason, limited by no expediency.

[*The Philosophy of Immanuel Kant*, trans. L. W. Beck (University of Chicago Press: Chicago, 1949), 346–9. First published in 1785.]

b. Criticism

RAE LANGTON

75 Maria von Herbert's Challenge to Kant

This is a paper about two philosophers who wrote to each other. One is famous; the other is not. It is about two practical standpoints, the strategic and the human, and what the famous philosopher said of them. And it is about friendship and deception, duty and despair. That is enough by way of preamble.[1]

Friendship

In 1791 Kant received a letter from an Austrian lady whom he had never met. She was Maria von Herbert, a keen and able student of Kant's philosophy, and sister to Baron Franz Paul von Herbert, another zealous Kantian disciple. The zeal of her brother the Baron was indeed so great that he had left his lead factory, and his wife, for two years in order to study Kant's philosophy in Weimar and Jena. Upon his return, the von Herbert household had become a centre, a kind of *salon*, where the critical philosophy was intensely debated, against the backdrop of vehement opposition to Kant in Austria as in many German states. The household was, in the words of a student of Fichte's, 'a new Athens', an oasis of Enlightenment spirit, devoted to preaching and propagating the Kantian gospel, reforming religion, and replacing dull unthinking piety with a morality based on reason.[2] Here is the letter.

1. *To Kant, from Maria von Herbert, August 1791*

Great Kant,

As a believer calls to his God, I call to you for help, for comfort, or for counsel to prepare me for death. Your writings prove that there is a future life. But as for this life, I have found nothing, nothing at all that could replace the good I have lost, for I loved someone who, in my eyes, encompassed within himself all that is worthwhile, so that I lived only for him, everything else was in comparison just rubbish, cheap trinkets. Well, I have offended this person, because of a long drawn out lie, which I have now disclosed to him, though there was nothing unfavourable to my character in it, I had no vice in my life that needed hiding. The lie was enough though, and his love vanished. As an honourable man, he doesn't refuse me friend-

[1] This paper is a shortened version of 'Duty and Desolation', which appeared in *Philosophy*, 67 (1992). As the original version makes evident, my interpretation of Kant owes a great debt to the work of P. F. Strawson ('Freedom and Resentment', in *Freedom and Resentment* (Methuen: London, 1974), 1–25), and Christine Korsgaard, whose views on Kant and lying are developed in 'The Right to Lie: Kant on Dealing with Evil', *Philosophy and Public Affairs*, 15, 4 (1986), 325–49; and, on Kant and friendship, in 'Creating the Kingdom of Ends: Responsibility and Reciprocity in Personal Relations', *Philosophical Perspectives 6: Ethics*, ed. James Tomberlin (The Ridgeview Publishing Company: Atascadero, Calif., 1992). 'Duty and Desolation' was first read at a conference on moral psychology at Monash, Aug. 1991, and has been read at the University of Queensland, the Australian National University, and the University of Delhi. I am indebted to those present on all these occasions for stimulating and searching comments. I am especially grateful to Philip Pettit and Richard Holton for helpful discussion, and to Margaret Wilson and Christine Korsgaard for written comments on an early draft.

[2] According to Arnulf Zweig, in his introduction to *Kant: Philosophical Correspondence, 1759–1799* (University of Chicago Press: Chicago, 1967), 24.

ship. But that inner feeling that once, unbidden, led us to each other, is no more—
oh my heart splinters into a thousand pieces! If I hadn't read so much of your work
I would certainly have put an end to my life. But the conclusion I had to draw from
your theory stops me—it is wrong for me to die because my life is tormented,
instead I'm supposed to live because of my being. Now put yourself in my place,
and either damn me or comfort me. I've read the metaphysic of morals, and the
categorical imperative, and it doesn't help a bit. My reason abandons me just when
I need it. Answer me, I implore you—or you won't be acting in accordance with
your own imperative.

My address is Maria Herbert of Klagenfurt, Carinthia, care of the white lead
factory, or perhaps you would rather send it via Reinhold because the mail is more
reliable there.

Kant, much impressed by this letter, sought advice from a friend as to
what he should do. The friend advised him strongly to reply, and to do his
best to distract his correspondent from 'the object to which she [was]
enfettered'.[1] We have the carefully prepared draft of Kant's response.

2. To Maria von Herbert, Spring 1792 (Kant's rough draft)

Your deeply felt letter comes from a heart that must have been created for the sake
of virtue and honesty, since it is so receptive to instruction in those qualities. I must
do as you ask, namely, put myself in your place, and prescribe for you a pure moral
sedative. I do not know whether your relationship is one of marriage or friendship,
but it makes no significant difference. For love, be it for one's spouse or for a friend,
presupposes the same mutual esteem for the other's character, without which it is
no more than perishable, sensual delusion.

A love like that wants to communicate itself completely, and it expects of its
respondent a similar sharing of heart, unweakened by distrustful reticence. That is
what the ideal of friendship demands. But there is something in us which puts limits
on such frankness, some obstacle to this mutual outpouring of the heart, which
makes one keep some part of one's thoughts locked within oneself, even when one
is most intimate. The sages of old complained of this secret distrust—'My dear
friends, there is no such thing as a friend!'

We can't expect frankness of people, since everyone fears that to reveal himself
completely would be to make himself despised by others. But this lack of frankness,
this reticence, is still very different from dishonesty. What the honest but reticent
man says is true, but not the whole truth. What the dishonest man says is something he knows to be false. Such an assertion is called, in the theory of virtue, a lie.

[1] Letter to Kant from Ludwig Ernst Borowski, probably Aug. 1791. The correspondence
between Kant and Maria von Herbert, and the related letters, are in volume 11 of the edition of
Kant's work published by the Prussian Academy of Sciences (Walter de Gruyter: Berlin, 1922).
The English translations given in this paper are closely based on those of Arnulf Zweig, partly
revised in the light of the Academy edition, and very much abridged. See Zweig, Kant: Philosophical Correspondence, 1759–99, © 1967 by the University of Chicago. All Rights Reserved. (I make
use of the translations with the kind permission of Prof. Zweig and the University of Chicago
Press. Readers who would like to see fuller versions of the letters should consult the Academy
edition, or the Zweig translations.)

It may be harmless, but it is not on that account innocent. It is a serious violation of a duty to oneself; it subverts the dignity of humanity in our own person, and attacks the roots of our thinking. As you see, you have sought counsel from a physician who is no flatterer. I speak for your beloved and present him with arguments that justify his having wavered in his affection for you.

Ask yourself whether you reproach yourself for the imprudence of confessing, or for the immorality intrinsic to the lie. If the former, then you regret having done your duty. And why? Because it has resulted in the loss of your friend's confidence. This regret is not motivated by anything moral, since it is produced by an awareness not of the act itself, but of its consequences. But if your reproach is grounded in a moral judgment of your behaviour, it would be a poor moral physician who would advise you to cast it from your mind.

When your change in attitude has been revealed to your beloved, only time will be needed to quench, little by little, the traces of his justified indignation, and to transform his coldness into a more firmly grounded love. If this doesn't happen, then the earlier warmth of his affection was more physical than moral, and would have disappeared anyway—a misfortune which we often encounter in life, and when we do, must meet with composure. For the value of life, insofar as it consists of the enjoyment we get from people, is vastly overrated.

Here then, my dear friend, you find the customary divisions of a sermon: instruction, penalty and comfort. Devote yourself to the first two; when they have had their effect, comfort will be found by itself.

Kant's letter has an enormously interesting and sensitive discussion of friendship and secrecy, much of which turns up word for word in *The Doctrine of Virtue*, published some six years later.[1] But what Kant's letter fails to say is as at least as interesting as what it says. Herbert writes that she has lost her love, that her heart is shattered, that there is nothing left to make life worth living, and that Kant's moral philosophy hasn't helped a bit. Kant's reply is to suggest that the love is deservedly lost, that misery is an appropriate response to one's own moral failure, and that the really interesting moral question here is the one that hinges on a subtle but necessary scope distinction: the distinction between telling a lie and failing to tell the truth, between *saying 'not-p'*, and *not saying 'p'*. Conspicuously absent is an acknowledgement of Herbert's more than theoretical interest in the question: is suicide compatible with the moral law? And perhaps this is just as well from a practical point of view. The sooner she gives up those morbid thoughts the better; the less said on the morbid subject, the less likely the morbid thoughts will arise. Perhaps it is also just as well, for Kant, from a theoretical point of view. Kant's conviction that suicide is incom-

---

[1] Immanuel Kant, *The Doctrine of Virtue*, (part II of *The Metaphysic of Morals*), trans. Mary Gregor (Harper and Row: London, 1964). One wonders whether these parts of *The Doctrine of Virtue* may have been influenced by Kant's thoughts about Herbert's predicament. An alternative explanation might be that *The Doctrine of Virtue* and Kant's letter to Herbert are both drawing on Kant's lecture notes.

patible with the moral law is not nearly as well founded as he liked to think; so here too, the less said, the better. Having posted his moral sedative off to Austria, and receiving no reply from the patient in more than a year, Kant enquired of a mutual friend who often saw her about the effect his letter had had. Herbert then wrote back, with apologies for her delay. This is her second letter.

3. To Kant, from Maria von Herbert, January 1793

Dear and revered sir,

Your kindness, and your exact understanding of the human heart, encourage me to describe to you, unshrinkingly, the further progress of my soul. The lie was no cloaking of a vice, but a sin of keeping something back out of consideration for the friendship (still veiled by love) that existed then. There was a struggle, I was aware of the honesty friendship demands, and at the same time I could foresee the terribly wounding consequences. Finally I had the strength and revealed the truth to my friend, but so late—and when I told him, the stone in my heart was gone, but his love was torn away in exchange. My friend hardened in his coldness, just as you said in your letter. But then afterwards he changed towards me, and offered me again the most intimate friendship. I'm glad enough about it, for his sake—but I'm not really content, because it's just amusement, it doesn't have any point.

My vision is clear now. I feel that a vast emptiness extends inside me, and all around me—so that I almost find my self to be superfluous, unnecessary. Nothing attracts me. I'm tormented by a boredom that makes life intolerable. Don't think me arrogant for saying this, but the demands of morality are too easy for me. I would eagerly do twice as much as they command. They only get their prestige from the attractiveness of sin, and it costs me almost no effort to resist that.

I comfort myself with the thought that, since the practice of morality is so bound up with sensuality, it can only count for this world. I can hope that the afterlife won't be yet another life ruled by these few, easy demands of morality, another empty and vegetating life. Experience wants to take me to task for this bad temper I have against life by showing me that nearly everyone finds his life ending much too soon, everyone is so glad to be alive. So as not to be a queer exception to the rule, I shall tell you of a remote cause of my deviation, namely my chronic poor health, which dates from the time I first wrote to you. I don't study the natural sciences or the arts any more, since I don't feel that I'm genius enough to extend them; and for myself, there's no need to know them. I'm indifferent to everything that doesn't bear on the categorical imperative, and my transcendental consciousness—although I'm all done with those thoughts too.

You can see, perhaps, why I only want one thing, namely to shorten this pointless life, a life which I am convinced will get neither better nor worse. If you consider that I am still young and that each day interests me only to the extent that it brings me closer to death, you can judge what a great benefactor you would be if you were to examine this question closely. I ask you, because my conception of morality is silent here, whereas it speaks decisively on all other matters. And if you cannot give me the answer I seek, I beg you to give me something that will get this intolerable emptiness out of my soul. Then I might become a useful part of nature, and, if my health permits, would make a trip to Königsberg in a few years. I want to ask permission, in advance, to visit you. You must tell me your story then, because I would like to know what kind of life your philosophy has led you to—whether it never seemed to you to be worth the bother to marry, or to give your whole heart to anyone, or to reproduce your likeness. I have an engraved portrait of you by Bause, from Leipzig. I see a profound calm there, and moral depth—but not the astuteness of which the *Critique of Pure Reason* is proof. And I'm dissatisfied not to be able to look you right in the face.

Please fulfill my wish, if it's not too inconvenient. And I need to remind you: if you do me this great favour and take the trouble to answer, please focus on specific details, not on the general points, which I understand, and already understood back when I happily studied your works at the side of my friend. You would like him, I'm sure. He is honest, goodhearted, and intelligent—and besides that, fortunate enough to fit this world.

I am with deepest respect and truth, Maria Herbert.

Herbert's letter speaks for itself. The passion, the turbulence, has vanished. Desolation has taken its place, a 'vast emptiness', a vision of the world and the self that is chilling in its clarity, chilling in its nihilism. Apathy reigns. Desire is dead. Nothing attracts. Bereft of inclination, the self is 'superfluous', as Herbert so starkly puts it. Nothing has any point—except of course the categorical imperative. But morality itself has become a torment, not because it is too difficult, but because it is too easy. Without the counterweight of opposing inclination, what course could there be but to obey? The moral life is the empty, vegetating life, where one sees at a glance what the moral law requires and simply does it, unhampered by the competing attractions of sin. Herbert concludes that morality must be bound up with sensuality, that moral credit depends on the battle of the will with the sensual passions, a battle which, when there are no passions, is won merely, and tediously, by default—and where can be the credit in that? The imperative requires us never to treat persons merely as means to one's own ends. But if one has no ends, if one is simply empty, what could be easier than to obey? Herbert draws hope from her conclusion: if morality is bound to sensuality, with luck the next life will not be thus accursed.

This sounds like heresy. Is it? If so, Kant is blind to it. But perhaps it is not heresy at all. What Kant fails to see—what Herbert herself fails to see—is that her life constitutes a profound challenge to his philosophy, at least construed one way. Consider Kant's views on duty and inclination.

An action has moral worth when it is done for the sake of duty; it is not sufficient that the action conforms with duty.[1] Now, inclinations are often sufficient to make us perform actions that conform with our duty. To preserve one's life is a duty; and most of us have strong inclinations to preserve our lives. To help others where one can is a duty; and most of us

---

[1] *The Groundwork of the Metaphysic of Morals*, trans. M. J. Paton (Harper and Row: London, 1964), 397.

are sympathetic enough and amiable enough to be inclined to help others, at least some of the time. But—if we take Kant at his word here—actions thus motivated have no moral worth. The action of moral worth is that of 'the wretched man . . . [for whom] disappointments and hopeless misery have quite taken away the taste for life, who longs for death' but who, notwithstanding, preserves his life. The action that has moral worth is that of the misanthropist, 'the man cold in temperament and indifferent to the sufferings of others' who nonetheless helps others 'not from inclination but from duty'.[1]

This looks as though moral credit depends on both the absence of coinciding inclinations, such as sympathy; and the presence of opposing inclinations, like misanthropy. If so, Herbert is right: morality depends on there being inclinations to defeat. It is important to see though that even here, what Kant says is not motivated by a kind of blind rule worship, but by a sense of the gulf between the two standpoints from which we must view ourselves. We are at once cogs in the grand machine of nature, and free agents in the Kingdom of Ends. We are persons, members of an intelligible world, authors of our actions; and at the same time animals, puppets of our genes and hormones, buffeted about by our lusts and loathings. Inclinations are *passions* in the sense that they *just happen* to us. And insofar as we let our actions be driven by them we allow ourselves to be puppets, not persons. We allow ourselves, to use Kant's own metaphors, to become marionettes or automatons, which may appear to be initiators of action, but whose freedom is illusory, 'no better than the freedom of a turnspit, which, when once wound up also carries out its motions by itself'.[2] The inclinations are effects on us, they are *pathe*, and for that reason pathological. If we let them be causes of our behaviour, we abandon our personhood.

Whether they lead us towards the action of duty or away from it, inclinations are among virtue's chief obstacles. When inclination opposes duty, it is an obstacle to duty's performance. When inclination coincides with duty, it is an obstacle at least to knowledge of the action's worth. 'Inclination, be it good-natured or otherwise, is blind and slavish . . . The feeling of sympathy and warmhearted fellow-feeling . . . is burdensome even to right-thinking persons, confusing their considered maxims and creating the wish to be free from them and subject only to law-giving reason.'[3] In the battle against the inclinations we can enlist the aid of that strange thing, respect, or reverence for the moral law. Reverence for the law serves to 'weaken the hindering influence of the inclinations'.[4] Reverence is a kind of feeling, but

---

[1] Ibid. 398.
[2] Immanuel Kant, *Critique of Practical Reason*, trans. L. W. Beck (Macmillan: London, 1956), 97, 101.
[3] Ibid. 119.   [4] Ibid. 80.

it is not something we 'passively feel', something inflicted upon us from outside. It is the sensible correlate of our own moral activity, the 'consciousness of the direct constraint of the will through law'.[1] Its function is not to motivate our moral actions, for that would still be motivation by feeling. Rather, its function is to remove the obstacles, to silence inclinations, something we should all look forward to. For inclinations are 'so far from having an absolute value . . . that it must . . . be the universal wish of every rational being to be wholly free from them'.[2]

Kant goes so far as to say we have a *duty of apathy*, a duty he is less than famous for. 'Virtue necessarily presupposes apathy', he says in *The Doctrine of Virtue*. 'The word "apathy" has fallen into disrepute', he continues, 'as if it meant lack of feeling and so subjective indifference regarding objects of choice: it has been taken for weakness. We can prevent this misunderstanding by giving the name "moral apathy" to that freedom from agitation which is to be distinguished from indifference, for in it the feelings arising from sensuous impressions lose their influence on moral feeling only because reverence for the law prevails over all such feelings'.[3] Something rather similar to apathy is described in the *Critique of Practical Reason*, but this time it is called not apathy, but 'bliss' (*Seligkeit*). Bliss is the state of 'complete independence from inclinations and desires'.[4] While it must be the universal wish of every rational being to achieve bliss, can we in fact achieve it? Apparently not, or not here. Bliss is 'the self-sufficiency which can be ascribed only to the Supreme Being'.[5] The Supreme Being has no passions and inclinations. His intuition is intellectual, and not sensible. He can be affected by nothing, not even our prayers. He can have no *pathe*. God is the being more apathetic than which cannot be conceived.

What of Kant's moral patient? She is well beyond the virtue of apathy that goes with mastery of the inclinations. She has no inclinations left to master. She respects the moral law, and obeys it. But she needn't battle her passions to do so. She has no passions. She is empty—but for the clear vision of the moral law and unshrinking obedience to it. She is well on the way to bliss, lucky woman, and, if Kant is right about bliss, well on the way to Godhead. No wonder she feels that she—unlike her unnamed friend—does not quite 'fit the world'. She obeys the moral law in her day to day dealings with people from the motive of duty alone. She has no other motives. She is no heretic. She is a Kantian saint. Oh brave new world, that has such moral saints in it.[6]

What should Kant have said about inclinations? I have no clear view about this, but some brief remarks may be in order. A saner view is

<hr />

[1] Ibid. 117. [2] *Groundwork*, 428. [3] *Doctrine of Virtue*, 407.
[4] *Critique of Practical Reason*, 118. [5] Ibid.
[6] See Susan Wolf, 'Moral Saints', *The Journal of Philosophy*, 79 (1982), 419–39, on the perils of sainthood.

arguably to be found in Kant's own writings. In the *Doctrine of Virtue*[1] Kant apparently advocates the cultivation of natural sentiment to back up the motive of duty. It is hard, though, to reconcile this with his other teachings, which tell us that inclinations, all inclinations, are to be abjured, as 'blind and slavish', in the graphic phrase from the *Critique of Practical Reason*. 'Blind' is an evocative word in the Kantian context, associated as it is with the blind workings of nature, with the sensual as opposed to the intellectual. It calls to mind the famous slogan of the first *Critique*: thoughts without content are empty, intuitions without concepts are *blind*. That slogan famously captures the synthesis of rationalism and empiricism Kant thought necessary for knowledge. It acknowledges the twin aspects of human creatures, as Kant sees us: we have a *sensible* intuition, a *passive* intuition, through which we are affected by the world; and an active intellect. *We need both.* If only Kant had effected a similar synthesis in the moral sphere: for if it is true, as he says, that inclinations without reasons are blind, it seems equally true that reasons without inclinations are empty. The moral life without inclinations is a life of 'intolerable emptiness', as Herbert found. We need both.

I said that Herbert has no inclinations: but there are two exceptions. She wants to die. And she wants to visit Kant. She is, it seems, like the would-be suicide Kant describes in *The Groundwork*: her persistence with life has moral worth, because it is so opposed to her inclinations. But is she really like him? Not quite. For she is not even sure that duty points to persistence with life. Notice the change here. In her first letter she believed that self-respect, respect for 'her own being' required her to persist with life. But as her 'being' has begun to contract, as the self has withered, sloughed off, become superfluous—as the emptiness has grown—so too has her doubt. Now her conception of morality is 'silent' on the question of suicide. She wants to die. She has almost no opposing inclinations. And morality is silent. It takes no expert to wonder if she is in danger.

Why does she want to visit Kant? She says (letter 3): 'I would like to know what kind of life your philosophy has led you to'. In the *Critique of Practical Reason* Kant cites approvingly what he took to be the practice of the ancients: no one was justified in calling himself a philosopher—a lover of wisdom—'unless he could show [philosophy's] infallible effect on his own person as an example'.[2] Kant thinks we are justified in inquiring after the effect of philosophy on the philosopher, daunting as the prospect seems today. But what does Herbert have in mind? She wonders, perhaps, whether Kant's life is as empty as her own, and for the same reason. She discovered that love is 'pointless' when inclinations have withered, when you have no passions of your own and therefore no passions to share. And she wonders

---

[1] See e.g. *Doctrine of Virtue*, 456.   [2] *Critique of Practical Reason*, 190.

whether Kant's life reflects this discovery. She wonders whether Kant's philosophy has led him to think that it was simply 'not worth the bother' to marry, or to 'give his whole heart' to anyone. Perhaps she is right to wonder.

Shipwreck

In reply to an enquiry, Kant received this explanatory letter from a mutual friend, Erhard.

4. To Kant, from J. B. Erhard, January 17, 1793

I can say little of Miss Herbert. She has capsized on the reef of romantic love. In order to realize an idealistic love, she gave herself to a man who misused her trust. And then, trying to achieve such love with another, she told her new lover about the previous one. That is the key to her letter. If my friend Herbert had more delicacy, I think she could still be saved.

Yours, Erhard.

Kant writes again, not to Herbert, but to someone about whom we know little:

5. From Kant, to Elisabeth Motherby, February 11, 1793

I have numbered the letters[1] which I have the honour of passing on to you, my dear mademoiselle, according to the dates I received them. The ecstatical little lady didn't think to date them. The third letter, from another source, provides an explanation of the lady's curious mental derangement. A number of expressions refer to writings of mine that she read, and are difficult to understand without an interpreter.

You have been so fortunate in your upbringing that I do not need to commend these letters to you as an example of warning, to guard you against the wanderings of a sublimated fantasy. But they may serve nonetheless to make your perception of that good fortune all the more lively.

I am, with the greatest respect, my honoured lady's most obedient servant, I. Kant.

Kant is unaware that he has received a letter from a Kantian saint. Indeed, it is hard to believe that he has read her second letter. He relies on the opinion of his friend, whose diagnosis of the patient resorts to that traditional and convenient malady of feminine hysteria. Herbert 'has capsized on the reef of romantic love'. The diagnosis is exactly wrong. Herbert has no passions. Her vision is clear. Her life is empty. But it is easier not to take this in, easier to suppose a simpler illness. She is at the mercy (aren't all women?) of irrational passions. She is evidently beyond the reach of in-

---

[1] Letters 1, 3, and 4 above. Elisabeth Motherby was the daughter of Kant's friend Robert Motherby, an English merchant in Königsberg.

struction, beyond the reach of his moral sedatives; so Kant abandons her. It is hard to imagine a more dramatic shift from the interactive stance to the objective.[1] In Kant's first letter, Herbert is 'my dear friend', she is the subject for moral instruction, and reprimand. She is responsible for some immoral actions, but she has a 'heart created for the sake of virtue', capable of seeing the good and doing it. Kant is doing his best to communicate, instruct, and console. He is not very good at it, hardly surprising if he believes—as I think he does—that he should master rather than cultivate his moral sentiments. But there is little doubt that the good will is there. He treats her as a human being, as an end, as a person. This is the standpoint of interaction.

But now? Herbert is *die kleine Schwärmerin*, the little dreamer, the ecstatical girl, suffering a 'curious mental derangement', lost in the 'wanderings of a sublimated fantasy', who doesn't think, especially about important things like dating letters. Kant is here forgetting an important aspect of the duty of respect, which requires something like a Davidsonian principle of charity. We have 'a duty of respect for man *even in the logical use of his reason*: a duty not to censure his error by calling it absurdity . . . but rather to suppose that his error must yet contain some truth and to seek this out.'[2] Herbert, now deranged, is no longer guilty. She is merely unfortunate. She is not responsible for what she does. She is the pitiful product of a poor upbringing. She is an item in the natural order, a ship wrecked on a reef. She is a thing.

And, true to Kant's picture, it now becomes appropriate to use her as a means to his own ends. He bundles up her letters, private communications from a 'dear friend', letters that express thoughts, philosophical and personal, some of them profound. He bundles them up and sends them to an acquaintance under the title, 'Example of Warning'. The end is obscure and contradictory: it seems it is to warn somebody who, on Kant's own view, needs no warning. Is it gossip? Ingratiation? But the striking thing is that the letters are no longer seen as human communications. Far from it: Kant's presumption is that they *will not be understood* by their new recipient. For the letters 'refer to writings of mine that she read, that are difficult to understand without an interpreter'. This is not the speech of persons, to be understood and debated; this is derangement, to be feared and avoided. These are not thoughts, but symptoms. Kant is doing something with her as one does something with a tool: Herbert cannot share the end of the action. She cannot be co-author. Kant's deceiving of her—neatly achieved by reticence—has made sure of that. Her action of pleading for help, asking

---

[1] This is Strawson's way of characterizing the two standpoints in Kant's moral philosophy ('Freedom and Resentment').

[2] *Doctrine of Virtue*, 462, my italics.

advice, arguing philosophy, her action of writing to a well-loved philosopher and then to a friend—these have become the action of warning of
the perils of romantic love. She did not choose to do *that*. Well may Kant
have warned 'My dear friends, there is no such thing as a friend'.

Strategy for the Kingdom's Sake

Enough. This is not a cautionary tale of the inability of philosophers to live
by their philosophy. What interests me is what interested Kant at the
outset: friendship and deception. What interests me is the very first problem: the 'long drawn out lie, disclosed'. Was it wrong for Herbert to
deceive? Is it always wrong to deceive? Apparently, yes, from the Kantian
perspective. In deceiving we treat our hearers as less than human. We act
from the objective standpoint. We force others to perform actions they
don't choose to perform. We make them things. If I reply to the murderer,
'No, my friend is not here', I deceive a human being, use his reasoning
ability as a tool, do something that has a goal (saving my friend) that I make
impossible for him to share, make him do something (abandon his prey)
that he did not choose to do. I have made him, in this respect, a thing.

But this is too simple. Recall that Herbert puts her dilemma like this: 'I
was aware of *the honesty friendship demands* and at the same time I could see
the terribly wounding consequences . . . The lie . . . was a . . . keeping
something back *out of consideration for the friendship*.'[1] She is torn. Friendship
demands honesty; and friendship demands dishonesty. Is she confused? Is
she in contradiction? Not at all. It is an old dilemma: having an ideal you
want to live by, and an ideal you want to seek and preserve. You owe
honesty to your friend; but the friendship will vanish if you are honest.
Friendship is a very great good: it is the Kingdom of Ends made real and
local. Kant says that the man who is without a friend is the man who 'must
shut himself up in himself', who must remain 'completely alone with his
thoughts, as in a prison'.[2] One of the goods of friendship is that it makes
possible the kind of relationship where one can unlock the prison of the
self, reveal oneself to the compassionate and understanding eye of the
other. But Kant sees true friendship to be a very rare thing, rare, he says as
a black swan.[3] And what threatens friendship most is asymmetry, inequality
with regard to love or respect, which can result in the partial breakdown of
the interactive stance. This asymmetry can be brought about by the very
act of self revelation: if one person 'reveals his failings while the other
person concealed his own, he would lose something of the other's respect

---

[1] Letter 3, my italics.
[2] *Doctrine of Virtue*, 471. This is a remarkable metaphor for a philosopher who finds in the
autonomous human self, and its self-legislating activity, the only source of intrinsic value.
[3] Ibid. 471. Kant's ignorance of Antipodean bird life is (just) forgivable.

by presenting himself so candidly'.[1] What Kant is pointing to is the very problem encountered, far more acutely, by Herbert: in being a friend, in acting in the way that friendship demands, one can sometimes threaten friendship. To act as a member of the Kingdom can make the Kingdom more, and not less, remote. How should we think of Kant's ideal: is the Kingdom an ideal to be lived by, or a goal to be sought? If it is ever the latter, then sometimes—in evil circumstances—it will be permissible, and even required, to act strategically for the Kingdom's sake.[2] There is a question about what evil is. But for Kant it must, above all, be this: the reduction of persons to things. Now consider Herbert's position. There is something we have been leaving out. Herbert is a *woman* in a society in which women start out on an unequal footing and then live out their lives that way, where women—especially women—must perpetually walk a tightrope between being treated as things and treated as persons. She must make her choices against a backdrop of social institutions and habits that strip her of the dignity due to persons, where what she does and what she says will always be interpreted in the light of that backdrop, so that even if she says 'my vision is clear', and speaks in a manner consistent with that claim, her speech will be read as the speech of the deranged, a mere plaything of the passions. Central among the institutions she must en-counter in her life is that of the sexual marketplace, where human beings are viewed as having a *price*, and not a dignity, and where the price of women is fixed in a particular way. Women, as things, as items in the sexual marketplace, have a market value that depends in part on whether they have been used. Virgins fetch a higher price than second hand goods. Such are the background circumstances in which Herbert finds herself. They are, I suggest, evil circumstances, evil by Kantian lights (though Kant himself never saw it).

Despite these handicaps, Herbert has achieved a great thing: she has achieved something like a friendship of mutual love and respect, found someone with whom she can share her activities and goals, become a partner in a relationship where ends are chosen in such a way that the ends of both agents coincide (prominent among which was, it seems, the happy study of Kant's works!). She has achieved a relationship where frankness and honesty prevail—with one exception. Her lie is the lie of 'keeping something back for the sake of the friendship'. If she tells the truth, evil circumstance will see to it that her action will not be taken as the honest self-revelation of a person, but the revelation of her thing-hood, her hither-to unrecognised status as used merchandise, as item with a price that is

---

[1] Ibid. 471.

[2] This development of Kant's philosophy is proposed by Korsgaard as a way of addressing the problem of lying to the murderer at the door (Korsgaard, 'The Right to Lie'). I discuss it in more detail in the original version of this paper.

lower than the usual. If she tells the truth, she becomes a thing, and the friendship—that small neighbourhood of the Kingdom—will vanish. Should she lie? Perhaps. If her circumstances are evil, she is permitted to have friendship as her goal, to be sought and preserved, rather than a law to be lived by. So she is permitted to lie. Then other considerations come in. She has a duty to 'humanity in her own person', of which Kant says: 'By virtue of this worth we are not for sale at any price; we possess an inalienable dignity which instils in us reverence for ourselves'. She has a duty of self esteem: she must respect her own person and demand such respect of others, abjuring the vice of servility.[1] I think she may have a duty to lie.

This is strategy, for the Kingdom's sake. Kant would not allow it. He thinks we should act as if the Kingdom of Ends is with us now. He thinks we should rely on God to make it all right in the end. But God will not make it all right in the end. And the Kingdom of Ends is not with us now. Perhaps we should do what we can to bring it about.

Coda

Kant never replied, and his correspondent, as far as I know, did not leave Austria.[2] In 1803 Maria von Herbert killed herself, having worked out at last an answer to that persistent and troubling question—the question to which Kant, and her own moral sense, had responded with silence. Was that a vicious thing to do? Not entirely. As Kant himself concedes, 'Self murder requires courage, and in this attitude there is always room for reverence for humanity in one's own person.'[3]

JONATHAN BENNETT

76 The Conscience of Huckleberry Finn

In this paper, I shall present not just the conscience of Huckleberry Finn but two others as well. One of them is the conscience of Heinrich Himmler. He became a Nazi in 1923; he served drably and quietly, but well, and was rewarded with increasing responsibility and power. At the peak of his career he held many offices and commands, of which the most powerful was that of leader of the SS—the principal police force of the Nazi regime. In this capacity, Himmler commanded the whole concentration-camp system, and was responsible for the execution of the so-called 'final solution of

---

[1] *Doctrine of Virtue*, 434, 435.
[2] There is one final letter from her on the record, dated early 1794, in which she expresses again a wish to visit Kant, and reflects upon her own desire for death.
[3] Ibid. 424.

the Jewish problem'. It is important for my purposes that this piece of social engineering should be thought of not abstractly but in concrete terms of Jewish families being marched to what they think are bath-houses, to the accompaniment of loud-speaker renditions of extracts from *The Merry Widow* and *Tales of Hoffman*, there to be choked to death by poisonous gases. Altogether, Himmler succeeded in murdering about four and a half million of them, as well as several million gentiles, mainly Poles and Russians.

The other conscience to be discussed is that of the Calvinist theologian and philosopher Jonathan Edwards. He lived in the first half of the eighteenth century, and has a good claim to be considered America's first serious and considerable philosophical thinker. He was for many years a widely-renowned preacher and Congregationalist minister in New England; in 1748 a dispute with his congregation led him to resign (he couldn't accept their view that unbelievers should be admitted to the Lord's Supper in the hope that it would convert them); for some years after that he worked as a missionary, preaching to Indians through an interpreter; then in 1758 he accepted the presidency of what is now Princeton University, and within two months died from a smallpox inoculation. Along the way he wrote some first-rate philosophy: his book attacking the notion of free will is still sometimes read. Why I should be interested in Edwards' *conscience* will be explained in due course.

I shall use Heinrich Himmler, Jonathan Edwards and Huckleberry Finn to illustrate different aspects of a single theme, namely the relationship between *sympathy* on the one hand and *bad morality* on the other.

All that I can mean by a 'bad morality' is a morality whose principles I deeply disapprove of. When I call a morality bad, I cannot prove that mine is better; but when I here call any morality bad, I think you will agree with me that it is bad; and that is all I need.

There could be dispute as to whether the springs of someone's actions constitute a *morality*. I think, though, that we must admit that someone who acts in ways which conflict grossly with our morality may nevertheless have a morality of his own—a set of principles of action which he sincerely assents to, so that for him the problem of acting well or rightly or in obedience to conscience is the problem of conforming to *those* principles. The problem of conscientiousness can arise as acutely for a bad morality as for any other: rotten principles may be as difficult to keep as decent ones.

As for 'sympathy': I use this term to cover every sort of fellow-feeling, as when one feels pity over someone's loneliness, or horrified compassion over his pain, or when one feels a shrinking reluctance to act in a way which will bring misfortune to someone else. These *feelings* must not be confused with *moral judgments*. My sympathy for someone in distress may lead me to help him, or even to think that I ought to help him; but in itself it is not a judgment about what I ought to do but just a *feeling* for him in his plight. We shall get some light on the difference between feelings and moral judgments when we consider Huckleberry Finn.

Obviously, feelings can impel one to action, and so can moral judgments; and in a particular case sympathy and morality may pull in opposite directions. This can happen not just with bad moralities, but also with good ones like yours and mine. For example, a small child, sick and miserable, clings tightly to his mother and screams in terror when she tries to pass him over to the doctor to be examined. If the mother gave way to her sympathy, that is to her feeling for the child's misery and fright, she would hold it close and not let the doctor come near; but don't we agree that it might be wrong for her to act on such a feeling? Quite generally, then, anyone's moral principles may apply to a particular situation in a way which runs contrary to the particular thrusts of fellow-feeling that he has in that situation. My immediate concern is with sympathy in relation to bad morality, but not because such conflicts occur only when the morality is bad.

Now, suppose that someone who accepts a bad morality is struggling to make himself act in accordance with it in a particular situation where his sympathies pull him another way. He sees the struggle as one between doing the right, conscientious thing, and acting wrongly and weakly, like the mother who won't let the doctor come near her sick, frightened baby. Since we don't accept this person's morality, we may see the situation very differently, thoroughly disapproving of the action he regards as the right one, and endorsing the action which from his point of view constitutes weakness and backsliding.

Conflicts between sympathy and bad morality won't always be like this, for we won't disagree with every single dictate of a bad morality. Still, it can happen in the way I have described, with the agent's right action being our wrong one, and vice versa. That is just what happens in a certain episode in chapter 16 of *The Adventures of Huckleberry Finn*, an episode which brilliantly illustrates how fiction can be instructive about real life.

Huck Finn has been helping his slave friend Jim to run away from Miss Watson, who is Jim's owner. In their raft-journey down the Mississippi river, they are near to the place at which Jim will become legally free. Now let Huck take over the story:

Jim said it made him all over trembly and feverish to be so close to freedom. Well, I can tell you it made me all over trembly and feverish, too, to hear him, because I begun to get it through my head that he *was* most free—and who was to blame for it? Why, *me*. I couldn't get that out of my conscience, no how nor no way. . . . It hadn't ever come home to me, before, what this thing was that I was doing. But now it did; and it stayed with me, and scorched me more and more. I tried to make out to myself that *I* warn't to blame, because *I* didn't run Jim off from his rightful owner; but it warn't no use, conscience up and say, every time: 'But you knowed he was running for his freedom, and you could a paddled ashore and told somebody.' That was so—I couldn't get around that, no way. That was where it pinched. Conscience says to me: 'What had poor Miss Watson done to you, that you could see her nigger go off right under your eyes and never say one single word? What did that poor old woman do to you, that you could treat her so mean? . . .' I got to feeling so mean and so miserable I most wished I was dead.

Jim speaks of his plan to save up to buy his wife, and then his children, out of slavery; and he adds that if the children cannot be bought he will arrange to steal them. Huck is horrified:

Thinks I, this is what comes of my not thinking. Here was this nigger which I had as good as helped to run away, coming right out flat-footed and saying he would steal his children—children that belonged to a man I didn't even know; a man that hadn't ever done me no harm.

I was sorry to hear Jim say that, it was such a lowering of him. My conscience got to stirring me up hotter than ever, until at last I says to it: 'Let up on me—it ain't too late, yet—I'll paddle ashore at first light, and tell.' I felt easy, and happy, and light as a feather, right off. All my troubles was gone.

This is bad morality all right. In his earliest years Huck wasn't taught any principles, and the only ones he has encountered since then are those of rural Missouri, in which slave-owning is just one kind of ownership and is not subject to critical pressure. It hasn't occurred to Huck to question those principles. So the action, to us abhorrent, of turning Jim in to the authorities presents itself *clearly* to Huck as the right thing to do.

For us, morality and sympathy would both dictate helping Jim to escape. If we felt any conflict, it would have both these on one side and something else on the other—greed for a reward, or fear of punishment. But Huck's morality conflicts with his sympathy, that is, with his unargued, natural feeling for his friend. The conflict starts when Huck sets off in the canoe towards the shore, pretending that he is going to reconnoitre, but really planning to turn Jim in:

As I shoved off, [Jim] says: 'Pooty soon I'll be a-shout'n for joy, en I'll say, it's all on accounts o' Huck I's a free man . . . Jim won't ever forget you, Huck; you's de bes' fren' Jim's ever had; en you's de *only* fren' old Jim's got now.'

I was paddling off, all in a sweat to tell on him; but when he says this, it seemed to kind of take the tuck all out of me. I went along slow then, and I warn't right down certain whether I was glad I started or whether I warn't. When I was fifty yards off, Jim says:

'Dah you goes, de ole true Huck; de on'y white genlman dat ever kep' his promise to ole Jim.' Well, I just felt sick. But I says, I *got* to do it—I can't get *out* of it.

In the upshot, sympathy wins over morality. Huck hasn't the strength of will to do what he sincerely thinks he ought to do. Two men hunting for runaway slaves ask him whether the man on his raft is black or white:

I didn't answer up prompt. I tried to, but the words wouldn't come. I tried, for a second or two, to brace up and out with it, but I warn't man enough—hadn't the spunk of a rabbit. I see I was weakening; so I just give up trying, and up and says: 'He's white.'

So Huck enables Jim to escape, thus acting weakly and wickedly—he thinks. In this conflict between sympathy and morality, sympathy wins.

One critic has cited this episode in support of the statement that Huck suffers 'excruciating moments of wavering between honesty and respectability'. That is hopelessly wrong, and I agree with the perceptive comment on it by another critic, who says:

The conflict waged in Huck is much more serious: he scarcely cares for respectability and never hesitates to relinquish it, but he does care for honesty and gratitude—and both honesty and gratitude require that he should give Jim up. It is not, in Huck, honesty at war with respectability but love and compassion for Jim struggling against his conscience. His decision is for Jim and hell: a right decision made in the mental chains that Huck never breaks. His concern for Jim is and remains *irrational*. Huck finds many reasons for giving Jim up and none for stealing him. To the end Huck sees his compassion for Jim as a weak, ignorant, and wicked felony.[1]

That is precisely correct—and it can have that virtue only because Mark Twain wrote the episode with such unerring precision. The crucial point concerns *reasons*, which all occur on one side of the conflict. On the side of conscience we have principles, arguments, considerations, ways of looking at things:

'It hadn't ever come home to me before what I was doing'
'I tried to make out that I warn't to blame'
'Conscience said "But you knowed . . ."—I couldn't get around that'
'What had poor Miss Watson done to you?'
'This is what comes of my not thinking'
'. . . children that belonged to a man I didn't even know'.

On the other side, the side of feeling, we get nothing like that. When Jim rejoices in Huck, as his only friend, Huck doesn't consider the claims of friendship or have the situation 'come home' to him in a different light. All that happens is: 'When he says this, it seemed to kind of take the tuck all out of me. I went along slow then, and I warn't right down certain whether I was glad I started or whether I warn't.' Again, Jim's words about Huck's 'promise' to him don't give Huck any *reason* for changing his plan: in his

---

[1] M. J. Sidnell, 'Huck Finn and Jim', *The Cambridge Quarterly*, 2, 205–6.

morality promises to slaves probably don't count. Their effect on him is of a different kind: 'Well, I just felt sick.' And when the moment for final decision comes, Huck doesn't weigh up pros and cons: he simply *fails* to do what he believes to be right—he isn't strong enough, hasn't 'the spunk of a rabbit'. This passage in the novel is notable not just for its finely wrought irony, with Huck's weakness of will leading him to do the right thing, but also for its masterly handling of the difference between general moral principles and particular unreasoned emotional pulls.

Consider now another case of bad morality in conflict with human sympathy: the case of the odious Himmler. Here, from a speech he made to some SS generals, is an indication of the content of his morality:

What happens to a Russian, to a Czech, does not interest me in the slightest. What the nations can offer in the way of good blood of our type, we will take, if necessary by kidnapping their children and raising them here with us. Whether nations live in prosperity or starve to death like cattle interests me only in so far as we need them as slaves to our *Kultur*; otherwise it is of no interest to me. Whether 10,000 Russian females fall down from exhaustion while digging an antitank ditch interests me only in so far as the antitank ditch for Germany is finished.[1]

But has this a moral basis at all? And if it has, was there in Himmler's own mind any conflict between morality and sympathy? Yes there was. Here is more from the same speech:

I also want to talk to you quite frankly on a very grave matter . . . I mean . . . the extermination of the Jewish race. . . . Most of you must know what it means when 100 corpses are lying side by side, or 500, or 1,000. To have stuck it out and at the same time—apart from exceptions caused by human weakness—to have remained decent fellows, that is what has made us hard. This is a page of glory in our history which has never been written and is never to be written.

Himmler saw his policies as being hard to implement while still retaining one's human sympathies—while still remaining a 'decent fellow'. He is saying that only the weak take the easy way out and just squelch their sympathies, and is praising the stronger and more glorious course of retaining one's sympathies while acting in violation of them. In the same spirit, he ordered that when executions were carried out in concentration camps, those responsible 'are to be influenced in such a way as to suffer no ill effect in their character and mental attitude'. A year later he boasted that the SS had wiped out the Jews

---

[1] Quoted in William L. Shirer, *The Rise and Fall of the Third Reich* (Simon and Schuster: New York, 1960), pp. 937–8. Next quotation: ibid. 966. All further quotations relating to Himmler are from Roger Manvell and Heinrich Fraenkel, *Heinrich Himmler* (Heinemann: London, 1965), 132, 197, 184 (twice), 187.

without our leaders and their men suffering any damage in their minds and souls. The danger was considerable, for there was only a narrow path between the Scylla of their becoming heartless ruffians unable any longer to treasure life, and the Charybdis of their becoming soft and suffering nervous breakdowns.

And there really can't be any doubt that the basis of Himmler's policies was a set of principles which constituted his morality—a sick, bad, wicked *morality*. He described himself as caught in 'the old tragic conflict between will and obligation'. And when his physician Kersten protested at the intention to destroy the Jews, saying that the suffering involved was 'not to be contemplated', Kersten reports that Himmler replied:

He knew that it would mean much suffering for the Jews. . . . 'It is the curse of greatness that it must step over dead bodies to create new life. Yet we must . . . cleanse the soil or it will never bear fruit. It will be a great burden for me to bear.'

This, I submit, is the language of morality.

So in this case, tragically, bad morality won out over sympathy. I am sure that many of Himmler's killers did extinguish their sympathies, becoming 'heartless ruffians' rather than 'decent fellows'; but not Himmler himself. Although his policies ran against the human grain to a horrible degree, he did not sandpaper down his emotional surfaces so that there was no grain there, allowing his actions to slide along smoothly and easily. He did, after all, bear his hideous burden, and even paid a price for it. He suffered a variety of nervous and physical disabilities, including nausea and stomach-convulsions, and Kersten was doubtless right in saying that these were 'the expression of a psychic division which extended over his whole life'.

This same division must have been present in some of those officials of the Church who ordered heretics to be tortured so as to change their theological opinions. Along with the brutes and the cold careerists, there must have been some who cared, and who suffered from the conflict between their sympathies and their bad morality.

In the conflict between sympathy and bad morality, then, the victory may go to sympathy as in the case of Huck Finn, or to morality as in the case of Himmler.

Another possibility is that the conflict may be avoided by giving up, or not ever having, those sympathies which might interfere with one's principles. That seems to have been the case with Jonathan Edwards. I am afraid that I shall be doing an injustice to Edwards' many virtues, and to his great intellectual energy and inventiveness; for my concern is only with the worst thing about him—namely his morality, which was worse than Himmler's.

According to Edwards, God condemns some men to an eternity of unimaginably awful pain, though he arbitrarily spares others—'arbitrarily' because none deserve to be spared:

Natural men are held in the hand of God over the pit of hell; they have deserved the fiery pit, and are already sentenced to it; and God is dreadfully provoked, his anger is as great towards them as to those that are actually suffering the executions of the fierceness of his wrath in hell . . .; the devil is waiting for them, hell is gaping for them, the flames gather and flash about them, and would fain lay hold on them . . .; and . . . there are no means within reach that can be any security to them. . . . All that preserves them is the mere arbitrary will, and uncovenanted unobliged forebearance of an incensed God.[1]

Notice that he says 'they have deserved the fiery pit'. Edwards insists that men *ought* to be condemned to eternal pain; and his position isn't that this is right because God wants it, but rather that God wants it because it is right. For him, moral standards exist independently of God, and God can be assessed in the light of them (and of course found to be perfect). For example, he says:

They deserve to be cast into hell; so that . . . justice never stands in the way, it makes no objection against God's using his power at any moment to destroy them. Yea, on the contrary, justice calls aloud for an infinite punishment of their sins.

Elsewhere, he gives elaborate arguments to show that God is acting justly in damning sinners. For example, he argues that a punishment should be exactly as bad as the crime being punished; God is infinitely excellent; so any crime against him is infinitely bad; and so eternal damnation is exactly right as a punishment—it is infinite, but, as Edwards is careful also to say, it is 'no more than infinite'.

Of course, Edwards himself didn't torment the demand; but the question still arises of whether his sympathies didn't conflict with his *approval* of eternal torment. Didn't he find it painful to contemplate any fellow-human's being tortured for ever? Apparently not:

The God that holds you over the pit of hell, much as one holds a spider or some loathsome insect over the fire, abhors you, and is dreadfully provoked; . . . he is of purer eyes than to bear to have you in his sight; you are ten thousand times so abominable in his eyes as the most hateful venomous serpent is in ours.

When God is presented as being as misanthropic as that, one suspects misanthropy in the theologian. This suspicion is increased when Edwards claims that 'the saints in glory will . . . understand how terrible the sufferings of the damned are; yet . . . will not be sorry for [them].'[2] He bases this partly on a view of human nature whose ugliness he seems not to notice:

[1] Vergilius Ferm (ed.), *Puritan Sage: Collected Writings of Jonathan Edwards* (Library Publishers: New York, 1953), 370. Next three quotations: ibid. 366, 294 ('no more than infinite'), 372.

[2] This and the next two quotations are from 'The End of the Wicked Contemplated by the Righteous: or, The Torments of the Wicked in Hell, no Occasion of Grief to the Saints in Heaven', from *The Works of President Edwards*, iv (London, 1817), 507–8, 511–12, and 509 respectively.

The seeing of the calamities of others tends to heighten the sense of our own enjoyments. When the saints in glory, therefore, shall see the doleful state of the damned, how will this heighten their sense of the blessedness of their own state . . . When they shall see how miserable others of their fellow-creatures are . . . ; when they shall see the smoke of their torment, . . . and hear their dolorous shrieks and cries, and consider that they in the mean time are in the most blissful state, and shall surely be in it to all eternity; how they will rejoice!

I hope this is less than the whole truth! His other main point about why the saints will rejoice to see the torments of the damned is that it is *right* that they should do so:

The heavenly inhabitants . . . will have no love nor pity to the damned. . . . [This will not show] a want of a spirit of love in them . . .; for the heavenly inhabitants will know that it is not fit that they should love [the damned] because they will know then, that God has no love to them, nor pity for them.

The implication that *of course* one can adjust one's feelings of pity so that they conform to the dictates of some authority—doesn't this suggest that ordinary human sympathies played only a small part in Edwards' life?

Huck Finn, whose sympathies are wide and deep, could never avoid the conflict in that way; but he is determined to avoid it, and so he opts for the only other alternative he can see—to give up morality altogether. After he has tricked the slave-hunters, he returns to the raft and undergoes a peculiar crisis:

I got aboard the raft, feeling bad and low, because I knowed very well I had done wrong, and I see it warn't no use for me to try to learn to do right; a body that don't get *started* right when he's little, ain't got no show—when the pinch comes there ain't nothing to back him up and keep him to his work, and so he gets beat. Then I thought a minute, and says to myself, hold on—s'pose you'd a done right and give Jim up; would you feel better than what you do now? No, says I, I'd feel bad—I'd feel just the same way I do now. Well, then, says I, what's the use you learning to do right, when it's troublesome to do right and ain't no trouble to do wrong, and the wages is just the same? I was stuck. I couldn't answer that. So I reckoned I wouldn't bother no more about it, but after this always do whichever come handiest at the time.

Huck clearly cannot conceive of having any morality except the one he has learned—too late, he thinks—from his society. He is not entirely a prisoner of that morality, because he does after all reject it; but for him that is a decision to relinquish morality as such; he cannot envisage revising his morality, altering its content in face of the various pressures to which it is subject, including pressures from his sympathies. For example, he does not begin to approach the thought that slavery should be rejected on moral grounds, or the thought that what he is doing is not theft because a person cannot be owned and therefore cannot be stolen.

The basic trouble is that he cannot or will not engage in abstract intellectual operations of any sort. In chapter 33 he finds himself 'feeling to blame, somehow' for something he knows he had no hand in; he assumes that this feeling is a deliverance of conscience; and this confirms him in his belief that conscience shouldn't be listened to:

> It don't make no difference whether you do right or wrong, a person's conscience ain't got no sense, and just goes for him *anyway*. If I had a yaller dog that didn't know no more than a person's conscience does, I would pison him. It takes up more room than all the rest of a person's insides, and yet ain't no good, nohow.

That brisk, incurious dismissiveness fits well with the comprehensive rejection of morality back on the raft. But this is a digression.

On the raft, Huck decides not to live by principles, but just to do whatever 'comes handiest at the time'—always acting according to the mood of the moment. Since the morality he is rejecting is narrow and cruel, and his sympathies are broad and kind, the results will be good. But moral principles are good to have, because they help to protect one from acting badly at moments when one's sympathies happen to be in abeyance. On the highest possible estimate of the role one's sympathies should have, one can still allow for principles as embodiments of one's best feelings, one's broadest and keenest sympathies. On that view, principles can help one across intervals when one's feelings are at less than their best, i.e. through periods of misanthropy or meanness or self-centredness or depression or anger.

What Huck didn't see is that one can live by principles and yet have ultimate control over their content. And one way such control can be exercised is by checking of one's principles in the light of one's sympathies. This is sometimes a pretty straightforward matter. It can happen that a certain moral principle becomes untenable—meaning literally that one cannot hold it any longer—because it conflicts intolerably with the pity or revulsion or whatever that one feels when one sees what the principle leads to. One's experience may play a large part here: experiences evoke feelings, and feelings force one to modify principles. Something like this happened to the English poet Wilfred Owen, whose experiences in the First World War transformed him from an enthusiastic soldier into a virtual pacifist. I can't document his change of conscience in detail; but I want to present something which he wrote about the way experience can put pressure on morality.

The Latin poet Horace wrote that it is sweet and fitting (or right) to die for one's country—*dulce et decorum est pro patria mori*—and Owen wrote a fine poem about how experience could lead one to relinquish that particular moral principle.[1] He describes a man who is too slow donning his gas

---

[1] I am grateful to the Executors of the Estate of Harold Owen, and to Chatto and Windus Ltd., for permission to quote from Wilfred Owen's 'Dulce et Decorum Est' and 'Insensibility'.

mask during a gas attack—'As under a green sea I saw him drowning,' Owen says. The poem ends like this:

> In all my dreams before my helpless sight
> He plunges at me, guttering, choking, drowning.
> If in some smothering dreams, you too could pace
> Behind the wagon that we flung him in,
> And watch the white eyes writhing in his face,
> His hanging face, like a devil's sick of sin;
> If you could hear, at every jolt, the blood
> Come gargling from the froth-corrupted lungs,
> Bitter as the cud
> Of vile, incurable sores on innocent tongues,—
> My friend, you would not tell with such high zest
> To children ardent for some desperate glory,
> The old Lie: Dulce et decorum est
> Pro patria mori.

There is a difficulty about drawing from all this a moral for ourselves. I imagine that we agree in our rejection of slavery, eternal damnation, genocide, and uncritical patriotic self-abnegation; so we shall agree that Huck Finn, Jonathan Edwards, Heinrich Himmler, and the poet Horace would all have done well to bring certain of their principles under severe pressure from ordinary human sympathies. But then we can say this because we can say that all those are bad moralities, whereas we cannot look at our own moralities and declare them bad. This is not arrogance: it is obviously incoherent for someone to declare the system of moral principles that he *accepts* to be *bad*, just as one cannot coherently say of anything that one *believes* it but it is *false*.

Still, although I can't point to any of my beliefs and say 'That is false', I don't doubt that some of my beliefs *are* false; and so I should try to remain open to correction. Similarly, I accept every single item in my morality—that is inevitable—but I am sure that my morality could be improved, which is to say that it could undergo changes which I should be glad of once I had made them. So I must try to keep my morality open to revision, exposing it to whatever valid pressures there are—including pressures from my sympathies.

I don't give my sympathies a blank cheque in advance. In a conflict between principle and sympathy, principles ought sometimes to win. For example, I think it was right to take part in the Second World War on the allied side; there were many ghastly individual incidents which might have led someone to doubt the rightness of his participation in that war; and I think it would have been right for such a person to keep his sympathies in a subordinate place on those occasions, not allowing them to modify his principles in such a way as to make a pacifist of him.

Still, one's sympathies should be kept as sharp and sensitive and aware as possible, and not only because they can sometimes affect one's principles or one's conduct or both. Owen, at any rate, says that feelings and sympathies are vital even when they can do nothing but bring pain and distress. In another poem he speaks of the blessings of being numb in one's feelings: 'Happy are the men who yet before they are killed/Can let their veins run cold,' he says. These are the ones who do not suffer from any compassion which, as Owen puts it, 'makes their feet/Sore on the alleys cobbled with their brothers'. He contrasts these 'happy' ones, who 'lose all imagination', with himself and others 'who with a thought besmirch/Blood over all our soul'. Yet the poem's verdict goes against the 'happy' ones. Owen does not say that they will act worse than the others whose souls are besmirched with blood because of their keen awareness of human suffering. He merely says that they are the losers because they have cut themselves off from the human condition:

> By choice they made themselves immune
> To pity and whatever moans in man
> Before the last sea and the hapless stars;
> Whatever mourns when many leave these shores;
> Whatever shares
> The eternal reciprocity of tears.

['The Conscience of Huckleberry Finn', *Philosophy*, 49 (1974), 123–34.]

This paper began life as the Potter Memorial Lecture, given at Washington State University in Pullman, Washington, in 1972.

iii. Consequentialism

a. The Theory

JEREMY BENTHAM

77   The Principle of Utility

I. Nature has placed mankind under the governance of two sovereign masters, *pain* and *pleasure*. It is for them alone to point out what we ought to do, as well as to determine what we shall do. On the one hand the standard of right and wrong, on the other the chain of causes and effects, are fastened to their throne. They govern us in all we do, in all we say, in all we think: every effort we can make to throw off our subjection, will serve but to demonstrate and confirm it. In words a man may pretend to abjure their empire: but in reality he will remain subject to it all the while. The *principle of utility*[1] recognises this subjection, and assumes it for the foundation of that system, the object of which is to rear the fabric of felicity by the hands of reason and of law. Systems which attempt to question it, deal in sounds instead of sense, in caprice instead of reason, in darkness instead of light.

But enough of metaphor and declamation: it is not by such means that moral science is to be improved.

II. The principle of utility is the foundation of the present work: it will be proper therefore at the outset to give an explicit and determinate account of what is meant by it. By the principle[2] of utility is meant that principle which approves or disapproves of every action whatsoever, according to the tendency which it appears to have to augment or diminish the happiness of the party whose interest is in question: or, what is the same thing

---

[1] Note by the Author, July 1822: To this denomination has of late been added, or substituted, the *greatest happiness* or *greatest felicity* principle: this for shortness, instead of saying at length *that principle* which states the greatest happiness of all those whose interest is in question, as being the right and proper, and only right and proper and universally desirable, end of human action: of human action in every situation, and in particular in that of a functionary or set of functionaries exercising the powers of Government. The word *utility* does not so clearly point to the ideas of *pleasure* and *pain* as the words *happiness* and *felicity* do: nor does it lead us to the consideration of the *number*, of the interests affected; to the *number*, as being the circumstance, which contributes, in the largest proportion, to the formation of the standard here in question; the *standard of right and wrong*, by which alone the propriety of human conduct, in every situation, can with propriety be tried. This want of a sufficiently manifest connexion between the ideas of *happiness* and *pleasure* on the one hand, and the idea of *utility* on the other, I have every now and then found operating, and with but too much efficiency, as a bar to the acceptance, that might otherwise have been given, to this principle.

in other words, to promote or to oppose that happiness. I say of every action whatsoever; and therefore not only of every action of a private individual, but of every measure of government.

III. By utility is meant that property in any object, whereby it tends to produce benefit, advantage, pleasure, good, or happiness, (all this in the present case comes to the same thing) or what comes again to the same thing) to prevent the happening of mischief, pain, evil, or unhappiness to the party whose interest is considered: if that party be the community in general, then the happiness of the community: if a particular individual, then the happiness of that individual.

IV. The interest of the community is one of the most general expressions that can occur in the phraseology of morals: no wonder that the meaning of it is often lost. When it has a meaning, it is this. The community is a fictitious *body*, composed of the individual persons who are considered as constituting as it were its *members*. The interest of the community then is, what?—the sum of the interests of the several members who compose it.

V. It is in vain to talk of the interest of the community, without understanding what is the interest of the individual. A thing is said to promote the interest, or to be *for* the interest, of an individual, when it tends to add to the sum total of his pleasures: or, what comes to the same thing, to diminish the sum total of his pains.

VI. An action then may be said to be conformable to the principle of utility, or, for shortness sake, to utility, (meaning with respect to the community at large) when the tendency it has to augment the happiness of the community is greater than any it has to diminish it.

VII. A measure of government (which is but a particular kind of action, performed by a particular person or persons) may be said to be conformable to or dictated by the principle of utility, when in like manner the tendency which it has to augment the happiness of the community is greater than any which it has to diminish it.

VIII. When an action, or in particular a measure of government, is supposed by a man to be conformable to the principle of utility, it may be convenient, for the purposes of discourse, to imagine a kind of law or

---

[2] The word principle is derived from the Latin *principium*: which seems to be compounded of the two words *primus*, first, or chief, and *cipium*, a termination which seems to be derived from *capio*, to take, as in *mancipium, municipium*; to which are analogous, *auceps, forceps*, and others. It is a term of very vague and very extensive signification: it is applied to any thing which is conceived to serve as a foundation or beginning to any series of operations: in some cases, of physical operations; but of mental operations in the present case.

The principle here in question may be taken for an act of the mind; a sentiment; a sentiment of approbation; a sentiment which, when applied to an action, approves of its utility, as that quality of it by which the measure of approbation or disapprobation bestowed upon it ought to be governed.

dictate, called a law or dictate of utility: and to speak of the action in question, as being conformable to such law or dictate.

IX. A man may be said to be a partizan of the principle of utility, when the approbation or disapprobation he annexes to any action, or to any measure, is determined by and proportioned to the tendency which he conceives it to have to augment or to diminish the happiness of the community: or in other words, to its conformity or unconformity to the laws or dictates of utility.

X. Of an action that is conformable to the principle of utility one may always say either that it is one that ought to be done, or at least that it is not one that ought not to be done. One may say also, that it is right it should be done; at least that it is not wrong it should be done: that it is a right action; at least that it is not a wrong action. When thus interpreted, the words *ought*, and *right* and *wrong*, and others of that stamp, have a meaning: when otherwise, they have none.

XI. Has the rectitude of this principle been ever formally contested? It should seem that it had, by those who have not known what they have been meaning. Is it susceptible of any direct proof? it should seem not: for that which is used to prove every thing else, cannot itself be proved: a chain of proofs must have their commencement somewhere. To give such proof is as impossible as it is needless.

XII. Not that there is or ever has been that human creature breathing, however stupid or perverse, who has not on many, perhaps on most occasions of his life, deferred to it. By the natural constitution of the human frame, on most occasions of their lives men in general embrace this principle, without thinking of it: if not for the ordering of their own actions, yet for the trying of their own actions, as well as of those of other men. There have been, at the same time, not many, perhaps, even of the most intelligent, who have been disposed to embrace it purely and without reserve. There are even few who have not taken some occasion or other to quarrel with it, either on account of their not understanding always how to apply it, or on account of some prejudice or other which they were afraid to examine into, or could not bear to part with. For such is the stuff that man is made of: in principle and in practice, in a right track and in a wrong one, the rarest of all human qualities is consistency.

XIII. When a man attempts to combat the principle of utility, it is with reasons drawn, without his being aware of it, from that very principle itself. His arguments, if they prove any thing, prove not that the principle is *wrong*, but that, according to the applications he supposes to be made of it, it is *misapplied*. Is it possible for a man to move the earth? Yes; but he must first find out another earth to stand upon.

XIV. To disprove the propriety of it by arguments is impossible; but, from the causes that have been mentioned, or from some confused or partial view of it, a man may happen to be disposed not to relish it. Where this is the case, if he thinks the settling of his opinions on such a subject worth the trouble, let him take the following steps, and at length, perhaps, he may come to reconcile himself to it.

1. Let him settle with himself, whether he would wish to discard this principle altogether; if so, let him consider what it is that all his reasonings (in matters of politics especially) can amount to?

2. If he would, let him settle with himself, whether he would judge and act without any principle, or whether there is any other he would judge and act by?

3. If there be, let him examine and satisfy himself whether the principle he thinks he has found is really any separate intelligible principle; or whether it be not a mere principle in words, a kind of phrase, which at bottom expresses neither more nor less than the mere averment of his own unfounded sentiments; that is, what in another person he might be apt to call caprice?

4. If he is inclined to think that his own approbation or disapprobation, annexed to the idea of an act, without any regard to its consequences, is a sufficient foundation for him to judge and act upon, let him ask himself whether his sentiment is to be a standard of right and wrong, with respect to every other man, or whether every man's sentiment has the same privilege of being a standard to itself?

5. In the first case, let him ask himself whether his principle is not despotical, and hostile to all the rest of human race?

6. In the second case, whether it is not anarchial, and whether at this rate there are not as many different standards of right and wrong as there are men? and whether even to the same man, the same thing, which is right to-day, may not (without the least change in its nature) be wrong to-morrow? and whether the same thing is not right and wrong in the same place at the same time? and in either case, whether all argument is not at an end? and whether, when two men have said, 'I like this,' and 'I don't like it,' they can (upon such a principle) have any thing more to say?

7. If he should have said to himself, No: for that the sentiment which he proposes as a standard must be grounded on reflection, let him say on what particulars the reflection is to turn? if on particulars having relation to the utility of the act, then let him say whether this is not deserting his own principle, and borrowing assistance from that very one in opposition to which he sets it up: or if not on those particulars, on what other particulars?

8. If he should be for compounding the matter, and adopting his own principle in part, and the principle of utility in part, let him say how far he will adopt it?

9. When he has settled with himself where he will stop, then let him ask himself how he justifies to himself the adopting it so far? and why he will not adopt it any farther?

10. Admitting any other principle than the principle of utility to be a right principle, a principle that it is right for a man to pursue; admitting (what is not true) that the word *right* can have a meaning without reference to utility, let him say whether there is any such thing as a *motive* that a man can have to pursue the dictates of it: if there is, let him say what that motive is, and how it is to be distinguished from those which enforce the dictates of utility: if not, then lastly let him say what it is this other principle can be good for?

* * * * * *

I. Pleasures then, and the avoidance of pains, are the *ends* which the legislator has in view: it behoves him therefore to understand their *value*. Pleasures and pains are the *instruments* he has to work with: it behoves him therefore to understand their force, which is again, in other words, their value.

II. To a person considered *by himself*, the value of a pleasure or pain considered *by itself*, will be greater or less, according to the four following circumstances[1]:

1. Its *intensity*.
2. Its *duration*.
3. Its *certainty* or *uncertainty*.
4. Its *propinquity* or *remoteness*.

III. These are the circumstances which are to be considered in estimating a pleasure or a pain considered each of them by itself. But when the value of any pleasure or pain is considered for the purpose of estimating the tendency of any *act* by which it is produced, there are two other circumstances to be taken into the account; these are,

5. Its *fecundity*, or the chance it has of being followed by sensations of the *same* kind: that is, pleasures, if it be a pleasure: pains, if it be a pain.

6. Its *purity*, or the chance it has of *not* being followed by sensations of the *opposite* kind: that is, pains, if it be a pleasure: pleasures, if it be a pain.

These two last, however, are in strictness scarcely to be deemed properties of the pleasure or the pain itself; they are not, therefore, in strictness to be taken into the account of the value of that pleasure or that pain. They

---

[1] These circumstances have since been denominated *elements* or *dimensions* of *value* in a pleasure or a pain. Not long after the publication of the first edition, the following memoriter verses were framed, in the view of lodging more effectually, in the memory, these points, on which the whole fabric of morals and legislation may be seen to rest.

> Intense, long, certain, speedy, fruitful, pure—
> Such marks in *pleasures* and in *pains* endure.
> Such pleasures seek if *private* be thy end:
> If it be *public*, wide let them *extend*.
> Such *pains* avoid, whichever be thy view:
> If pains *must* come, let them *extend* to few.

are in strictness to be deemed properties only of the act, or other event, by which such pleasure or pain has been produced; and accordingly are only to be taken into the account of the tendency of such act or such event.

IV. To a *number* of persons, with reference to each of whom the value of a pleasure or a pain is considered, it will be greater or less, according to seven circumstances: to wit, the six preceding ones; *viz.*

1. Its *intensity.*
2. Its *duration.*
3. Its *certainty* or *uncertainty.*
4. Its *propinquity* or *remoteness.*
5. Its *fecundity.*
6. Its *purity.*

And one other; to wit:

7. Its *extent*; that is, the number of persons to whom it *extends*; or (in other words) who are affected by it.

V. To take an exact account then of the general tendency of any act, by which the interests of a community are affected, proceed as follows. Begin with any one person of those whose interests seem most immediately to be affected by it: and take an account,

1. Of the value of each distinguishable *pleasure* which appears to be produced by it in the *first* instance.

2. Of the value of each *pain* which appears to be produced by it in the *first* instance.

3. Of the value of each pleasure which appears to be produced by it *after* the first. This constitutes the *fecundity* of the first *pleasure* and the *impurity* of the first *pain.*

4. Of the value of each *pain* which appears to be produced by it after the first. This constitutes the *fecundity* of the first *pain*, and the *impurity* of the first pleasure.

5. Sum up all the values of all the *pleasures* on the one side, and those of all the pains on the other. The balance, if it be on the side of pleasure, will give the *good* tendency of the act upon the whole, with respect to the interests of that *individual* person; if on the side of pain, the *bad* tendency of it upon the whole.

6. Take an account of the *number* of persons whose interests appear to be concerned; and repeat the above process with respect to each. *Sum up* the numbers expressive of the degrees of *good* tendency, which the act has, with respect to each individual, in regard to whom the tendency of it is *good* upon the whole: do this again with respect to each individual, in regard to whom the tendency of it is *good* upon the whole: do this again with respect to each individual, in regard to whom the tendency of it is *bad* upon the whole. Take the *balance*; which, if on the side of *pleasure*, will give the general *good tendency* of the act, with respect to the total number or

community of individuals concerned; if on the side of pain, the general *evil tendency*, with respect to the same community.

VI. It is not to be expected that this process should be strictly pursued previously to every moral judgment, or to every legislative or judicial operation. It may, however, be always kept in view: and as near as the process actually pursued on these occasions approaches to it, so near will such process approach to the character of an exact one.

[*Introduction to the Principles of Morals and Legislation* (Hafner: New York, 1948), 1–7, 29–31. First published in 1789.]

WILLIAM GODWIN

78 The Archbishop and the Chambermaid

Justice is a rule of conduct originating in the connection of one percipient being with another. A comprehensive maxim which has been laid down upon the subject is 'that we should love our neighbour as ourselves.' But this maxim, though possessing considerable merit as a popular principle, is not modelled with the strictness of philosophical accuracy.

In a loose and general view I and my neighbour are both of us men, and of consequence entitled to equal attention. But in reality it is probable that one of us is a being of more worth and importance than the other. A man is of more worth than a beast, because, being possessed of higher faculties, he is capable of a more refined and genuine happiness. In the same manner the illustrious archbishop of Cambrai was of more worth than his chambermaid, and there are few of us that would hesitate to pronounce, if his palace were in flames and the life of only one of them could be preserved, which of the two ought to be preferred.

But there is another ground of preference beside the private consideration of one of them being farther removed from the state of a mere animal. We are not connected with one or two percipient beings, but with a society, a nation, and in some sense with the whole family of mankind. Of consequence that life ought to be preferred which will be most conducive to the general good. In saving the life of Fenelon, suppose at the moment when he was conceiving the project of his immortal *Telemachus*, I should be promoting the benefit of thousands who have been cured by the perusal of it of some error, vice and consequent unhappiness. Nay, my benefit would extend farther than this, for every individual thus cured has become a better member of society and has contributed in his turn to the happiness, the information and improvement of others.

Supposing I had been myself the chambermaid, I ought to have chosen to die rather than that Fenelon should have died. The life of Fenelon was really preferable to that of the chambermaid. But understanding is the faculty that perceives the truth of this and similar propositions; and justice is the principle that regulates my conduct accordingly. It would have been just in the chambermaid to have preferred the archbishop to herself. To have done otherwise would have been a breach of justice.

Supposing the chambermaid had been my wife, my mother or my bene-factor. This would not alter the truth of the proposition. The life of Fenelon would still be more valuable than that of the chambermaid; and justice—pure, unadulterated justice—would still have preferred that which was most valuable. Justice would have taught me to save the life of Fenelon at the expense of the other. What magic is there in the pronoun 'my' to overturn the decisions of everlasting truth? My wife or my mother may be a fool or a prostitute, malicious, lying or dishonest. If they be, of what consequence is it that they are mine?

'But my mother endured for me the pains of child bearing, and nourished me in the helplessness of infancy.' When she first subjected herself to the necessity of these cares, she was probably influenced by no particular motives of benevolence to her future offspring. Every voluntary benefit however entitles the bestower to some kindness and retribution. But why so? Because a voluntary benefit is an evidence of benevolent intention; that is, of virtue. It is the disposition of the mind, not the external action, that entitles to respect. But the merit of this disposition is equal whether the benefit was conferred upon me or upon another. I and another man cannot both be right in preferring our own individual benefactor, for no man can be at the same time both better and worse than his neighbour. My benefac-tor ought to be esteemed, not because he bestowed a benefit upon me, but because he bestowed it upon a human being. His desert will be in exact proportion to the degree in which that human being was worthy of the distinction conferred. Thus every view of the subject brings us back to the consideration of my neighbour's moral worth and his importance to the general weal as the only standard to determine the treatment to which he is entitled. Gratitude therefore, a principle which has so often been the theme of the moralist and the poet, is no part either of justice or virtue.

[*An Enquiry concerning Political Justice* (Alfred Knopf: New York, 1926), 40–3. First published in 1793.]

79 **Issues for Utilitarians**

By Utilitarianism is here meant the ethical theory, that the conduct which, under any given circumstances, is objectively right, is that which will produce the greatest amount of happiness on the whole; that is, taking into account all whose happiness is affected by the conduct. [. . .]

We have next to consider who the 'all' are, whose happiness is to be taken into account. Are we to extend our concern to all the beings capable of pleasure and pain whose feelings are affected by our conduct? or are we to confine our view to human happiness? The former view is the one adopted by Bentham and Mill, and (I believe) by the Utilitarian school generally: and is obviously most in accordance with the universality that is characteristic of their principle. It is the Good *Universal*, interpreted and defined as 'happiness' or 'pleasure,' at which a Utilitarian considers it his duty to aim: and it seems arbitrary and unreasonable to exclude from the end, as so conceived, any pleasure of any sentient being.

It may be said that by giving this extension to the notion, we considerably increase the scientific difficulties of the hedonistic comparison: for if it be difficult to compare the pleasures and pains of other men accurately with our own, a comparison of either with the pleasures and pains of brutes is obviously still more obscure. Still, the difficulty is at least not greater for Utilitarians than it is for any other moralists who recoil from the paradox of disregarding altogether the pleasures and pains of brutes. But even if we limit our attention to human beings, the extent of the subjects of happiness is not yet quite determinate. In the first place, it may be asked, How far we are to consider the interests of posterity when they seem to conflict with those of existing human beings? It seems, however, clear that the time at which a man exists cannot affect the value of his happiness from a universal point of view; and that the interests of posterity must concern a Utilitarian as much as those of his contemporaries, except in so far as the effect of his actions on posterity—and even the existence of human beings to be affected—must necessarily be more uncertain. But a further question arises when we consider that we can to some extent influence the number of future human (or sentient) beings. We have to ask how, on Utilitarian principles, this influence is to be exercised. Here I shall assume that, for human beings generally, life on the average yields a positive balance of pleasure over pain. This has been denied by thoughtful persons: but the denial seems to me clearly opposed to the common experience of mankind, as expressed in their commonly accepted principles of action. The great majority of men, in the great majority of conditions under which human life is lived, certainly act as if death were one of the worst of evils, for themselves and for those whom they love: and the administration of criminal justice proceeds on a similar assumption.

Assuming, then, that the average happiness of human beings is a positive quantity, it seems clear that, supposing the average happiness enjoyed remains undiminished, Utilitarianism directs us to make the number enjoying it as great as possible. But if we foresee as possible that an increase in numbers will be accompanied by a decrease in average happiness or *vice versa*, a point arises which has not only never been formally noticed, but which seems to have been substantially overlooked by many Utilitarians. For if we take Utilitarianism to prescribe, as the ultimate end of action, happiness on the whole, and not any individual's happiness, unless considered as an element of the whole, it would follow that, if the additional population enjoy on the whole positive happiness, we ought to weigh the amount of happiness gained by the extra number against the amount lost by the remainder. So that, strictly conceived, the point up to which, on Utilitarian principles, population ought to be encouraged to increase, is not that at which average happiness is the greatest possible,—as appears to be often assumed by political economists of the school of Malthus—but that at which the product formed by multiplying the number of persons living into the amount of average happiness reaches its maximum.

It may be well here to make a remark which has a wide application in Utilitarian discussion. The conclusion just given wears a certain air of absurdity to the view of Common Sense; because its show of exactness is grotesquely incongruous with our consciousness of the inevitable inexactness of all such calculations in actual practice. But, that our practical Utilitarian reasonings must necessarily be rough, is no reason for not making them as accurate as the case admits; and we shall be more likely to succeed in this if we keep before our mind as distinctly as possible the strict type of the calculation that we should have to make, if all the relevant considerations could be estimated with mathematical precision.

We have hitherto supposed that the innovator is endeavouring to introduce a new rule of conduct, not for himself only, but for others also, as more conducive to the general happiness than the rule recognised by Common Sense. It may perhaps be thought that this is not the issue most commonly raised between Utilitarianism and Common Sense: but rather whether exceptions should be allowed to rules which both sides accept as generally valid. For no one doubts that it is, *generally speaking*, conducive to the common happiness that men should be veracious, faithful to promises, obedient to law, disposed to satisfy the normal expectations of others, having their malevolent impulses and their sensual appetites under strict control: but it is thought that an exclusive regard to pleasurable and painful consequences would frequently admit exceptions to rules which Common Sense imposes as absolute. It should, however, be observed that the admission of an exception on general grounds is merely the establishment of a more complex and delicate rule, instead of one that is broader and simpler; for if it is conducive to the general good that such an exception be admitted in one case, it will be equally so in all similar cases. Suppose (*e.g.*) that a Utilitarian thinks it on general grounds right to answer falsely a question as to the manner in which he has voted at a political election where the voting is by secret ballot. His reasons will probably be that the Utilitarian prohibition of falsehood is based on (1) the harm done by misleading particular individuals, and (2) the tendency of false statements to diminish the mutual confidence that men ought to have in each other's assertions: and that in this exceptional case it is (1) expedient that the questioner should be misled; while (2), in so far as the falsehood tends to produce a general distrust of all assertions as to the manner in which a man has voted, it only furthers the end for which voting has been made secret. It is evident, that if these reasons are valid for any person, they are valid for all persons; in fact, that they establish the expediency of a new general rule in respect of truth and falsehood, more complicated than the old one; a rule which the Utilitarian, as such, should desire to be universally obeyed. [. . .]

[T]he Utilitarian may have no doubt that in a community consisting generally of enlightened Utilitarians, these grounds for exceptional ethical treatment would be regarded as valid; still he may, as I have said, doubt whether the more refined and complicated rule which recognises such exceptions is adapted for the community in which he is actually living; and whether the attempt to introduce it is not likely to do more harm by weakening current morality than good by improving its quality. Supposing such a doubt to arise, [. . .] it becomes necessary that the Utilitarian should consider carefully the extent to which his advice or example are likely to influence persons to whom they would be dangerous: and it is evident that the result of this consideration may depend largely on the degree of publicity which he gives to either advice or example. Thus, on Utilitarian principles, it may be right to do and privately recommend, under certain circumstances, what it would not be right to advocate openly; it may be right to teach openly to one set of persons what it would be wrong to teach to others; it may be conceivably right to do, if it can be done with comparative secrecy, what it would be wrong to do in the face of the world; and even, if perfect secrecy can be reasonably expected, what it would be wrong to recommend by private advice or example. These conclusions are all of a paradoxical character:[1] there is no doubt that the moral consciousness of a plain man broadly repudiates the general notion of an esoteric morality, differing from that popularly taught; and it would be commonly agreed that an action which would be bad if done openly is not rendered good by secrecy. We may observe, however, that there are strong utilitarian reasons for maintaining generally this latter common opinion; for it is obviously advantageous, generally speaking, that acts which it is expedient

---

[1] In particular cases, however, they seem to be admitted by Common Sense to a certain extent. For example, it would be commonly thought wrong to express in public speeches disturbing religious or political opinions which may be legitimately published in books.

to repress by social disapprobation should become known, as otherwise the disapprobation cannot operate; so that it seems inexpedient to support by any moral encouragement the natural disposition of men in general to conceal their wrong doings; besides that the concealment would in most cases have importantly injurious effects on the agent's habits of veracity. Thus the Utilitarian conclusion, carefully stated, would seem to be this; that the opinion that secrecy may render an action right which would not otherwise be so should itself be kept comparatively secret; and similarly it seems expedient that the doctrine that esoteric morality is expedient should itself be kept esoteric. Or if this concealment be difficult to maintain, it may be desirable that Common Sense should repudiate the doctrines which it is expedient to confine to an enlightened few. And thus a Utilitarian may reasonably desire, on Utilitarian principles, that some of his conclusions should be rejected by mankind generally; or even that the vulgar should keep aloof from his system as a whole, in so far as the inevitable indefiniteness and complexity of its calculations render it likely to lead to bad results in their hands.

Of course, as I have said, in an ideal community of enlightened Utilitarians this swarm of perplexities and paradoxes would vanish; as in such a society no one can have any ground for believing that other persons will act on moral principles different from those which he adopts. And any enlightened Utilitarian must of course desire this consummation; as all conflict of moral opinion must *pro tanto* be regarded as an evil, as tending to impair the force of morality generally in its resistance to seductive impulses. Still such conflict may be a necessary evil in the actual condition of civilised communities, in which there are so many different degrees of intellectual and moral development.

[*The Methods of Ethics*, 7th edn. (Macmillan: London, 1907), 411, 414–16, 485, 489–90.]

J. J. C. SMART

80   Desert Island Promises

The chief persuasive argument in favour of utilitarianism has been that the dictates of any deontological ethics will always, on some occasions, lead to the existence of misery that could, on utilitarian principles, have been prevented. Thus if the deontologist says that promises always should be kept (or even if, like Ross, he says that there is a *prima facie* duty to keep them) we may confront him with a situation like the following, the well-known 'desert island promise': I have promised a dying man on a desert island, from which subsequently I alone am rescued, to give his hoard of gold to the South Australian Jockey Club. On my return I give it to the

Royal Adelaide Hospital, which, we may suppose, badly needs it for a new X-ray machine. Could anybody deny that I had done rightly without being open to the charge of heartlessness? (Remember that the promise was known only to me, and so my action will not in this case weaken the general confidence in the social institution of promising.) Think of the persons dying of painful tumours who could have been saved by the desert island gold!

'But', the deontologist may still object, 'it is my doctrine which is the humane one. You have accused me of inhumanity because I sometimes cause avoidable misery for the sake of keeping a rule. But it is these very rules, which you regard as so cold and inhuman, which safeguard mankind from the most awful atrocities. In the interests of future generations are we to allow millions to die of starvation, or still more millions to be sent to forced labour? Is it not this very consequentialist mentality which is at the root of the vast injustices which we see in the world today?' Two replies are relevant. In the first place the man who says this sort of thing may or may not be interested in the welfare of future generations. It is perfectly possible not to have the sentiment of generalized benevolence but to be moved by a localized benevolence. When this is localized in space we get the ethics of the tribe or the race: when it is localized in time we get an ethics of the present day and generation. It may well be that atrocities carried out for the sake of a Utopian future repel some people *simply* because they mortgage the present for the sake of the future. Here we have a difference about ultimate ends, and in this case I cannot accuse my opponent of being either confused or superstitious, though I may accuse him of being limited in his vision. Why should not future generations matter as much as present ones? To deny it is to be temporally parochial. If it is objected that future generations will only *probably* exist, I reply: would not the objector take into account a probably existing *present* population on a strange island before using it for bomb tests?

In the second place, however, the opponent of utilitarianism may have a perfectly disinterested benevolence, save for his regard for the observance of rules as such. Future generations may in fact mean as much to him as present ones. To him the utilitarian may reply as follows. If it were known to be true, as a question of fact, that measures which caused misery and death to tens of millions today *would* result in saving from greater misery and from death hundreds of millions in the future, and if this were the only way in which it could be done, then it *would* be right to cause these necessary atrocities. The case is surely no different in principle from that of the battalion commander who sacrifices a patrol to save a company. Where the tyrants who cause atrocities for the sake of Utopia are wrong is, surely, on the plain question of fact, and on confusing probabilities with certainties. After all, one would have to be *very sure* that future generations would be saved still greater misery before one embarked on such a tyrannical programme. One thing we should now know about the future is that large-scale predictions are impossible. Could Jeremy Bentham or Karl Marx (to take two very different political theorists) have foreseen the atom bomb? Could they have foreseen automation? Can we foresee the technology of the next century? Where the future is so dim a man must be mad who would sacrifice the present in a big way for the sake of it. Moreover even if the future were clear to us, it is very improbable that large scale atrocities could be beneficial. We must not forget the immense side effects: the brutalization of the people who ordered the atrocities and carried them out. We can, in fact, agree with the most violent denouncer of atrocities carried out in the name of Utopia without sacrificing our act-utilitarian principles. Indeed there are the best of act-utilitarian reasons for denouncing atrocities. But it is empirical facts, and empirical facts only, which will lead the utilitarian to say this.

['An Outline of a System of Utilitarian Ethics', in J. J. C. Smart and Bernard Williams, *Utilitarianism for and against* (Cambridge University Press: Cambridge, 1973), 62–4.]

R. M. HARE

81 The Structure of Ethics and Morals

I must start by saying what I think is the object of the enterprise called moral philosophy. It is to find a way of thinking better—that is, more rationally—about moral questions. The first step towards this is: *Understand the questions you are asking.* That might seem obvious; but hardly anybody tries to do it. We have to understand what we mean by expressions like 'I ought'. And to understand the meaning of a word like this involves understanding its logical properties, or in other words what it implies or what saying it commits us to. Then, if we find that we cannot accept what it commits us to, we shall have to give up saying it. And that is what moral argument essentially is. Ethics, the study of moral argument, is thus a branch of logic. This is one of the levels of thinking that are the concern of the moral philosopher. The others are about more substantial questions; but this first one, the logical or, as it is sometimes called, meta-ethical level is the foundation of the others.

Since the kind of ethics we are doing is a kind of logic, it has to use the methods of logic. But what are these? How do we find out what follows from what, what implies what, or what saying, for example, 'I ought to join the Army' or 'I ought to join the Revolution' commits me to? That is partly a general question about logical method, into which I shall not have room to go at all deeply. I can only declare what side I am on as regards some crucial questions. First, I think it is useful and indeed essential, and I hope it will not be thought pedantic, to distinguish between two kinds of questions. I am going to call the first kind *formal* questions, and the second kind *substantial* questions. Formal questions are questions that can be answered solely by appeal to the form—that is, the purely logical properties—of proposed answers to them. That is the sort of question we are concerned with in meta-ethics. In this part of our work we are not allowed to bring in any substantial assumptions.

I will illustrate the distinction by an example which has nothing to do with ethics, because it is a clearer example and does not beg any ethical questions. It comes from a well-known paper by Professors Strawson and Grice refuting (in my view successfully) a claim made in an even better-known paper by Professor Quine (some of Quine's claims may be all right, but it is pretty clear that Strawson and Grice have refuted this one).[1] Suppose I say 'My three-year-old child understands Russell's Theory of Types'. Everyone will be sure that what I have said is false. But logically it could be true. On the other hand, suppose I say 'My three-year-old child is an adult'. We know that I cannot consistently say this, if we know what the words mean and nothing else; and this is obviously not the case with the first proposition.

This illustrates the distinction between what I am calling formal questions and what I am calling substantial questions. It applies equally to moral questions, which can also be divided into these two kinds. Suppose I say 'There is nothing wrong with flogging people for fun'. People's reasons for disagreeing with me (and I will come later to what these reasons might be) are of a quite different sort from what they would be if I had said 'There is nothing wrong in doing what one ought not to do'. We know that I cannot consistently say the latter if we just know the meanings of the words 'ought' and 'wrong'; whereas I could *consistently* utter the first proposition; we all think it is a dreadful thing to say—only a very wicked person would say it—but in saying it he would not be being *logically* inconsistent.

It is not necessary here to discuss Quine's rejection of the notion of analyticity and of that of synonymy. Strawson and Grice may be right in defending these notions; but even if they are not, the formal claims that I need to make about moral concepts do not have to be stated in terms of them, but only in terms of the notion of logical truth, which Quine in that paper accepts. This is because the moral concepts are formal in an even stricter sense than I have so far claimed. That is, they require for their explanation no material semantic stipulations but only reference to their purely logical properties. The semantic properties of moral words have to

---

[1] See Sir Peter Strawson, 'Truth', *Aristotelian Society*, suppl. 24, (1950), and H. P. Grice, 'In Defense of a Dogma', *Philosophical Review*, 65 (1956); W. V. Quine, 'Two Dogmas of Empiricism', *Philosophical Review*, 60 (1951).

do with their particular descriptive meanings only, which are not part of their meaning in the narrow sense and do not affect their logic, though the fact that they have to have some descriptive meaning does affect it.[1]

It will be noticed that the example I have just given of a moral statement which we should all reject on logical grounds, 'There is nothing wrong in doing what we ought not to do', is one whose contradictory ('There is something wrong in doing what we ought not to do') is a logical truth. This is because 'ought' and 'wrong' are interdefinable in terms purely of their logical properties without bringing in their descriptive meanings or semantics, just as are 'all' and 'some' in most systems of quantificational logic.

Next, I must mention a point which will turn out to be of fundamental importance for moral argument. When we are settling questions of the second kind in each case (that is, formal questions) we are not allowed to appeal to any other kind of consideration except those which can be established on the basis of our understanding of the words or concepts used. To take our two examples: we know that we cannot say 'There is nothing wrong in doing what one ought not to do' because we know what 'wrong' and 'ought' mean; and we know that we cannot say 'My three-year-old child is an adult' because we know what 'child' and 'adult' mean. If, in order to establish that we could not say these things, we had to appeal to any other considerations than these, the questions of whether we could say them would not be formal questions.

In general, we establish theses in logic (or in the kind of logic I am speaking of, which includes the kind we use in ethics) by appeal to our understanding of the uses of words, and nothing else. It is because this logic is the foundation of moral argument that it is so important to understand the words. We must notice that this is a feature of the method I am advocating which distinguishes it quite radically from almost all the ethical theories which we find being proposed at the present time. All these theories appeal at some point or other, and often very frequently, to the substantial moral convictions which their proponents have, and which they hope their readers will share. Although I recognize that many people do not believe in the distinction that I have been making between formal and substantial moral questions, and therefore feel at liberty to use what I would call substantial convictions of theirs to support their theories, I still think that my way of proceeding provides a firmer basis for ethics.

Let me give very briefly my reasons for this confidence. If we are arguing about some moral question (for example about the question 'Ought I to join the Army?' or 'Ought I to join the Revolution?'), one of the things we

---

[1] On this, see R. M. Hare, *Moral Thinking: Its Levels, Method, and Point* (Oxford University Press: Oxford, 1981), 2 f., and *The Language of Morals* (Oxford University Press: Oxford, 1952), 122 f.

have to get clear about at the beginning is what the *question* is. That is to say, if we are not to talk at cross purposes, we have to be meaning the same things by the words in which we are asking our question. But if we *are* meaning the same by the words, we have a solid basis of agreement (albeit formal and not substantial agreement) on which we can found our future arguments. If the distinction between formal and substantial holds, then we can have this formal agreement in spite of our substantial disagreement. We can then, as I hope to show, use the formal agreement to test the arguments either of us uses to support his views. We can ask, 'Can he consistently *say* this?', or 'Can he consistently say *this*, if he also says *that*?'.

On the other hand, if people import their own substantial convictions into the very foundations of their moral arguments, they will not be able to argue cogently against anybody who does not share those convictions. This is what the philosophers called *intuitionists* do; and I say with some confidence that my own position is much stronger than theirs, because I do not rely on anything except what everybody has to agree to who is asking the same questions as I am trying to answer. That was why I said that before an argument begins we have to agree on the meaning we attach to our questions. That is *all* I require to start off with.

So much, then, for the question of ethical method. I could say, and in order to plug all the holes would have to say, a great deal more about it, and have done this elsewhere;[1] but now I wish to go on, and say what I hope to establish by this method and how it helps with real substantial questions. At the formal or meta-ethical level I need to establish just two theses; and for the sake of simplicity I shall formulate them as theses about the word 'ought' and its logic. I could have spoken instead about other words, such as 'right' and 'good'. But I prefer to talk about 'ought', because it is the simplest word that we use in our moral questionings.

Here, then, are two logical features of the word 'ought', as it occurs in the questions 'Ought I to join the Army?' and 'Ought I to join the Revolution?'. They are parts of what I commit myself to if I say 'Yes, I ought'. The first is sometimes called the *prescriptivity* of moral judgements. If I say, 'Yes, I ought to join the Army', and mean it sincerely, and in its full sense—if I really think I ought—I shall join the Army. Of course there are plenty of less than full-blooded senses of 'ought', or of 'think that I ought', in which I could say 'I think that I ought, but I'm not going to', or 'I ought, but so what?'. But anyone who has been in this situation (as I have—it was one of the things that made me take up philosophy) will know that the whole point of asking 'Ought I?' is to help us decide the question 'Shall I?', and the answer to the first question, when asked in this sense, implies an answer to the second question. If it did not, what would have been the point of asking it?

---

[1] Hare, *Moral Thinking*, ch. 1.

The second feature of the word 'ought' that I shall be relying on is usually called *universalizability*. When I say that I ought, I commit myself to more than that *I* ought. Prescriptivity demands that the man who says 'I ought' should himself act accordingly, if the judgement applies to him and if he can so act. Universalizability means that, by saying 'I ought', he commits himself to agreeing that *anybody* ought who is in just those circumstances. If I say 'I ought, but there is someone else in exactly the same circumstances, doing it to someone who is just like the person I should be doing it to, but he ought not to do it', then logical eyebrows will be raised; it is *logically inconsistent* to say, of two exactly similar people in exactly similar situations, that the first ought to do something and the second ought not. I must explain that the similarity of the situations extends to the personal characteristics, and in particular to the likes and dislikes, of the people in them. If, for example, the person I was flogging actually liked being flogged (some people do) that would mean that the situation was not exactly similar to the normal case, and the difference might be relevant.

So, putting together these two features of prescriptivity and universalizability, we see that if I say 'I ought to do it to him', I commit myself to saying, not just that I should do it to him (and accordingly doing it), but that he should do it to me were our roles precisely reversed. That is, as we shall see, how moral argument gets its grip. I must repeat that it is not an essential part of my argument that *all* uses of 'ought' have these features. All I am maintaining now is that we do sometimes, when asking 'Ought I?', use the word in this way. I am addressing myself to those who are asking such questions, as I am sure many people do. If anybody wished to ask *different* questions, he might have to use a different logic. But I am quite sure that we do sometimes find ourselves asking, and disagreeing about, universal prescriptive questions—that is, about what to prescribe universally for all situations of a given kind, no matter who is the agent or the victim. I shall be content if I can show how we can validly argue about such questions, whose logical character is determined by their being *those* questions, i.e. universal prescriptive ones.

I might add that the whole point of having a moral language with these features—a language whose meaning is determined by its logical characteristics alone, and which can therefore be used in discussion by two people who have very different substantial moral convictions, is that then the words will mean the same to both of them, and they will be bound by the same logical rules in their argument. If their different moral convictions had somehow got written into the very meanings of their moral words (as does happen with *some* moral words, and as some philosophers mistakenly think happens with all of them[1]—then they would be at cross purposes

---

[1] See R. M. Hare, *Essays in Ethical Theory* (Oxford University Press: Oxford, 1989), 121.

from the start; their moral argument would very quickly break down, and they would just have to fight it out. It is because of this formal character of my theory about the moral words that I think it more helpful than the theories of other philosophers who try to write their own moral convictions into the meanings of the words or the rules of argument. This is especially true when we come to deal with the kinds of moral problems about which people have radically different convictions. If the convictions have infected the words, they will not be able to communicate rationally with one another. That is indeed what we see happening all over the world (think of South Africa, for example). In this situation the theories I am criticizing are of no help at all, because people will appeal to their opposing convictions, and serious, fruitful argument cannot even begin.

The next thing that I have to make clear is the place in moral argument of appeal to *facts*. If I ask 'Ought I to join the Army?', the first thing, as I said, is to be clear about what I mean by 'ought'. But that is not enough. I have to be clear what I am asking; but another important part of this is what the words 'join the Army' imply. In other words, what should I be doing if I joined the Army? There are some philosophers who use the word 'consequentialist' as a term of abuse for their opponents. Now I readily agree that there may be a sense in which we ought to do what is right and damn the consequences. But these philosophers are really very confused if they think that in deciding what we ought to do we can ignore what we should be doing if we did one or other of the things we could do. If someone thinks he ought not to join the Army, or that it would be wrong to do it, his reason (what in his view makes it wrong), must have something to do with what he would be doing if he joined the Army. That is the act or series of acts about whose morality we are troubled. Joining the Army means, in his circumstances (if that is the sort of regime he lives in, as in South Africa), committing himself to shooting people in the streets if the Government tells him to. That is what becoming a soldier involves in his present situation. Anyone who thinks that in this sense consequences are irrelevant to moral decisions cannot have understood what morality is about: it is about actions; that is, about what we do; and that is, what we are bringing about—the difference we are making to the course of events. These are the facts we have to know.

There are some ethical theories, known generally as *naturalistic* theories, which make facts relevant to moral decisions in a very direct way. They do it by saying that what moral words *mean* is something factual. To give a very crude example: if 'wrong' *meant* 'such as would endanger the State', then obviously it would be wrong to do anything that would endanger the State, and we ought not to do it. The trouble with such theories is the same, in effect, as with those I mentioned earlier. It makes a theory useless for the purposes of moral argument if its author writes his own moral convictions into the theory itself; and *one* of the ways of doing this is to write them into the meanings of the moral words. This makes communication and rational argument between people of different moral convictions impossible.[1] If 'wrong' did mean what has just been suggested, somebody who thought that there were some things more important morally than the preservation of the State could not use the word to argue with a supporter of the regime. One of them would just have to join the Army and the other the Revolution; they would just have to fight.

I am not saying what naturalists say, because the account I have given of the meaning of 'ought' in terms of prescriptivity and universalizability does *not* incorporate any substantial moral convictions; it is *neutral* between the two participants in such a dispute, and both of them can therefore use the words, if I am right, in discussing their disagreement. I therefore have to give, and have already partly given a different account of how facts are relevant to moral decisions. This goes via an account of rationality itself—of the notion of a reason.

It may be helpful if we start with something simpler than moral judgements: with plain imperatives. These two sorts of speech acts must not be confused, because there are important differences; but imperatives like 'Join the Army' do illustrate in a much simpler way the point I am trying to explain. They are the simplest kind of prescriptions (moral judgements are a much more complex kind because of universalizability). To take an even simpler example: suppose I say 'Give me tea' and not 'Give me coffee'. I say this because of *something about* drinking tea or drinking coffee just then. That is my reason for saying it. If drinking tea were of a different character, I might not have said it. I want, or choose, to drink tea not coffee because I believe that that is what drinking tea would be like, i.e. because of a (supposed) fact about it. I hope that, if it is clear that, even in the case of simple imperatives like this, facts can be reasons for uttering them, it will be equally clear that moral judgements too can be uttered for reasons, even though they are not *themselves* (or not just) statements of fact, but are prescriptive. It would be irrational to ask for tea in complete disregard of what, in fact, it would be like to drink tea.[2] Note that what I have just said in no way depends on universalizability; I have deliberately taken the case of plain simple imperatives which are *not* universalizable. We shall later be making a move which depends on universalizability; but it is not necessary at this stage.

Now I wish to introduce another move, which does not depend on universalizability either, and indeed is independent of everything I have said so far. It too is a logical move, which depends on the meanings of words. It concerns the relation between *knowing* what it is to experience

[1] Ibid. 102, 121.   [2] Ibid. 37.

something, and experiencing it. The relevance of this to what I have been saying so far is that, if we are to know the facts about what we should be doing if we did something, one of the things we have to know is what we, or others, would experience if we did it. For example, if we are thinking of flogging somebody for fun, it is important that what we should be doing if we flogged him would be giving him *that* extremely unpleasant experience. If he did not mind it, or even liked it, our act would be different in a morally relevant respect. So it is important to consider what are the conditions for being said really to know what an experience (our own or somebody else's) which would be the result of our proposed act would be like.

Suppose that the experience in question is (as in this case) *suffering* of some kind. I wish to claim that we cannot suffer without knowing that we are suffering, nor know that we are suffering without suffering. The relation between having experiences and knowing that we are having them was noticed already by Aristotle.[1] There are two distinct reasons for the last half of the thesis I have just put forward. The first is that we cannot know *anything* without its being the case (that is the sort of word that 'know' is). The second reason is a particular one, and more important for our argument: if we did not have the experience of suffering, there would be nothing to know, and no means of knowing it. The knowledge that we are having the experience of suffering is *direct* knowledge, not any kind of knowledge by inference, and so cannot exist without the object of knowledge (that is, the suffering) being present in our experience. That, indeed, is why it is so difficult to know what the sufferings of other people are like. As we shall see, imagination has to fill, in an inadequate way, the place of experience.

Next, we cannot be suffering without having the preference, *pro tanto*, so far as that goes, that we should not be. If we did not prefer, other things being equal, that it should stop, it is not suffering. The preference that it should stop is what would be expressed, if it were expressed in language, by means of a prescription that it should stop. So, putting all this together, if we are suffering, and therefore know that we are, we are bound to assent to the prescription that, other things being equal, it should stop. We must want it to stop, or it is not suffering.

So much for our own present sufferings. We have now to consider what is implied by the knowledge that we *shall*, or *would* under certain conditions, be suffering, or that *somebody else* is suffering. Let us take the last-mentioned case first. What am I committed to if I truly claim that I know how somebody else is suffering, or what it is like for him to suffer like that? The touchstone for this is, it seems to me, the question 'What are my preferences (or in other words, to what prescriptions do I assent) regarding

---

[1] Aristotle, *Nicomachean Ethics*, 1120–29.

a situation in which *I* was forthwith to be put into *his* exact situation, suffering just like that?' If he is suffering like that, he knows that he is, and has the preference that it should stop (a preference of a determinate strength, depending on how severe the suffering is). He thus assents, with a determinate strength of assent, to the prescription that it should stop. This preference and this assent are part of his situation, and therefore part of what I have to imagine myself experiencing, were I to be transferred forthwith into it.

I asked just now, 'What am I committed to if I truly claim that I know how he is suffering?' My thesis is going to be that I am committed to having myself a preference that, if I were myself to be transferred forthwith into his situation with his preferences, the suffering should stop; and the strength of this preference that I am committed to having is the same as the strength of his preference.

I said that that was going to be my thesis. But I have not yet argued for it, and the argument for it will be, I am sure, controversial. The move I am going to make is this: whether I am really thinking of the person who would be put forthwith into that situation as *myself* depends on whether I associate myself with, or take to myself, the preferences which that person (i.e. I myself) would have. Of course, as before, we have to add 'other things being equal'; there may well be other things which I prefer so strongly that they outweigh my preference that that person's preference (the person who I imagine myself being) should be satisfied.[1] But *other things being equal* I have to be preferring that it be satisfied, with the same strength of preference as I should have were I in that situation with those preferences. If I am not, then either I do not really know what it is like to be in that situation with those preferences (I am not really fully representing it to myself), or I am not really thinking of the person who would be in that situation as myself.

Let me give an example to illustrate all this.[2] Suppose that somebody has been tied up and a tyre put round his neck, and the tyre ignited with petrol. He is suffering to a certain extreme degree, and therefore knows that he is suffering. What is it for *me* to know what it is like for him to suffer like that? Or, to put it in terms of preferences: he prefers very much that he should stop being burnt in that way; what it is for me to know what it is like to have a preference like that for that outcome, or of that strength (to be saying 'Oh, stop! Stop!' with that degree of anguish)? And suppose then that I claim to know just what it is like for him to have such a preference and to be suffering like that; and then suppose that somebody offers to do the same to me without further delay, and I say 'I don't mind; it's all the same to me'. That would surely show that I do not know what it is like for

---

[1] See Hare, *Essays in Ethical Theory*, 247.   [2] Ibid. 40.

him. This presumes that if I had it done to me, I should have the same experiences and the same preferences as the person to whom it is being done. I think that the same could be shown in less dramatic examples, and that, when we have made due allowance for other things not being equal (that is, for competing preferences), I could show convincingly that the thesis stands up; but I am not going to go on defending it now, because I want to draw conclusions from it for my main argument.

Let me first sum up the theses that I have advanced so far. We have the prescriptivity and the universalizability of moral judgements, which, I claim, can be established by arguments based on the meanings of words— logical arguments. Then we have the necessity, if we are to assent rationally to prescriptions, including prescriptions expressed with 'ought', of correct factual information. Lastly we have the thesis that we are *not* in possession of correct factual information about someone else's suffering, or in general about his preference, unless we ourselves have preferences that, were *we* in his situation with his preferences, those preferences should be satisfied. Note, again, that although I claimed to be able to establish universalizability, I have not yet used it in the argument. That is what I am going to do now, in conjunction with the other theses.

Let us suppose that it is I who am causing the victim to suffer. He very much wants me to untie him. That is to say, he assents with a certain very high strength of assent to the prescription that I should untie him. Already, without bringing in universalizability, we can say, on the strength of our previous theses, that I, if I know what it is like, for him, to be in that state (and if I do not know that, my moral judgement is faulted for lack of information)—I must myself have a preference that if I were in that state they should untie me. That is, I must be prescribing that they should, in those hypothetical circumstances, untie me. Now suppose that I ask myself what *universal* prescription I am prepared to assent to with regard to my present conduct which is causing him to suffer; that is, what I am prepared to say that I *ought* now to do to him. The 'ought' here expresses a universal prescription, so that, if I say 'I ought not to untie him', I am committed to the prescription that they should not untie me in similar circumstances.

I can of course say that I am not prepared to assent to *any* universal prescription. That is the position of the person whom I have elsewhere called the *amoralist*, and indicated how I would deal with him.[1] But suppose I am not an amoralist, and am therefore prepared to assent to some universal prescription for people in precisely the present situation. The question is what this is going to be. If I universalize the prescription to go on making him suffer, then this entails prescribing that, if anybody were making me suffer in a precisely analogous situation, he should carry on doing it. But

[1] See *Moral Thinking*, 182 ff.

this runs counter to a prescription which, as we have seen, I already must be assenting to if I know what it is like to be in the situation of my victim: the prescription that if I were in that situation they should *not* carry on doing it, but should untie me. Thus I am in the predicament that Kant called a contradiction in the will.[1]

How is the contradiction to be resolved? The answer becomes obvious if we notice that what is happening (what has to happen if I am trying to universalize my prescriptions) is that I am being constrained to treat other people's preferences as if they were my own. This is just another way of putting the requirement to universalize my prescriptions. But if in this situation the two preferences which have come into contradiction were both my own, what I would do would be to let the stronger of them override the weaker. And that is what I am constrained to do in the present case, where, as a result of the attempt to universalize, I have landed myself with two mutually contradictory preferences or prescriptions as to what should be done to me in the hypothetical situation in which I was in the other person's shoes. So the answer is that if my victim's preference that I should desist from tormenting him is stronger than my own preference that I should not desist (as it certainly will be), I should desist.

We have thus, in this simple bilateral case involving only two people, arrived at what is essentially a utilitarian answer to our moral problem; and we have arrived at it by a Kantian route. People talk as if Kant and the utilitarians were at opposite poles in moral philosophy; but this just shows how little they have understood either the utilitarians or Kant.[2] We are led to give weight to the preferences of all the affected parties (in this case, two) in proportion to their strengths, and to say that we ought to act on the stronger. I could, if there were room, show how, by generalizing this argument to cover multilateral situations in which the preferences of many parties are affected, we should also adopt utilitarian answers, namely that we ought in each case so to act as to maximize the satisfactions of the preferences of all affected parties, treated impartially. But I am not going to attempt this now; I have done it elsewhere,[3] and I have to go on to explain how this way of thinking is going to work out in the course of our actual moral lives, when we have to decide practical issues. I shall be able to do this only in very general terms.

It might be thought that what we have arrived at is a kind of act-utilitarianism; and this is in fact true. But it is not the kind of act-utilitarianism to which all beginner philosophy students are taught the standard objections.

---

[1] I. Kant (1785) *The Groundwork of the Metaphysic of Morals*, trans H. J. Paton (Hutchinson: London, 1948).
[2] See R. M. Hare, 'Philosophy of Language in Ethics', in *Sprachphilosophie*, ed. M. Dascal *et al.* (De Gruyter: Berlin 1989).
[3] See *Moral Thinking*, 115 ff.

I will now try to explain how the kind of act-utilitarianism that I am advocating differs from the crude kind. The difference is not, strictly speaking, a theoretical one. It derives rather from a consideration of our actual human predicament when we are doing our moral thinking. To see this, let us think what it would be like if we had no human limitations. Suppose, that is to say, that we had infinite knowledge and clarity of thought and no partiality to self or other human weaknesses. Elsewhere I have called a being who has these superhuman powers the *archangel*.[1] He really could think in an act-utilitarian way. But it would often be disastrous if we humans tried to do it, for obvious reasons. First of all, we lack the necessary information nearly always; in particular, we are very bad at putting ourselves in other people's shoes and imagining what it is like to be them. Secondly, we lack the time for acquiring and thinking about this information; and then we lack the ability to think clearly. These three handicaps make it all too easy for us to pretend to ourselves that some act is likely to be for the best (to satisfy preferences maximally and impartially) when in fact what commends it to us is our own self-interest. One sees this kind of special pleading going on all the time.

Suppose that, conscious of these handicaps, we went to an archangel for advice, not about a particular situation (for we shall not always have access to him, and therefore want him to give us advice for the future) but about how in general to minimize their bad effects. People think that they can appeal to God in this way; though what they say he tells them varies from one person to another. But let us suppose that we *had* immediate access to some supreme or at least superior being who could advise us. He would point out that the best we can do is on each occasion to make as great as possible the expectation of preference-satisfaction resulting from our actions. I am sure that this is what God would do, because he loves his creatures, and he wants us to do the best we can for them.

The expectation of preference-satisfaction (of utility, for short) is the sum of the products of the utility and the probability of the outcome for all the alternative possible outcomes of the action. This is what I mean by 'Acting for the best'. The question is, How shall we achieve this? Given our limitations, we shall not achieve it by doing a utilitarian calculation or a cost-benefit analysis on each occasion. The archangel will tell us, rather, to cultivate in ourselves a set of dispositions or principles, together with the attitudes or feelings or, if anybody wishes to use the word, intuitions that go with them: a set such that the cultivation of them is most likely on the whole to lead to the maximization of preference-satisfaction. The archangel, who can get the right answer on every single occasion, can do better than us; but that is the best that we can do.

[1] Ibid., ch. 3.

It will be noticed that this, although in a sense it is a form of rule-utilitarianism, is a form which is not incompatible with act-utilitarianism. For what the archangel is advising us to do is to perform certain acts, namely acts of cultivating dispositions; and his reason for advising this is that these acts are the most likely to be for the best—which is exactly what an act-utilitarian would advise. However, this version of utilitarianism secures the advantages which older forms of rule-utilitarianism claimed, in particular the advantage of making our proposed system immune to objections based on the counter-intuitiveness of its consequences. For the intuitions which the act-utilitarian archangel will bid us cultivate are the *same* intuitions as those to which the objectors are appealing.

The effect of this move is to divide moral thinking into two levels (in addition to the third or meta-ethical level which is concerned, not with substantial moral thinking, but with the form of moral thinking (that is, with the logic of the moral language). I call these two levels the *intuitive* level and the *critical* level. If we follow the archangel's advice, we shall do nearly all our moral thinking at the intuitive level; in fact, for nearly all the time, we shall behave just as the intuitionists say we do and should. The difference, however, will be that because, as everyone realizes, the good dispositions and principles and attitudes that we rightly cultivate are to some degree general and simple and unspecific (if they were not, they would be unmanageable and unhelpful and unteachable), they will come into conflict in particular hard cases; and then, unlike intuitionists, we shall know what we have to try to do, difficult and dangerous as it is. Since we do not in fact have archangels on call, we have to do the best we can to think critically like archangels on those problematic occasions. But when our intuitions give us clear guidance, we shall follow them—at least that is what our utilitarian archangel will advise us during our once-for-all counselling session with him.

But, it will be said, this presumes that our intuitions are the right ones. Indeed it does. This gives us another reason for using critical thinking. It is dangerous to use it in crises; but when they are over, or in anticipation of them, it may be essential. Otherwise how shall we have any confidence that the intuitions we happen to have grown up with are the best ones? Intuitions about how Whites should treat Blacks, for example, or men women? So what the wise archangel will advise, and what wise human educators and self-educators will practise, will be a judicious admixture of intuitive and critical thinking, each employed on appropriate occasions. And this is what wise people do already.

[*Essays in Moral Theory* (Oxford University Press: Oxford, 1989), 175–90.]

b. Criticism

FYODOR DOSTOEVSKY

82 Ivan's Challenge

Tell me honestly, I challenge you—answer me: imagine that you are charged with building the edifice of human destiny, the ultimate aim of which is to bring people happiness, to give them peace and contentment at last, but that in order to achieve this it is essential and unavoidable to torture just one little speck of creation, that same little child beating her chest with her little fists, and imagine that this edifice, has to be erected on her unexpiated tears. Would you agree to be the architect under those conditions? Tell me honestly!'

[*The Karamazov Brothers*, trans. Ignat Avsey (Oxford University Press: Oxford, 1994), i, part 2, bk. 5, ch. 4. First published in 1879–80.]

W. D. ROSS

83 The Personal Character of Duty

The real point at issue between hedonism and utilitarianism on the one hand and their opponents on the other is not whether 'right' means 'productive of so and so'; for it cannot with any plausibility be maintained that it does. The point at issue is that to which we now pass, viz. whether there is any general character which makes right acts right, and if so, what it is. Among the main historical attempts to state a single characteristic of all right actions which is the foundation of their rightness are those made by egoism and utilitarianism. But I do not propose to discuss these, not because the subject is unimportant, but because it has been dealt with so often and so well already, and because there has come to be so much agreement among moral philosophers that neither of these theories is satisfactory. A much more attractive theory has been put forward by Professor Moore: that what makes actions right is that they are productive of more *good* than could have been produced by any other action open to the agent.[1]

This theory is in fact the culmination of all the attempts to base rightness on productivity of some sort of result. The first form this attempt takes is

---

[1] I take the theory which, as I have tried to show, seems to be put forward in *Ethics* rather than the earlier and less plausible theory put forward in *Principia Ethica*.

the attempt to base rightness on conduciveness to the advantage or pleasure of the agent. This theory comes to grief over the fact, which stares us
in the face, that a great part of duty consists in an observance of the rights
and a furtherance of the interests of others, whatever the cost to ourselves
may be. Plato and others may be right in holding that a regard for the rights
of others never in the long run involves a loss of happiness for the agent,
that 'the just life profits a man'. But this, even if true, is irrelevant to the
rightness of the act. As soon as a man does an action *because* he thinks he
will promote his own interests thereby, he is acting not from a sense of its
rightness but from self-interest.

To the egoistic theory hedonistic utilitarianism supplies a much-needed
amendment. It points out correctly that the fact that a certain pleasure will
be enjoyed by the agent is no reason why he *ought* to bring it into being
rather than an equal or greater pleasure to be enjoyed by another, though,
human nature being what it is, it makes it not unlikely that he *will* try to
bring it into being. But hedonistic utilitarianism in its turn needs a correction. On reflection it seems clear that pleasure is not the only thing in life
that we think good in itself, that for instance we think the possession of a
good character, or an intelligent understanding of the world, as good or
better. A great advance is made by the substitution of 'productive of the
greatest good' for 'productive of the greatest pleasure'.

Not only is this theory more attractive than hedonistic utilitarianism, but
its logical relation to that theory is such that the latter could not be true
unless *it* were true, while it might be true though hedonistic utilitarianism
were not. It is in fact one of the logical bases of hedonistic utilitarianism.
For the view that what produces the maximum pleasure is right has for its
bases the views (1) that what produces the maximum good is right, and (2)
that pleasure is the only thing good in itself. If they were not assuming that
what produces the maximum *good* is right, the utilitarians' attempt to show
that pleasure is the only thing good in itself, which is in fact the point they
take most pains to establish, would have been quite irrelevant to their
attempt to prove that only what produces the maximum *pleasure* is right. If,
therefore, it can be shown that productivity of the maximum good is not
what makes all right actions right, we shall *a fortiori* have refuted hedonistic
utilitarianism.

When a plain man fulfils a promise because he thinks he ought to do so,
it seems clear that he does so with no thought of its total consequences, still
less with any opinion that these are likely to be the best possible. He thinks
in fact much more of the past than of the future. What makes him think it
right to act in a certain way is the fact that he has promised to do so—that
and, usually, nothing more. That his act will produce the best possible
consequences is not his reason for calling it right. What lends colour to the
theory we are examining, then, is not the actions (which form probably a

great majority of our actions) in which some such reflection as 'I have promised' is the only reason we give ourselves for thinking a certain action right, but the exceptional cases in which the consequences of fulfilling a promise (for instance) would be so disastrous to others that we judge it right not to do so. It must of course be admitted that such cases exist. If I have promised to meet a friend at a particular time for some trivial purpose, I should certainly think myself justified in breaking my engagement if by doing so I could prevent a serious accident or bring relief to the victims of one. And the supporters of the view we are examining hold that my thinking so is due to my thinking that I shall bring more good into existence by the one action than by the other. A different account may, however, be given of the matter, an account which will, I believe, show itself to be the true one. It may be said that besides the duty of fulfilling promises I have and recognize a duty of relieving distress,[1] and that when I think it right to do the latter at the cost of not doing the former, it is not because I think I shall produce more good thereby but because I think it the duty which is in the circumstances more of a duty. This account surely corresponds much more closely with what we really think in such a situation. If, so far as I can see, I could bring equal amounts of good into being by fulfilling my promise and by helping some one to whom I had made no promise, I should not hesitate to regard the former as my duty. Yet on the view that what is right is right because it is productive of the most good I should not so regard it.

There are two theories, each in its way simple, that offer a solution of such cases of conscience. One is the view of Kant, that there are certain duties of perfect obligation, such as those of fulfilling promises, of paying debts, of telling the truth, which admit of no exception whatever in favour of duties of imperfect obligation, such as that of relieving distress. The other is the view of, for instance, Professor Moore and Dr Rashdall, that there is only the duty of producing good, and that all 'conflicts of duties' should be resolved by asking 'by which action will most good be produced?' But it is more important that our theory fit the facts than that it be simple, and the account we have given above corresponds (it seems to me) better than either of the simpler theories with what we really think, viz. that normally promise-keeping, for example, should come before benevolence, but that when and only when the good to be produced by the benevolent act is very great and the promise comparatively trivial, the act of benevolence becomes our duty.

In fact the theory of 'ideal utilitarianism', if I may for brevity refer so to the theory of Professor Moore, seems to simplify unduly our relations to

---

[1] These are not strictly speaking duties, but things that tend to be our duty, or *prima facie* duties.

our fellows. It says, in effect, that the only morally significant relation in which my neighbours stand to me is that of being possible beneficiaries by my action.[1] They do stand in this relation to me, and this relation is morally significant. But they may also stand to me in the relation of promisee to promiser, of creditor to debtor, of wife to husband, of child to parent, of friend to friend, of fellow countryman to fellow countryman, and the like; and each of these relations is the foundation of a *prima facie* duty, which is more or less incumbent on me according to the circumstances of the case. When I am in a situation, as perhaps I always am, in which more than one of these *prima facie* duties is incumbent on me, what I have to do is to study the situation as fully as I can until I form the considered opinion (it is never more) that in the circumstances one of them is more incumbent than any other; then I am bound to think that to do this *prima facie* duty is my duty *sans phrase* in the situation.

I suggest '*prima facie* duty' or 'conditional duty' as a brief way of referring to the characteristic (quite distinct from that of being a duty proper) which an act has, in virtue of being of a certain kind (e.g. the keeping of a promise), of being an act which would be a duty proper if it were not at the same time of another kind which is morally significant. Whether an act is a duty proper or actual duty depends on *all* the morally significant kinds it is an instance of. The phrase '*prima facie* duty' must be apologized for, since (1) it suggests that what we are speaking of is a certain kind of duty, whereas it is in fact not a duty, but something related in a special way to duty. Strictly speaking, we want not a phrase in which duty is qualified by an adjective, but a separate noun. (2) '*Prima*' *facie* suggests that one is speaking only of an appearance which a moral situation presents at first sight, and which may turn out to be illusory; whereas what I am speaking of is an objective fact involved in the nature of the situation, or more strictly in an element of its nature, though not, as duty proper does, arising from its *whole* nature. I can, however, think of no term which fully meets the case. 'Claim' has been suggested by Professor Prichard. The word 'claim' has the advantage of being quite a familiar one in this connexion, and it seems to cover much of the ground. It would be quite natural to say, 'a person to whom I have made a promise has a claim on me', and also, 'a person whose distress I could relieve (at the cost of breaking the promise) has a claim on me'. But (1) while 'claim' is appropriate from *their* point of view, we want a word to express the corresponding fact from the agent's point of view—the fact of his being subject to claims that can be made against him; and ordinary language provides us with no such correlative to

---

[1] Some will think it, apart from other considerations, a sufficient refutation of this view to point out that I also stand in that relation to myself, so that for this view the distinction of oneself from others is morally insignificant.

'claim'. And (2) (what is more important) 'claim' seems inevitably to suggest two persons, one of whom might make a claim on the other; and while this covers the ground of social duty, it is inappropriate in the case of that important part of duty which is the duty of cultivating a certain kind of character in oneself. It would be artificial, I think, and at any rate metaphorical, to say that one's character has a claim on oneself.

There is nothing arbitrary about these *prima facie* duties. Each rests on a definite circumstance which cannot seriously be held to be without moral significance. Of *prima facie* duties I suggest, without claiming completeness or finality for it, the following division.[1]

(1) Some duties rest on previous acts of my own. These duties seem to include two kinds, (a) those resting on a promise or what may fairly be called an implicit promise, such as the implicit undertaking not to tell lies which seems to be implied in the act of entering into conversation (at any rate by civilized men), or of writing books that purport to be history and not fiction. These may be called the duties of fidelity. (b) Those resting on a previous wrongful act. These may be called the duties of reparation. (2) Some rest on previous acts of other men, i.e. services done by them to me. These may be loosely described as the duties of gratitude. (3) Some rest on the fact or possibility of a distribution of pleasure or happiness (or of the means thereto) which is not in accordance with the merit of the persons concerned; in such cases there arises a duty to upset or prevent such a distribution. These are the duties of justice. (4) Some rest on the mere fact that there are other beings in the world whose condition we can make better in respect of virtue, or of intelligence, or of pleasure. These are the duties of beneficence. (5) Some rest on the fact that we can improve our own condition in respect of virtue or of intelligence. These are the duties of self-improvement. (6) I think that we should distinguish from (4) the duties that may be summed up under the title of 'not injuring others'. No doubt to injure others is incidentally to fail to do them good; but it seems to me clear that non-maleficence is apprehended as a duty distinct from that of beneficence, and as a duty of a more stringent character. It will be noticed that this alone among the types of duty has been stated in a negative way.

---

[1] I should make it plain at this stage that I am *assuming* the correctness of some of our main convictions as to *prima facie* duties, or, more strictly, am claiming that we *know* them to be true. To me it seems as self-evident as anything could be, that to make a promise, for instance, is to create a moral claim on us in someone else. Many readers will perhaps say that they do *not* know this to be true. If so, I certainly cannot prove it to them; I can only ask them to reflect again, in the hope that they will ultimately agree that they also know it to be true. The main moral convictions of the plain man seem to me to be, not opinions which it is for philosophy to prove or disprove, but knowledge from the start; and in my own case I seem to find little difficulty in distinguishing these essential convictions from other moral convictions which I also have, which are merely fallible opinions based on an imperfect study of the working for good or evil of certain institutions or types of action.

An attempt might no doubt be made to state this duty, like the others, in a positive way. It might be said that it is really the duty to prevent ourselves from acting either from an inclination to harm others or from an inclination to seek our own pleasure, in doing which we should incidentally harm them. But on reflection it seems clear that the primary duty here is the duty not to harm others, this being a duty whether or not we have an inclination that if followed would lead to our harming them; and that when we have such an inclination the primary duty not to harm others gives rise to a consequential duty to resist the inclination. The recognition of this duty of non-maleficence is the first step on the way to the recognition of the duty of beneficence; and that accounts for the prominence of the commands 'thou shalt not kill', 'thou shalt not commit adultery', 'thou shalt not steal', 'thou shalt not bear false witness', in so early a code as the Decalogue. But even when we have come to recognize the duty of beneficence, it appears to me that the duty of non-maleficence is recognized as a distinct one, and as *prima facie* more binding. We should not in general consider it justifiable to kill one person in order to keep another alive, or to steal from one in order to give alms to another.

The essential defect of the 'ideal utilitarian' theory is that it ignores, or at least does not do full justice to, the highly personal character of duty. If the only duty is to produce the maximum of good, the question who is to have the good—whether it is myself, or my benefactor, or a person to whom I have made a promise to confer that good on him, or a mere fellow man to whom I stand in no such special relation—should make no difference to my having a duty to produce that good. But we are all in fact sure that it makes a vast difference.

[*The Right and the Good* (Oxford University Press: Oxford, 1930), 16–22.]

JOHN RAWLS

84   The Separateness of Persons

The striking feature of the utilitarian view of justice is that it does not matter, except indirectly, how this sum of satisfactions is distributed among individuals any more than it matters, except indirectly, how one man distributes his satisfactions over time. The correct distribution in either case is that which yields the maximum fulfillment. Society must allocate its means of satisfaction whatever these are, rights and duties, opportunities and privileges, and various forms of wealth, so as to achieve this maximum if it can. But in itself no distribution of satisfaction is better than another except that the more equal distribution is to be preferred to break ties. It is true that certain common sense precepts of justice, particularly those

which concern the protection of liberties and rights, or which express the
claims of desert, seem to contradict this contention. But from a utilitarian
standpoint the explanation of these precepts and of their seemingly stringent character is that they are those precepts which experience shows
should be strictly respected and departed from only under exceptional
circumstances if the sum of advantages is to be maximized. Yet, as with all
other precepts, those of justice are derivative from the one end of attaining
the greatest balance of satisfaction. Thus there is no reason in principle why
the greater gains of some should not compensate for the lesser losses of
others; or more importantly, why the violation of the liberty of a few might
not be made right by the greater good shared by many. It simply happens
that under most conditions, at least in a reasonably advanced stage of
civilization, the greatest sum of advantages is not attained in this way. No
doubt the strictness of common sense precepts of justice has a certain
usefulness in limiting men's propensities to injustice and to socially injurious actions, but the utilitarian believes that to affirm this strictness as a first
principle of morals is a mistake. For just as it is rational for one man to
maximize the fulfillment of his system of desires, it is right for a society to
maximize the net balance of satisfaction taken over all of its members.

The most natural way, then, of arriving at utilitarianism (although not,
of course, the only way of doing so) is to adopt for society as a whole the
principle of rational choice for one man. Once this is recognized, the place
of the impartial spectator and the emphasis on sympathy in the history of
utilitarian thought is readily understood. For it is by the conception of the
impartial spectator and the use of sympathetic identification in guiding our
imagination that the principle for one man is applied to society. It is this
spectator who is conceived as carrying out the required organization of the
desires of all persons into one coherent system of desire; it is by this
construction that many persons are fused into one. Endowed with ideal
powers of sympathy and imagination, the impartial spectator is the perfectly rational individual who identifies with and experiences the desires of
others as if these desires were his own. In this way he ascertains the
intensity of these desires and assigns them their appropriate weight in the
one system of desire the satisfaction of which the ideal legislator then tries
to maximize by adjusting the rules of the social system. On this conception
of society separate individuals are thought of as so many different lines
along which rights and duties are to be assigned and scarce means of
satisfaction allocated in accordance with rules so as to give the greatest
fulfillment of wants. The nature of the decision made by the ideal legislator
is not, therefore, materially different from that of an entrepreneur deciding
how to maximize his profit by producing this or that commodity, or that of
a consumer deciding how to maximize his satisfaction by the purchase of
this or that collection of goods. In each case there is a single person whose

system of desires determines the best allocation of limited means. The correct decision is essentially a question of efficient administration. This view of social cooperation is the consequence of extending to society the principle of choice for one man, and then, to make this extension work, conflating all persons into one through the imaginative acts of the impartial sympathetic spectator. Utilitarianism does not take seriously the distinction between persons.

[*A Theory of Justice* (Harvard University Press: Cambridge, Mass.: 1972), 26–7.]

85 Jim and the Indians

Let us look more concretely at two examples, to see what utilitarianism might say about them, what we might say about utilitarianism and, most importantly of all, what would be implied by certain ways of thinking about the situation. [. . .]

(1) George, who has just taken his Ph.D. in chemistry, finds it extremely difficult to get a job. He is not very robust in health, which cuts down the number of jobs he might be able to do satisfactorily. His wife has to go out to work to keep them, which itself causes a great deal of strain, since they have small children and there are severe problems about looking after them. The results of all this, especially on the children, are damaging. An older chemist, who knows about this situation, says that he can get George a decently paid job in a certain laboratory, which pursues research into chemical and biological warfare. George says that he cannot accept this, since he is opposed to chemical and biological warfare. The older man replies that he is not too keen on it himself, come to that, but after all George's refusal is not going to make the job or the laboratory go away; what is more, he happens to know that if George refuses the job, it will certainly go to a contemporary of George's who is not inhibited by any such scruples and is likely if appointed to push along the research with greater zeal than George would. Indeed, it is not merely concern for George and his family, but (to speak frankly and in confidence) some alarm about this other man's excess of zeal, which has led the older man to offer to use his influence to get George the job . . . George's wife, to whom he is deeply attached, has views (the details of which need not concern us) from which it follows that at least there is nothing particularly wrong with research into CBW. What should he do?

(2) Jim finds himself in the central square of a small South American town. Tied up against the wall are a row of twenty Indians, most terrified, a few defiant, in front of them several armed men in uniform. A heavy man

in a sweat-stained khaki shirt turns out to be the captain in charge and, after a good deal of questioning of Jim which establishes that he got there by accident while on a botanical expedition, explains that the Indians are a random group of the inhabitants who, after recent acts of protest against the government, are just about to be killed to remind other possible protestors of the advantages of not protesting. However, since Jim is an honoured visitor from another land, the captain is happy to offer him a guest's privilege of killing one of the Indians himself. If Jim accepts, then as a special mark of the occasion, the other Indians will be let off. Of course, if Jim refuses, then there is no special occasion, and Pedro here will do what he was about to do when Jim arrived, and kill them all. Jim, with some desperate recollection of schoolboy fiction, wonders whether if he got hold of a gun, he could hold the captain, Pedro and the rest of the soldiers to threat, but it is quite clear from the set-up that nothing of that kind is going to work: any attempt at that sort of thing will mean that all the Indians will be killed, and himself. The men against the wall, and the other villagers, understand the situation, and are obviously begging him to accept. What should he do?

To these dilemmas, it seems to me that utilitarianism replies, in the first case, that George should accept the job, and in the second, that Jim should kill the Indian. Not only does utilitarianism give these answers but, if the situations are essentially as described and there are no further special factors, it regards them, it seems to me, as *obviously* the right answers. But many of us would certainly wonder whether, in (1), that could possibly be the right answer at all; and in the case of (2), even one who came to think that perhaps that was the answer, might well wonder whether it was obviously the answer. Nor is it just a question of the rightness or obviousness of these answers. It is also a question of what sort of considerations come into finding the answer. A feature of utilitarianism is that it cuts out a kind of consideration which for some others makes a difference to what they feel about such cases: a consideration involving the idea, as we might first and very simply put it, that each of us is specially responsible for what *he* does, rather than for what other people do. This is an idea closely connected with the value of integrity. It is often suspected that utilitarianism, at least in its direct forms, makes integrity as a value more or less unintelligible. I shall try to show that this suspicion is correct. Of course, even if that is correct, it would not necessarily follow that we should reject utilitarianism; perhaps, as utilitarians sometimes suggest, we should just forget about integrity, in favour of such things as a concern for the general good. However, if I am right, we cannot merely do that, since the reason why utilitarianism cannot understand integrity is that it cannot coherently describe the relations between a man's projects and his actions. [. . .]

What projects does a utilitarian agent have? As a utilitarian, he has the general project of bringing about maximally desirable outcomes; how he is to do this at any given moment is a question of what causal levers, so to speak, are at that moment within reach. The desirable outcomes, however, do not just consist of agents carrying out *that* project; there must be other more basic or lower-order projects which he and other agents have, and the desirable outcomes are going to consist, in part, of the maximally harmonious realization of those projects ('in part', because one component of a utilitarianly desirable outcome may be the occurrence of agreeable experiences which are not the satisfaction of anybody's projects). Unless there were first-order projects, the general utilitarian project would have nothing to work on, and would be vacuous. What do the more basic or lower-order projects comprise? Many will be the obvious kinds of desires for things for oneself, one's family, one's friends, including basic necessities of life, and in more relaxed circumstances, objects of taste. Or there may be pursuits and interests of an intellectual, cultural or creative character. I introduce those as a separate class not because the objects of them lie in a separate class, and provide—as some utilitarians, in their churchy way, are fond of saying—'higher' pleasures. I introduce them separately because the agent's identification with them may be of a different order. It does not have to be: cultural and aesthetic interests just belong, for many, along with any other taste; but some people's commitment to these kinds of interests just is at once more thoroughgoing and serious than their pursuit of various objects of taste, while it is more individual and permeated with character than the desire for the necessities of life.

Beyond these, someone may have projects connected with his support of some cause: Zionism, for instance, or the abolition of chemical and biological warfare. Or there may be projects which flow from some more general disposition towards human conduct and character, such as a hatred of injustice, or of cruelty, or of killing.

It may be said that this last sort of disposition and its associated project do not count as (logically) 'lower-order' relative to the higher-order project of maximizing desirable outcomes; rather, it may be said, it is itself a 'higher-order' project. The vital question is not, however, how it is to be classified, but whether it and similar projects are to count among the projects whose satisfaction is to be included in the maximizing sum, and, correspondingly, as contributing to the agent's happiness. If the utilitarian says 'no' to that, then he is almost certainly committed to a version of utilitarianism as absurdly superficial and shallow as Benthamite versions have often been accused of being. For this project will be discounted, presumably, on the ground that it involves, in the specification of its object, the mention of other people's happiness or interests: thus it is the kind of project which (unlike the pursuit of food for myself) presupposes a reference to other people's projects. But that criterion would eliminate any desire at all which was not blankly and in the most straightforward sense egoistic. Thus we should be reduced to frankly egoistic first-order projects, and—for all essential purposes—the one second-order utilitarian project of maximally satisfying first-order projects. Utilitarianism has a tendency to slide in this direction, and to leave a vast hole in the range of human desires, between egoistic inclinations and necessities at one end, and impersonally benevolent happiness-management at the other. But the utilitarianism which has to leave this hole is the most primitive form, which offers a quite rudimentary account of desire. Modern versions of the theory are supposed to be neutral with regard to what sorts of things make people happy or what their projects are. Utilitarianism would do well then to acknowledge the evident fact that among the things that make people happy is not only making other people happy, but being taken up or involved in any of a vast range of projects, or—if we waive the evangelical and moralizing associations of the word—commitments. One can be committed to such things as a person, a cause, an institution, a career, one's own genius, or the pursuit of danger.

Now none of these is itself the *pursuit of happiness*: by an exceedingly ancient platitude, it is not at all clear that there could be anything which was just that, or at least anything that had the slightest chance of being successful. Happiness, rather, requires being involved in, or at least content with, something else.[1] It is not impossible for utilitarianism to accept that point: it does not have to be saddled with a naïve and absurd philosophy of mind about the relation between desire and happiness. What it does have to say is that if such commitments are worth while, then pursuing the projects that flow from them, and realizing some of those projects, will make the person for whom they are worth while, happy. It may be that to claim that is still wrong: it may well be that a commitment can make sense to a man (can make sense of his life) without his supposing that it will make him *happy*. But that is not the present point; let us grant to utilitarianism that all worthwhile human projects must conduce, one way or another, to happiness. The point is that even if that is true, it does not follow, nor could it possibly be true, that those projects are themselves projects of pursuing happiness. One has to believe in, or at least want, or quite minimally, be content with, other things, for there to be anywhere that happiness can come from.

---

[1] This does not imply that there is no such thing as the project of pursuing pleasure. Some writers who have correctly resisted the view that all desires are desires for pleasure, have given an account of pleasure so thoroughly adverbial as to leave it quite unclear how there could be a distinctively hedonist way of life at all. Some room has to be left for that, though there are important difficulties both in defining it and living it. Thus (particularly in the case of the very rich) it often has highly ritual aspects, apparently part of a strategy to counter boredom.

Utilitarianism, then, should be willing to agree that its general aim of maximizing happiness does not imply that what everyone is doing is just pursuing happiness. On the contrary, people have to be pursuing other things. What those other things may be, utilitarianism, sticking to its professed empirical stance, should be prepared just to find out. No doubt some possible projects it will want to discourage, on the grounds that their being pursued involves a negative balance of happiness to others: though even there, the unblinking accountant's eye of the strict utilitarian will have something to put in the positive column, the satisfactions of the destructive agent. Beyond that, there will be a vast variety of generally beneficent or at least harmless projects; and some no doubt, will take the form not just of tastes or fancies, but of what I have called 'commitments'. It may even be that the utilitarian researcher will find that many of those with commitments, who have really identified themselves with objects outside themselves, who are thoroughly involved with other persons, or institutions, or activities or causes, are actually happier than those whose projects and wants are not like that. If so, that is an important piece of utilitarian empirical lore.

When I say 'happier' here, I have in mind the sort of consideration which any utilitarian would be committed to accepting: as for instance that such people are less likely to have a break-down or commit suicide. Of course that is not all that is actually involved, but the point in this argument is to use to the maximum degree utilitarian notions, in order to locate a breaking point in utilitarian thought. In appealing to this strictly utilitarian notion, I am being more consistent with utilitarianism than Smart is. In his struggles with the problem of the brain-electrode man, Smart commends the idea that 'happy' is a partly evaluative term, in the sense that we call 'happiness' those kinds of satisfaction which, as things are, we approve of. But *by what standard* is this surplus element of approval supposed, from a utilitarian point of view, to be allocated? There is no source for it, on a strictly utilitarian view, except further degrees of satisfaction, but there are none of those available, or the problem would not arise. Nor does it help to appeal to the fact that we dislike in prospect things which we like when we get there, for from a utilitarian point of view it would seem that the original dislike was merely irrational or based on an error. Smart's argument at this point seems to be embarrassed by a well-known utilitarian uneasiness, which comes from a feeling that it is not respectable to ignore the 'deep', while not having anywhere left in human life to locate it.[1]

Let us now go back to the agent as utilitarian, and his higher-order project of maximizing desirable outcomes. At this level, he is committed

---

[1] One of many resemblances in spirit between utilitarianism and high-minded evangelical Christianity.

only to that: what the outcome will actually consist of will depend entirely on the facts, on what persons with what projects and what potential satisfactions there are within calculable reach of the causal levers near which he finds himself. His own substantial projects and commitments come into it, but only as one lot among others—they potentially provide one set of satisfactions among those which he may be able to assist from where he happens to be. He is the agent of the satisfaction system who happens to be at a particular point at a particular time: in Jim's case, our man in South America. His own decisions as a utilitarian agent are a function of all the satisfactions which he can affect from where he is: and this means that the projects of others, to an indeterminately great extent, determine his decision.

This may be so either positively or negatively. It will be so positively if agents within the causal field of his decision have projects which are at any rate harmless, and so should be assisted. It will equally be so, but negatively, if there is an agent within the causal field whose projects are harmful, and have to be frustrated to maximize desirable outcomes. So it is with Jim and the soldier Pedro. On the utilitarian view, the undesirable projects of other people as much determine, in this negative way, one's decisions as the desirable ones do positively: if those people were not there, or had different projects, the causal nexus would be different, and it is the actual state of the causal nexus which determines the decision. The determination to an indefinite degree of my decisions by other people's projects is just another aspect of my unlimited responsibility to act for the best in a causal framework formed to a considerable extent by their projects.

The decision so determined is, for utilitarianism, the right decision. But what if it conflicts with some project of mine? This, the utilitarian will say, has already been dealt with: the satisfaction to you of fulfilling your project, and any satisfactions to others of your so doing, have already been through the calculating device and have been found inadequate. Now in the case of many sorts of projects, that is a perfectly reasonable sort of answer. But in the case of projects of the sort I have called 'commitments', those with which one is more deeply and extensively involved and identified, this cannot just by itself be an adequate answer, and there may be no adequate answer at all. For, to take the extreme sort of case, how can a man, as a utilitarian agent, come to regard as one satisfaction among others, and a dispensable one, a project or attitude round which he has built his life, just because someone else's projects have so structured the causal scene that that is how the utilitarian sum comes out?

The point here is not, as utilitarians may hasten to say, that if the project or attitude is that central to his life, then to abandon it will be very disagreeable to him and great loss of utility will be involved. I have already argued that it is not like that; on the contrary, once he is prepared to look at it like that, the argument in any serious case is over anyway. The point is that he is identified with his actions as flowing from projects and attitudes which in some cases he takes seriously at the deepest level, as what his life is about (or, in some cases, this section of his life—seriousness is not necessarily the same as persistence). It is absurd to demand of such a man, when the sums come in from the utility network which the projects of others have in part determined, that he should just step aside from his own project and decision and acknowledge the decision which utilitarian calculation requires. It is to alienate him in a real sense from his actions and the source of his action in his own convictions. It is to make him into a channel between the input of everyone's projects, including his own, and an output of optimific decision; but this is to neglect the extent to which *his* actions and *his* decisions have to be seen as the actions and decisions which flow from the projects and attitudes with which he is most closely identified. It is thus, in the most literal sense, an attack on his integrity.

These sorts of considerations do not in themselves give solutions to practical dilemmas such as those provided by our examples; but I hope they help to provide other ways of thinking about them. In fact, it is not hard to see that in George's case, viewed from this perspective, the utilitarian solution would be wrong. Jim's case is different, and harder. But if (as I suppose) the utilitarian is probably right in this case, that is not to be found out just by asking the utilitarian's questions. Discussions of it—and I am not going to try to carry it further here—will have to take seriously the distinction between my killing someone, and its coming about because of what I do that someone else kills them: a distinction based, not so much on the distinction between action and inaction, as on the distinction between my projects and someone else's projects. At least it will have to start by taking that seriously, as utilitarianism does not; but then it will have to build out from there by asking why that distinction seems to have less, or a different, force in this case than it has in George's. One question here would be how far one's powerful objection to killing people just is, in fact, an application of a powerful objection to their being killed. Another dimension of that is the issue of how much it matters that the people at risk are actual, and there, as opposed to hypothetical, or future, or merely elsewhere.

['A Critique of Utilitarianism', in J. J. C. Smart and Bernard Williams, *Utilitarianism for and against* (Cambridge University Press: Cambridge, 1973), 96–100, 110–17.]

SUSAN WOLF

86 Moral Saints

I don't know whether there are any moral saints. But if there are, I am glad that neither I nor those about whom I care most are among them. By *moral saint* I mean a person whose every action is as morally good as possible, a person, that is, who is as morally worthy as can be. Though I shall in a moment acknowledge the variety of types of person that might be thought to satisfy this description, it seems to me that none of these types serve as unequivocally compelling personal ideals. In other words, I believe that moral perfection, in the sense of moral saintliness, does not constitute a model of personal well-being toward which it would be particularly rational or good or desirable for a human being to strive.

Outside the context of moral discussion, this will strike many as an obvious point. But, within that context, the point, if it be granted, will be granted with some discomfort. For within that context it is generally assumed that one ought to be as morally good as possible and that what limits there are to morality's hold on us are set by features of human nature of which we ought not to be proud. If, as I believe, the ideals that are derivable from common sense and philosophically popular moral theories do not support these assumptions, then something has to change. Either we must change our moral theories in ways that will make them yield more palatable ideals, or, as I shall argue, we must change our conception of what is involved in affirming a moral theory.

In this paper, I wish to examine the notion of a moral saint, first, to understand what a moral saint would be like and why such a being would be unattractive, and, second, to raise some questions about the significance of this paradoxical figure for moral philosophy. I shall look first at the model(s) of moral sainthood that might be extrapolated from the morality or moralities of common sense. Then I shall consider what relations these have to conclusions that can be drawn from utilitarian and Kantian moral theories. Finally, I shall speculate on the implications of these considerations for moral philosophy.

Moral Saints and Common Sense

Consider first what, pretheoretically, would count for us—contemporary members of Western culture—as a moral saint. A necessary condition of moral sainthood would be that one's life be dominated by a commitment to improving the welfare of others or of society as a whole. As to what role this commitment must play in the individual's motivational system, two contrasting accounts suggest themselves to me which might equally be thought to qualify a person for moral sainthood.

First, a moral saint might be someone whose concern for others plays the role that is played in most of our lives by more selfish, or, at any rate, less morally worthy concerns. For the moral saint, the promotion of the welfare of others might play the role that is played for most of us by the enjoyment of material comforts, the opportunity to engage in the intellectual and physical activities of our choice, and the love, respect, and companionship of people whom we love, respect, and enjoy. The happiness of the moral saint, then, would truly lie in the happiness of others, and so he would devote himself to others gladly, and with a whole and open heart.

On the other hand, a moral saint might be someone for whom the basic ingredients of happiness are not unlike those of most of the rest of us. What makes him a moral saint is rather that he pays little or no attention to his own happiness in light of the overriding importance he gives to the wider concerns of morality. In other words, this person sacrifices his own interests to the interests of others, and feels the sacrifice as such.

Roughly, these two models may be distinguished according to whether one thinks of the moral saint as being a saint out of love or one thinks of the moral saint as being a saint out of duty (or some other intellectual appreciation and recognition of moral principles). We may refer to the first model as the model of the Loving Saint; to the second, as the model of the Rational Saint.

The two models differ considerably with respect to the qualities of the motives of the individuals who conform to them. But this difference would have limited effect on the saints' respective public personalities. The shared content of what these individuals are motivated to be—namely, as morally good as possible—would play the dominant role in the determination of their characters. Of course, just as a variety of large-scale projects, from tending the sick to political campaigning, may be equally and maximally morally worthy, so a variety of characters are compatible with the ideal of moral sainthood. One moral saint may be more or less jovial, more or less garrulous, more or less athletic than another. But, above all, a moral saint must have and cultivate those qualities which are apt to allow him to treat others as justly and kindly as possible. He will have the standard moral virtues to a nonstandard degree. He will be patient, considerate, even-tempered, hospitable, charitable in thought as well as in deed. He will be very reluctant to make negative judgments of other people. He will be careful not to favor some people over others on the basis of properties they could not help but have.

Perhaps what I have already said is enough to make some people begin to regard the absence of moral saints in their lives as a blessing. For there comes a point in the listing of virtues that a moral saint is likely to have where one might naturally begin to wonder whether the moral saint isn't, after all, too good—if not too good for his own good, at least too good for his own well-being. For the moral virtues, given that they are, by hypothesis, *all* present in the same individual, and to an extreme degree, are apt to crowd out the nonmoral virtues, as well as many of the interests and personal characteristics that we generally think contribute to a healthy, well-rounded, richly developed character.

In other words, if the moral saint is devoting all his time to feeding the hungry or healing the sick or raising money for Oxfam, then necessarily he is not reading Victorian novels, playing the oboe, or improving his backhand. Although no one of the interests or tastes in the category containing these latter activities could be claimed to be a necessary element in a life well lived, a life in which *none* of these possible aspects of character are developed may seem to be a life strangely barren.

The reasons why a moral saint cannot, in general, encourage the discovery and development of significant nonmoral interests and skills are not logical but practical reasons. There are, in addition, a class of nonmoral characteristics that a moral saint cannot encourage in himself for reasons that are not just practical. There is a more substantial tension between having any of these qualities unashamedly and being a moral saint. These qualities might be described as going against the moral grain. For example, a cynical or sarcastic wit, or a sense of humor that appreciates this kind of wit in others, requires that one take an attitude of resignation and pessimism toward the flaws and vices to be found in the world. A moral saint, on the other hand, has reason to take an attitude in opposition to this—he should try to look for the best in people, give them the benefit of the doubt as long as possible, try to improve regrettable situations as long as there is any hope of success. This suggests that, although a moral saint might well enjoy a good episode of *Father Knows Best*, he may not in good conscience be able to laugh at a Marx Brothers movie or enjoy a play by George Bernard Shaw.

An interest in something like gourmet cooking will be, for different reasons, difficult for a moral saint to rest easy with. For it seems to me that no plausible argument can justify the use of human resources involved in producing a *paté de canard en croute* against possible alternative beneficent ends to which these resources might be put. If there is a justification for the institution of haute cuisine, it is one which rests on the decision *not* to justify every activity against morally beneficial alternatives, and this is a decision a moral saint will never make. Presumably, an interest in high fashion or interior design will fare much the same, as will, very possibly, a cultivation of the finer arts as well.

A moral saint will have to be very, very nice. It is important that he not be offensive. The worry is that, as a result, he will have to be dull-witted or humorless or bland.

This worry is confirmed when we consider what sorts of characters, taken and refined both from life and from fiction, typically form our ideals. One would hope they would be figures who are morally good—and by this I mean more than just not morally bad—but one would hope, too, that they are not just morally good, but talented or accomplished or attractive in nonmoral ways as well. We may make ideals out of athletes, scholars, artists—more frivolously, out of cowboys, private eyes, and rock stars. We may strive for Katharine Hepburn's grace, Paul Newman's "cool"; we are attracted to the high-spirited passionate nature of Natasha Rostov; we admire the keen perceptiveness of Lambert Strether. Though there is certainly nothing immoral about the ideal characters or traits I have in mind, they cannot be superimposed upon the ideal of a moral saint. For although it is a part of many of these ideals that the characters set high, and not merely acceptable, moral standards for themselves, it is also essential to their power and attractiveness that the moral strengths go, so to speak, alongside of specific, independently admirable, nonmoral ground projects and dominant personal traits.

When one does finally turn one's eyes toward lives that are dominated by explicitly moral commitments, moreover, one finds oneself relieved at the discovery of idiosyncrasies or eccentricities not quite in line with the picture of moral perfection. One prefers the blunt, tactless, and opinionated Betsy Trotwood to the unfailingly kind and patient Agnes Copperfield; one prefers the mischievousness and the sense of irony in Chesterton's Father Brown to the innocence and undiscriminating love of St. Francis.

It seems that, as we look in our ideals for people who achieve nonmoral varieties of personal excellence in conjunction with or colored by some version of high moral tone, we look in our paragons of moral excellence for people whose moral achievements occur in conjunction with or colored by some interests or traits that have low moral tone. In other words, there seems to be a limit to how much morality we can stand.

One might suspect that the essence of the problem is simply that there is a limit to how much of *any* single value, or any single type of value, we can stand. Our objection then would not be specific to a life in which one's dominant concern is morality, but would apply to any life that can be so completely characterized by an extraordinarily dominant concern. The objection in that case would reduce to the recognition that such a life is incompatible with well-roundedness. If that were the objection, one could fairly reply that well-roundedness is no more supreme a virtue than the totality of moral virtues embodied by the ideal it is being used to criticize. But I think this misidentifies the objection. For the way in which a concern for morality may dominate a life, or, more to the point, the way in which it may dominate an ideal of life, is not easily imagined by analogy to the dominance an aspiration to become an Olympic swimmer or a concert pianist might have.

A person who is passionately committed to one of these latter concerns might decide that her attachment to it is strong enough to be worth the sacrifice of her ability to maintain and pursue a significant portion of what else life might offer which a proper devotion to her dominant passion would require. But a desire to be as morally good as possible is not likely to take the form of one desire among others which, because of its peculiar psychological strength, requires one to forego the pursuit of other weaker and separately less demanding desires. Rather, the desire to be as morally good as possible is apt to have the character not just of a stronger, but of a higher desire, which does not merely successfully compete with one's other desires but which rather subsumes or demotes them. The sacrifice of other interests for the interest in morality, then, will have the character, not of a choice, but of an imperative.

Moreover, there is something odd about the idea of morality itself, or moral goodness, serving as the object of a dominant passion in the way that a more concrete and specific vision of a goal (even a concrete *moral* goal) might be imagined to serve. Morality itself does not seem to be a suitable object of passion. Thus, when one reflects, for example, on the Loving Saint easily and gladly giving up his fishing trip or his stereo or his hot fudge sundae at the drop of the moral hat, one is apt to wonder not at how much he loves morality, but at how little he loves these other things. One thinks that, if he can give these up so easily, he does not know what it *is* to truly love them. There seems, in other words, to be a kind of joy which the Loving Saint, either by nature or by practice, is incapable of experiencing. The Rational Saint, on the other hand, might retain strong nonmoral and concrete desires—he simply denies himself the opportunity to act on them. But this is no less troubling. The Loving Saint one might suspect of missing a piece of perceptual machinery, of being blind to some of what the world has to offer. The Rational Saint, who sees it but foregoes it, one suspects of having a different problem—a pathological fear of damnation, perhaps, or an extreme form of self-hatred that interferes with his ability to enjoy the enjoyable in life.

In other words, the ideal of a life of moral sainthood disturbs not simply because it is an ideal of a life in which morality unduly dominates. The normal person's direct and specific desires for objects, activities, and events that conflict with the attainment of moral perfection are not simply sacrificed but removed, suppressed, or subsumed. The way in which morality, unlike other possible goals, is apt to dominate is particularly disturbing, for it seems to require either the lack or the denial of the existence of an identifiable, personal self.

This distinctively troubling feature is not, I think, absolutely unique to the ideal of the moral saint, as I have been using that phrase. It is shared by the conception of the pure aesthete, by a certain kind of religious ideal, and, somewhat paradoxically, by the model of the thorough-going, self-conscious egoist. It is not a coincidence that the ways of comprehending the world of which these ideals are the extreme embodiments are sometimes described as "moralities" themselves. At any rate, they compete with what we ordinarily mean by 'morality'. Nor is it a coincidence that these ideals are naturally described as fanatical. But it is easy to see that these other types of perfection cannot serve as satisfactory personal ideals; for the realization of these ideals would be straightforwardly immoral. It may come as a surprise to some that there may in addition be such a thing as a *moral* fanatic.

Some will object that I am being unfair to "common-sense morality"— that it does not really require a moral saint to be either a disgusting goody-goody or an obsessive ascetic. Admittedly, there is no logical inconsistency between having any of the personal characteristics I have mentioned and being a moral saint. It is not morally wrong to notice the faults and shortcomings of others or to recognize and appreciate nonmoral talents and skills. Nor is it immoral to be an avid Celtics fan or to have a passion for caviar or to be an excellent cellist. With enough imagination, we can always contrive a suitable history and set of circumstances that will embrace such characteristics in one or another specific fictional story of a perfect moral saint.

If one turned onto the path of moral sainthood relatively late in life, one may have already developed interests that can be turned to moral purposes. It may be that a good golf game is just what is needed to secure that big donation to Oxfam. Perhaps the cultivation of one's exceptional artistic talent will turn out to be the way one can make one's greatest contribution to society. Furthermore, one might stumble upon joys and skills in the very service of morality. If, because the children are short a ninth player for the team, one's generous offer to serve reveals a natural fielding arm or if one's part in the campaign against nuclear power requires accepting a lobbyist's invitation to lunch at Le Lion d'Or, there is no moral gain in denying the satisfaction one gets from these activities. The moral saint, then, may, by happy accident, find himself with nonmoral virtues on which he can capitalize morally or which make psychological demands to which he has no choice but to attend. The point is that, for a moral saint, the existence of these interests and skills can be given at best the status of happy accidents— they cannot be encouraged for their own sakes as distinct, independent aspects of the realization of human good.

It must be remembered that from the fact that there is a tension between having any of these qualities and being a moral saint it does not follow that having any of these qualities is immoral. For it is not part of common-sense morality that one ought to be a moral saint. Still, if someone just happened to want to be a moral saint, he or she would not have or encourage these qualities, and, on the basis of our common-sense values, this counts as a reason not to want to be a moral saint.

One might still wonder what kind of reason this is, and what kind of conclusion this properly allows us to draw. For the fact that the models of moral saints are unattractive does not necessarily mean that they are unsuitable ideals. Perhaps they are unattractive because they make us feel uncomfortable—they highlight our own weaknesses, vices, and flaws. If so, the fault lies not in the characters of the saints, but in those of our unsaintly selves.

To be sure, some of the reasons behind the disaffection we feel for the model of moral sainthood have to do with a reluctance to criticize our selves and a reluctance to committing ourselves to trying to give up activities and interests that we heartily enjoy. These considerations might provide an *excuse* for the fact that we are not moral saints, but they do not provide a basis for criticizing sainthood as a possible ideal. Since these considerations rely on an appeal to the egoistic, hedonistic side of our natures, to use them as a basis for criticizing the ideal of the moral saint would be at best to beg the question and at worst to glorify features of ourselves that ought to be condemned.

The fact that the moral saint would be without qualities which we have and which, indeed, we like to have, does not in itself provide reason to condemn the ideal of the moral saint. The fact that some of these qualities are good qualities, however, and that they are qualities we *ought* to like, does provide reason to discourage this ideal and to offer other ideals in its place. In other words, some of the qualities the moral saint necessarily lacks are virtues, albeit nonmoral virtues, in the unsaintly characters who have them. The feats of Groucho Marx, Reggie Jackson, and the head chef at Lutèce are impressive accomplishments that it is not only permissible but positively appropriate to recognize as such. In general, the admiration of and striving toward achieving any of a great variety of forms of personal excellence are character traits it is valuable and desirable for people to have. In advocating the development of these varieties of excellence, we advocate nonmoral reasons for acting, and in thinking that it is good for a person to strive for an ideal that gives a substantial role to the interests and values that correspond to these virtues, we implicitly acknowledge the goodness of ideals incompatible with that of the moral saint. Finally, if we think that it is *as* good, or even better for a person to strive for one of these ideals than it is for him or her to strive for and realize the ideal of the moral saint, we express a conviction that it is good not to be a moral saint.

Moral Saints and Moral Theories

I have tried so far to paint a picture—or, rather, two pictures—of what a moral saint might be like, drawing on what I take to be the attitudes and beliefs about morality prevalent in contemporary, common-sense thought. To my suggestion that common-sense morality generates conceptions of moral saints that are unattractive or otherwise unacceptable, it is open to someone to reply, "so much the worse for common-sense morality." After all, it is often claimed that the goal of moral philosophy is to correct and improve upon common-sense morality, and I have as yet given no attention to the question of what conceptions of moral sainthood, if any, are generated from the leading moral theories of our time.

A quick, breezy reading of utilitarian and Kantian writings will suggest the images, respectively, of the Loving Saint and the Rational Saint. A utilitarian, with his emphasis on happiness, will certainly prefer the Loving Saint to the Rational one, since the Loving Saint will himself be a happier person than the Rational Saint. A Kantian, with his emphasis on reason, on the other hand, will find at least as much to praise in the latter as in the former. Still, both models, drawn as they are from common sense, appeal to an impure mixture of utilitarian and Kantian intuitions. A more careful examination of these moral theories raises questions about whether either model of moral sainthood would really be advocated by a believer in the explicit doctrines associated with either of these views.

Certainly, the utilitarian in no way denies the value of self-realization. He in no way disparages the development of interests, talents, and other personally attractive traits that I have claimed the moral saint would be without. Indeed, since just these features enhance the happiness both of the individuals who possess them and of those with whom they associate, the ability to promote these features both in oneself and in others will have considerable positive weight in utilitarian calculations.

This implies that the utilitarian would not support moral sainthood as a universal ideal. A world in which everyone, or even a large number of people, achieved moral sainthood—even a world in which they *strove* to achieve it—would probably contain less happiness than a world in which people realized a diversity of ideals involving a variety of personal and perfectionist values. More pragmatic considerations also suggest that, if the utilitarian wants to influence more people to achieve more good, then he would do better to encourage them to pursue happiness-producing goals that are more attractive and more within a normal person's reach.

These considerations still leave open, however, the question of what kind of an ideal the committed utilitarian should privately aspire to himself. Utilitarianism requires him to want to achieve the greatest general happiness, and this would seem to commit him to the ideal of the moral saint.

One might try to [claim] that a utilitarian should choose to give up utilitarianism. If, as I have said, a moral saint would be a less happy person both to be and to be around than many other possible ideals, perhaps one could create more total happiness by not trying too hard to promote the total happiness. But this argument is simply unconvincing in light of the empirical circumstances of our world. The gain in happiness that would accrue to oneself and one's neighbors by a more well-rounded, richer life than that of the moral saint would be pathetically small in comparison to the amount by which one could increase the general happiness if one devoted oneself explicitly to the care of the sick, the downtrodden, the starving, and the homeless. Of course, there may be psychological limits to the extent to which a person can devote himself to such things without going crazy. But the utilitarian's individual limitations would not thereby become a positive feature of his personal ideals.

The unattractiveness of the moral saint, then, ought not rationally convince the utilitarian to abandon his utilitarianism. It may, however, convince him to take efforts not to wear his saintly moral aspirations on his sleeve. If it is not too difficult, the utilitarian will try not to make those around him uncomfortable. He will not want to appear 'holier than thou'; he will not want to inhibit others' ability to enjoy themselves. In practice, this might make the perfect utilitarian a less nauseating companion than the moral saint. But insofar as this kind of reasoning produces a more bearable public personality, it is at the cost of giving him a personality that must be evaluated as hypocritical and condescending when his private thoughts and attitudes are taken into account.

Still, the criticisms I have raised against the saint of common-sense morality should make some difference to the utilitarian's conception of an ideal which neither requires him to abandon his utilitarian principles nor forces him to fake an interest he does not have or a judgment he does not make. For it may be that a limited and carefully monitored allotment of time and energy to be devoted to the pursuit of some nonmoral interests or to the development of some nonmoral talents would make a person a better contributor to the general welfare than he would be if he allowed himself no indulgences of this sort. The enjoyment of such activities in no way compromises a commitment to utilitarian principles as long as the involvement with these activities is conditioned by a willingness to give them up whenever it is recognized that they cease to be in the general interest.

This will go some way in mitigating the picture of the loving saint that an understanding of utilitarianism will on first impression suggest. But I think it will not go very far. For the limitations on time and energy will have to be rather severe, and the need to monitor will restrict not only the extent but also the quality of one's attachment to these interests and traits. They are only weak and somewhat peculiar sorts of passions to which one can consciously remain so conditionally committed. Moreover, the way in which the utilitarian can enjoy these 'extra-curricular' aspects of his life is simply not the way in which these aspects are to be enjoyed insofar as they figure into our less saintly ideals.

The problem is not exactly that the utilitarian values these aspects of his life only as a means to an end, for the enjoyment he and others get from these aspects are not a means to, but a part of, the general happiness. Nonetheless, he values these things only because of and insofar as they *are* a part of the general happiness. He values them, as it were, under the description 'a contribution to the general happiness'. This is to be contrasted with the various ways in which these aspects of life may be valued by nonutilitarians. A person might love literature because of the insights into human nature literature affords. Another might love the cultivation of roses because roses are things of great beauty and delicacy. It may be true that these features of the respective activities also explain why these activities are happiness-producing. But, to the nonutilitarian, this may not be to the point. For if one values these activities in these more direct ways, one may not be willing to exchange them for others that produce an equal, or even a greater amount of happiness. From that point of view, it is not because they produce happiness that these activities are valuable; it is because these activities are valuable in more direct and specific ways that they produce happiness.

To adopt a phrase of Bernard Williams', the utilitarian's manner of valuing the not explicitly moral aspects of his life 'provides (him) with one thought too many.'[1] The requirement that the utilitarian have this thought—periodically, at least—is indicative of not only a weakness but a shallowness in his appreciation of the aspects in question. Thus, the ideals toward which a utilitarian could acceptably strive would remain too close to the model of the common-sense moral saint to escape the criticisms of that model which I earlier suggested. [. . .]

Despite my claim that all-consuming moral saintliness is not a particularly healthy and desirable ideal, it seems perverse to insist that, were moral saints to exist, they would not, in their way, be remarkably noble and admirable figures. Despite my conviction that it is as rational and as good for a person to take Katharine Hepburn or Jane Austen as her role model instead of Mother Teresa, it would be absurd to deny that Mother Teresa is a morally better person.

I can think of two ways of viewing morality as having an upper bound. First, we can think that altruism and impartiality are indeed positive moral interests, but that they are moral only if the degree to which these interests are actively pursued remains within certain fixed limits. Second, we can think that these positive interests are only incidentally related to morality and that the essence of morality lies elsewhere, in, say, an implicit social contract or in the recognition of our own dignified rationality. According to the first conception of morality, there is a cut-off line to the amount of altruism or to the extent of devotion to justice and fairness that is worthy

---

[1] 'Persons, Character and Morality' in Amelie Rorty, (ed.), *The Identities of Persons* (University of California Press: Berkeley, Calif., 1976), 214.

of moral praise. But to draw this line earlier than the line that brings the altruist in question into a worse-off position than all those to whom he devotes himself seems unacceptably artificial and gratuitous. According to the second conception, these positive interests are not essentially related to morality at all. But then we are unable to regard a more affectionate and generous expression of good will toward others as a natural and reasonable extension of morality, and we encourage a cold and unduly self-centered approach to the development and evaluation of our motivations and concerns.

A moral theory that does not contain the seeds of an all-consuming ideal of moral sainthood thus seems to place false and unnatural limits on our opportunity to do moral good and our potential to deserve moral praise. Yet the main thrust of the arguments of this paper has been leading to the conclusion that, when such ideals are present, they are not ideals to which it is particularly reasonable or healthy or desirable for human beings to aspire. These claims, taken together, have the appearance of a dilemma from which there is no obvious escape. In a moment, I shall argue that, despite appearances, these claims should not be understood as constituting a dilemma. But, before I do, let me briefly describe another path which those who are convinced by my above remarks may feel inclined to take.

If the above remarks are understood to be implicitly critical of the views on the content of morality which seem most popular today, an alternative that naturally suggests itself is that we revise our views about the content of morality. More specifically, my remarks may be taken to support a more Aristotelian, or even a more Nietzschean, approach to moral philosophy. Such a change in approach involves substantially broadening or replacing our contemporary intuitions about which character traits constitute moral virtues and vices and which interests constitute moral interests. If, for example, we include personal bearing, or creativity, or sense of style, as features that contribute to one's *moral* personality, then we can create moral ideals which are incompatible with and probably more attractive than the Kantian and utilitarian ideals I have discussed. Given such an alteration of our conception of morality, the figures with which I have been concerned above might, far from being considered to be moral saints, be seen as morally inferior to other more appealing or more interesting models of individuals.

This approach seems unlikely to succeed, if for no other reason, because it is doubtful that any single, or even any reasonably small number of substantial personal ideals could capture the full range of possible ways of realizing human potential or achieving human good which deserve encouragement and praise. Even if we could provide a sufficiently broad characterization of the range of positive ways for human beings to live, however, I think there are strong reasons not to want to incorporate such a characterization more centrally into the framework of morality itself. For, in claiming that a character trait or activity is morally good, one claims that there is a certain kind of reason for developing that trait or engaging in that activity. Yet, lying behind our criticism of more conventional conceptions of moral sainthood, there seems to be a recognition that among the immensely valuable traits and activities that a human life might positively embrace are some of which we hope that, if a person does embrace them, he does so *not* for moral reasons. In other words, no matter how flexible we make the guide to conduct which we choose to label 'morality,' no matter how rich we make the life in which perfect obedience to this guide would result, we will have reason to hope that a person does not wholly rule and direct his life by the abstract and impersonal consideration that such a life would be morally good.

Once it is recognized that morality itself should not serve as a comprehensive guide to conduct, moreover, we can see reasons to retain the admittedly vague contemporary intuitions about what the classification of moral and nonmoral virtues, interests, and the like should be. That is, there seem to be important differences between the aspects of a person's life which are currently considered appropriate objects of moral evaluation and the aspects that might be included under the altered conception of morality we are now considering, which the latter approach would tend wrongly to blur or to neglect. Moral evaluation now is focused primarily on features of a person's life over which that person has control; it is largely restricted to aspects of his life which are likely to have considerable effect on other people. These restrictions seem as they should be. Even if responsible people could reach agreement as to what constituted good taste or a healthy degree of well-roundedness, for example, it seems wrong to insist that everyone try to achieve these things or to blame someone who fails or refuses to conform.

If we are not to respond to the unattractiveness of the moral ideals that contemporary theories yield either by offering alternative theories with more palatable ideals or by understanding these theories in such a way as to prevent them from yielding ideals at all, how, then, are we to respond? Simply, I think, by admitting that moral ideals do not, and need not, make the best personal ideals. Earlier I mentioned one of the consequences of regarding as a test of an adequate moral theory that perfect obedience to its laws and maximal devotion to its interests be something we can wholeheartedly strive for in ourselves and wish for in those around us. Drawing out the consequences somewhat further should, I think, make us more doubtful of the proposed test than of the theories which, on this test, would fail. Given the empirical circumstances of our world, it seems to be an ethical fact that we have unlimited potential to be morally good, and endless opportunity to promote moral interests. But this is not incompatible with the not-so-ethical fact that we have sound, compelling, and not particularly selfish reasons to choose not to devote ourselves univocally to realizing this potential or to taking up this opportunity.

Thus, in one sense at least, I am not really criticizing either Kantianism or utilitarianism. Insofar as the point of view I am offering bears directly on recent work in moral philosophy, in fact, it bears on critics of these theories who, in a spirit not unlike the spirit of most of this paper, point out that the perfect utilitarian would be flawed in this way or the perfect Kantian flawed in that.[1] The assumption lying behind these claims, implicitly or explicitly, has been that the recognition of these flaws shows us something wrong with utilitarianism as opposed to Kantianism, or something wrong with Kantianism as opposed to utilitarianism, or something wrong with both of these theories as opposed to some nameless third alternative. The claims of this paper suggest, however, that this assumption is unwarranted. The flaws of a perfect master of a moral theory need not reflect flaws in the intramoral content of the theory itself.

Moral Saints and Moral Philosophy

In pointing out the regrettable features and the necessary absence of some desirable features in a moral saint, I have not meant to condemn the moral saint or the person who aspires to become one. Rather, I have meant to insist that the ideal of moral sainthood should not be held as a standard against which any other ideal must be judged or justified, and that the posture we take in response to the recognition that our lives are not as morally good as they might be need not be defensive.[2] It is misleading to insist that one is *permitted* to live a life in which the goals, relationships, activities, and interests that one pursues are not maximally morally good. For our lives are not so comprehensively subject to the requirement that we apply for permission, and our nonmoral reasons for the goals we set ourselves are not excuses, but may rather be positive, good reasons which do not exist *despite* any reasons that might threaten to outweigh them. In other words, a person may be *perfectly wonderful* without being *perfectly moral*.

---

[1] See e.g. Bernard Williams, 'Persons, Character', and J. J. C. Smart and Bernard Williams, *Utilitarianism: For and Against* (Cambridge University Press: New York, 1973). Also, Michael Stocker, 'The Schizophrenia of Modern Ethical Theories,' *Journal of Philosophy*, 63 14 (12 Aug. 1976), 453–66.

[2] George Orwell makes a similar point in 'Reflections on Gandhi', in *A Collection of Essays by George Orwell* (Harcourt Brace Jovanovich: New York, 1945), 176: 'sainthood is . . . a thing that human beings must avoid. . . . It is too readily assumed that . . . the ordinary man only rejects it because it is too difficult; in other words, that the average human being is a failed saint. It is doubtful whether this is true. Many people genuinely do not wish to be saints, and it is probable that some who achieve or aspire to sainthood have never felt much temptation to be human beings.'

Recognizing this requires a perspective which contemporary moral philosophy has generally ignored. This perspective yields judgments of a type that is neither moral nor egoistic. Like moral judgments, judgments about what it would be good for a person to be are made from a point of view outside the limits set by the values, interests, and desires that the person might actually have. And, like moral judgments, these judgments claim for themselves a kind of objectivity or a grounding in a perspective which any rational and perceptive being can take up. Unlike moral judgments, however, the good with which these judgments are concerned is not the good of anyone or any group other than the individual himself.

Nonetheless, it would be equally misleading to say that these judgments are made for the sake of the individual himself. For these judgments are not concerned with what kind of life it is in a person's interest to lead, but with what kind of interests it would be good for a person to have, and it need not be in a person's interest that he acquire or maintain objectively good interests. Indeed, the model of the Loving Saint, whose interests are identified with the interests of morality, is a model of a person for whom the dictates of rational self-interest and the dictates of morality coincide. Yet, I have urged that we have reason not to aspire to this ideal and that some of us would have reason to be sorry if our children aspired to and achieved it.

The moral point of view, we might say, is the point of view one takes up insofar as one takes the recognition of the fact that one is just one person among others equally real and deserving of the good things in life as a fact with practical consequences, a fact the recognition of which demands expression in one's actions and in the form of one's practical deliberations. Competing moral theories offer alternative answers to the question of what the most correct or the best way to express this fact is. In doing so, they offer alternative ways to evaluate and to compare the variety of actions, states of affairs, and so on that appear good and bad to agents from other, nonmoral points of view. But it seems that alternative interpretations of the moral point of view do not exhaust the ways in which our actions, characters, and their consequences can be comprehensively and objectively evaluated. Let us call the point of view from which we consider what kinds of lives are good lives, and what kinds of persons it would be good for ourselves and others to be, the *point of view of individual perfection*.

Since either point of view provides a way of comprehensively evaluating a person's life, each point of view takes account of, and, in a sense, subsumes the other. From the moral point of view, the perfection of an individual life will have some, but limited, value—for each individual remains, after all, just one person among others. From the perfectionist point of view, the moral worth of an individual's relation to his world will likewise have some, but limited, value—for, as I have argued, the (perfectionist) goodness of an individual's life does not vary proportionally with the degree to which it exemplifies moral goodness.

It may not be the case that the perfectionist point of view is like the moral point of view in being a point of view we are ever *obliged* to take up and express in our actions. Nonetheless, it provides us with reasons that are independent of moral reasons for wanting ourselves and others to develop our characters and live our lives in certain ways. When we take up this point of view and ask how much it would be good for an individual to act from the moral point of view, we do not find an obvious answer.[1]

The considerations of this paper suggest, at any rate, that the answer is not 'as much as possible.' This has implications both for the continued development of moral theories and for the development of metamoral views and for our conception of moral philosophy more generally. From the moral point of view, we have reasons to want people to live lives that seem good from outside that point of view. If, as I have argued, this means that we have reason to want people to live lives that are not morally perfect, then any plausible moral theory must make use of some conception of supererogation.[2]

If moral philosophers are to address themselves at the most basic level to the question of how people should live, however, they must do more than adjust the content of their moral theories in ways that leave room for the affirmation of nonmoral values. They must examine explicitly the range and nature of these nonmoral values, and, in light of this examination, they must ask how the acceptance of a moral theory is to be understood and acted upon. For the claims of this paper do not so much conflict with the content of any particular currently popular moral theory as they call into question a metamoral assumption that implicitly surrounds discussions of

---

[1] A similar view, which has strongly influenced mine, is expressed by Thomas Nagel in 'The Fragmentation of Value', in *Mortal Questions* (Cambridge University Press: Cambridge, 1979), 128–41. Nagel focuses on the difficulties such apparently incommensurable points of view create for specific, isolable practical decisions that must be made both by individuals and by societies. In focusing on the way in which these points of view figure into the development of individual personal ideals, the questions with which I am concerned are more likely to lurk in the background of any individual's life.

[2] The variety of forms that a conception of supererogation might take, however, has not generally been noticed. Moral theories that make use of this notion typically do so by identifying some specific set of principles as universal moral requirements and supplement this list with a further set of directives which it is morally praiseworthy but not required for an agent to follow. [See e.g. Charles Fried, *Right and Wrong* (Harvard University Press: Cambridge, Mass., 1979).] But it is possible that the ability to live a morally blameless life cannot be so easily or definitely secured as this type of theory would suggest. The fact that there are some situations in which an agent is morally required to do something and other situations in which it would be good but not required for an agent to do something does not imply that there are specific principles such that, in any situation, an agent is required to act in accordance with these principles and other specific principles such that, in any situation, it would be good but not required for an agent to act in accordance with those principles.

moral theory more generally. Specifically, they call into question the assumption that it is always better to be morally better.

The role morality plays in the development of our characters and the shape of our practical deliberations need be neither that of a universal medium into which all other values must be translated nor that of an ever-present filter through which all other values must pass. This is not to say that moral value should not be an important, even the most important, kind of value we attend to in evaluating and improving ourselves and our world. It is to say that our values cannot be fully comprehended on the model of a hierarchical system with morality at the top.

The philosophical temperament will naturally incline, at this point, toward asking, 'What, then, *is* at the top—or, if there is no top, how *are* we to decide when and how much to be moral?' In other words, there is a temptation to seek a metamoral—though not, in the standard sense, metaethical—theory that will give us principles, or, at least, informal directives on the basis of which we can develop and evaluate more comprehensive personal ideals. Perhaps a theory that distinguishes among the various roles a person is expected to play within a life—as professional, as citizen, as friend, and so on—might give us some rules that would offer us, if nothing else, a better framework in which to think about and discuss these questions. I am pessimistic, however, about the chances of such a theory to yield substantial and satisfying results. For I do not see how a metamoral theory could be constructed which would not be subject to considerations parallel to those which seem inherently to limit the appropriateness of regarding moral theories as ultimate comprehensive guides for action.

This suggests that, at some point, both in our philosophizing and in our lives, we must be willing to raise normative questions from a perspective that is unattached to a commitment to any particular well-ordered system of values. It must be admitted that, in doing so, we run the risk of finding normative answers that diverge from the answers given by whatever moral theory one accepts. This, I take it, is the grain of truth in G. E. Moore's 'open question' argument. In the background of this paper, then, there lurks a commitment to what seems to me to be a healthy form of intuitionism. It is a form of intuitionism which is not intended to take the place of more rigorous, systematically developed, moral theories—rather, it is intended to put these more rigorous and systematic moral theories in their place.[1]

['Moral Saints', *Journal of Philosophy*, 79 (1982), 419–39.]

[1] I have benefited from the comments of many people who have heard or read an earlier draft of this paper. I wish particularly to thank Douglas MacLean, Robert Nozick, Martha Nussbaum, and the Society for Ethics and Legal Philosophy.

iv. Contract Ethics

a. The Theory

JOHN RAWLS

87   The Main Idea of the Theory of Justice

My aim is to present a conception of justice which generalizes and carries to a higher level of abstraction the familiar theory of the social contract as found, say, in Locke, Rousseau, and Kant.[1] In order to do this we are not to think of the original contract as one to enter a particular society or to set up a particular form of government. Rather, the guiding idea is that the principles of justice for the basic structure of society are the object of the original agreement. They are the principles that free and rational persons concerned to further their own interests would accept in an initial position of equality as defining the fundamental terms of their association. These principles are to regulate all further agreements; they specify the kinds of social cooperation that can be entered into and the forms of government that can be established. This way of regarding the principles of justice I shall call justice as fairness.

Thus we are to imagine that those who engage in social cooperation choose together, in one joint act, the principles which are to assign basic rights and duties and to determine the division of social benefits. Men are to decide in advance how they are to regulate their claims against one another and what is to be the foundation charter of their society. Just as each person must decide by rational reflection what constitutes his good, that is, the system of ends which it is rational for him to pursue, so a group of persons must decide once and for all what is to count among them as just and unjust. The choice which rational men would make in this hypothetical situation of equal liberty, assuming for the present that this choice problem has a solution, determines the principles of justice.

---

[1] As the text suggests, I shall regard Locke's *Second Treatise of Government*, Rousseau's *The Social Contract*, and Kant's ethical works beginning with *The Foundations of the Metaphysics of Morals* as definitive of the contract tradition. For all of its greatness, Hobbes's *Leviathan* raises special problems. A general historical survey is provided by J. W. Gough, *The Social Contract*, 2nd ed. (Clarendon Press: Oxford, 1957), and Otto Gierke, *Natural Law and the Theory of Society*, trans. with an introduction by Ernest Barker (Cambridge University Press: Cambridge, 1934). A presentation of the contract view as primarily an ethical theory is to be found in G. R. Grice, *The Grounds of Moral Judgment* (Cambridge University Press: Cambridge, 1967).

In justice as fairness the original position of equality corresponds to the state of nature in the traditional theory of the social contract. This original position is not, of course, thought of as an actual historical state of affairs, much less as a primitive condition of culture. It is understood as a purely hypothetical situation characterized so as to lead to a certain conception of justice.[1] Among the essential features of this situation is that no one knows his place in society, his class position or social status, nor does any one know his fortune in the distribution of natural assets and abilities, his intelligence, strength, and the like. I shall even assume that the parties do not know their conceptions of the good or their special psychological propensities. The principles of justice are chosen behind a veil of ignorance. This ensures that no one is advantaged or disadvantaged in the choice of principles by the outcome of natural chance or the contingency of social circumstances. Since all are similarly situated and no one is able to design principles to favor his particular condition, the principles of justice are the result of a fair agreement or bargain. For given the circumstances of the original position, the symmetry of everyone's relations to each other, this initial situation is fair between individuals as moral persons, that is, as rational beings with their own ends and capable, I shall assume, of a sense of justice. The original position is, one might say, the appropriate initial status quo, and thus the fundamental agreements reached in it are fair. This explains the propriety of the name 'justice as fairness': it conveys the idea that the principles of justice are agreed to in an initial situation that is fair. The name does not mean that the concepts of justice and fairness are the same, any more than the phrase 'poetry as metaphor' means that the concepts of poetry and metaphor are the same.

Justice as fairness begins, as I have said, with one of the most general of all choices which persons might make together, namely, with the choice of the first principles of a conception of justice which is to regulate all subsequent criticism and reform of institutions. Then, having chosen a conception of justice, we can suppose that they are to choose a constitution and a legislature to enact laws, and so on, all in accordance with the principles of justice initially agreed upon. Our social situation is just if it is such that by this sequence of hypothetical agreements we would have contracted into the general system of rules which defines it. Moreover, assuming that the original position does determine a set of principles (that is, that a particular

---

[1] Kant is clear that the original agreement is hypothetical. See *The Metaphysics of Morals*, pt. I (*Rechtslehre*), especially §§ 47, 52; and pt. II of the essay 'Concerning the Common Saying: This May Be True in Theory but It Does Not Apply in Practice', in *Kant's Political Writings*, ed. Hans Reiss and trans. H. B. Nisbet (Cambridge University Press: Cambridge, 1970), 73–87. See Georges Vlachos, *La Pensée politique de Kant* (Presses Universitaires de France: Paris, 1962), 326–35; and J. G. Murphy, *Kant: The Philosophy of Right* (Macmillan: London, 1970), 109–12, 133–6, for a further discussion.

conception of justice would be chosen), it will then be true that whenever social institutions satisfy these principles those engaged in them can say to one another that they are cooperating on terms to which they would agree if they were free and equal persons whose relations with respect to one another were fair. They could all view their arrangements as meeting the stipulations which they would acknowledge in an initial situation that embodies widely accepted and reasonable constraints on the choice of principles. The general recognition of this fact would provide the basis for a public acceptance of the corresponding principles of justice. No society can, of course, be a scheme of cooperation which men enter voluntarily in a literal sense; each person finds himself placed at birth in some particular position in some particular society, and the nature of this position materially affects his life prospects. Yet a society satisfying the principles of justice as fairness comes as close as a society can to being a voluntary scheme, for it meets the principles which free and equal persons would assent to under circumstances that are fair. In this sense its members are autonomous and the obligations they recognize self-imposed.

One feature of justice as fairness is to think of the parties in the initial situation as rational and mutually disinterested. This does not mean that the parties are egoists, that is, individuals with only certain kinds of interests, say in wealth, prestige, and domination. But they are conceived as not taking an interest in one another's interests. They are to presume that even their spiritual aims may be opposed, in the way that the aims of those of different religions may be opposed. Moreover, the concept of rationality must be interpreted as far as possible in the narrow sense, standard in economic theory, of taking the most effective means to given ends. I shall modify this concept to some extent, but one must try to avoid introducing into it any controversial ethical elements. The initial situation must be characterized by stipulations that are widely accepted.

In working out the conception of justice as fairness one main task clearly is to determine which principles of justice would be chosen in the original position. To do this we must describe this situation in some detail and formulate with care the problem of choice which it presents. These matters I shall take up in the immediately succeeding chapters. It may be observed, however, that once the principles of justice are thought of as arising from an original agreement in a situation of equality, it is an open question whether the principle of utility would be acknowledged. Offhand it hardly seems likely that persons who view themselves as equals, entitled to press their claims upon one another, would agree to a principle which may require lesser life prospects for some simply for the sake of a greater sum of advantages enjoyed by others. Since each desires to protect his interests, his capacity to advance his conception of the good, no one has a reason to acquiesce in an enduring loss for himself in order to bring about a greater net balance of satisfaction. In the absence of strong and lasting benevolent impulses, a rational man would not accept a basic structure merely because it maximized the algebraic sum of advantages irrespective of its permanent effects on his own basic rights and interests. Thus it seems that the principle of utility is incompatible with the conception of social cooperation among equals for mutual advantage. It appears to be inconsistent with the idea of reciprocity implicit in the notion of a well-ordered society. Or, at any rate, so I shall argue.

I shall maintain instead that the persons in the initial situation would choose two rather different principles: the first requires equality in the assignment of basic rights and duties, while the second holds that social and economic inequalities, for example inequalities of wealth and authority, are just only if they result in compensating benefits for everyone, and in particular for the least advantaged members of society. These principles rule out justifying institutions on the grounds that the hardships of some are offset by a greater good in the aggregate. It may be expedient but it is not just that some should have less in order that others may prosper. But there is no injustice in the greater benefits earned by a few provided that the situation of persons not so fortunate is thereby improved. The intuitive idea is that since everyone's well-being depends upon a scheme of cooperation without which no one could have a satisfactory life, the division of advantages should be such as to draw forth the willing cooperation of everyone taking part in it, including those less well situated. Yet this can be expected only if reasonable terms are proposed. The two principles mentioned seem to be a fair agreement on the basis of which those better endowed, or more fortunate in their social position, neither of which we can be said to deserve, could expect the willing cooperation of others when some workable scheme is a necessary condition of the welfare of all.[1] Once we decide to look for a conception of justice that nullifies the accidents of natural endowment and the contingencies of social circumstance as counters in quest for political and economic advantage, we are led to these principles. They express the result of leaving aside those aspects of the social world that seem arbitrary from a moral point of view.

The problem of the choice of principles, however, is extremely difficult. I do not expect the answer I shall suggest to be convincing to everyone. It is, therefore, worth noting from the outset that justice as fairness, like other contract views, consists of two parts: (1) an interpretation of the initial situation and of the problem of choice posed there, and (2) a set of principles which, it is argued, would be agreed to. One may accept the first part of the theory (or some variant thereof), but not the other, and conversely. The concept of the initial contractual situation may seem reasonable

---

[1] For the formulation of this intuitive idea I am indebted to Allan Gibbard.

although the particular principles proposed are rejected. To be sure, I want to maintain that the most appropriate conception of this situation does lead to principles of justice contrary to utilitarianism and perfectionism, and therefore that the contract doctrine provides an alternative to these views. Still, one may dispute this contention even though one grants that the contractarian method is a useful way of studying ethical theories and of setting forth their underlying assumptions.

Justice as fairness is an example of what I have called a contract theory. Now there may be an objection to the term 'contract' and related express-ions, but I think it will serve reasonably well. Many words have misleading connotations which at first are likely to confuse. The terms 'utility' and 'utilitarianism' are surely no exception. They too have unfortunate sugges-tions which hostile critics have been willing to exploit; yet they are clear enough for those prepared to study utilitarian doctrine. The same should be true of the term 'contract' applied to moral theories. As I have men-tioned, to understand it one has to keep in mind that it implies a certain level of abstraction. In particular, the content of the relevant agreement is not to enter a given society or to adopt a given form of government, but to accept certain moral principles. Moreover, the undertakings referred to are purely hypothetical: a contract view holds that certain principles would be accepted in a well-defined initial situation.

The merit of the contract terminology is that it conveys the idea that principles of justice may be conceived as principles that would be chosen by rational persons, and that in this way conceptions of justice may be ex-plained and justified. The theory of justice is a part, perhaps the most significant part, of the theory of rational choice. Furthermore, principles of justice deal with conflicting claims upon the advantages won by social cooperation; they apply to the relations among several persons or groups. The word 'contract' suggests this plurality as well as the condition that the appropriate division of advantages must be in accordance with principles acceptable to all parties. The condition of publicity for principles of justice is also connoted by the contract phraseology. Thus, if these principles are the outcome of an agreement, citizens have a knowledge of the principles that others follow. It is characteristic of contract theories to stress the public nature of political principles. Finally there is the long tradition of the contract doctrine. Expressing the tie with this line of thought helps to define ideas and accords with natural piety. There are then several advant-ages in the use of the term 'contract.' With due precautions taken, it should not be misleading.

A final remark. Justice as fairness is not a complete contract theory. For it is clear that the contractarian idea can be extended to the choice of more or less an entire ethical system, that is, to a system including principles for all the virtues and not only for justice. Now for the most part I shall consider only principles of justice and others closely related to them; I make no attempt to discuss the virtues in a systematic way. Obviously if justice as fairness succeeds reasonably well, a next step would be to study the more general view suggested by the name 'rightness as fairness.' But even this wider theory fails to embrace all moral relationships, since it would seem to include only our relations with other persons and to leave out of account how we are to conduct ourselves toward animals and the rest of nature. I do not contend that the contract notion offers a way to approach these questions which are certainly of the first importance; and I shall have to put them aside. We must recognize the limited scope of justice as fairness and of the general type of view that it exemplifies. How far its conclusions must be revised once these other matters are understood cannot be decided in advance.

[*A Theory of Justice* (Harvard University Press: Cambridge, Mass., 1972), 11–17.]

DAVID GAUTHIER

88   Why Contractarianism?

[L]et me sketch briefly those features of deliberative rationality that enable it to constrain maximizing choice. The key idea is that in many situations, if each person chooses what, given the choices of the others, would maximize her expected utility, then the outcome will be mutually disadvantageous in comparison with some alternative—everyone could do better.[1] Equilibrium, which obtains when each person's action is a best response to the others' actions, is incompatible with (Pareto-)optimality, which obtains when no one could do better without someone else doing worse. Given the ubiquity of such situations, each person can see the benefit, to herself, of participating with her fellows in practices requiring each to refrain from the direct endeavor to maximize her own utility, when such mutual restraint is mutually advantageous. No one, of course, can have reason to accept any unilateral constraint on her maximizing behavior; each benefits from, and only from, the constraint accepted by her fellows. But if one benefits more from a constraint on others than one loses by being constrained oneself, one may have reason to accept a practice requiring everyone, including oneself, to exhibit such a constraint. We may represent such a practice as capable of gaining unanimous agreement among rational persons who

---

[1] The now-classic example of this type of situation is the Prisoner's Dilemma. More generally, such situations may be said, in economists' parlance, to exhibit market failure. See, for example, 'Market Contractarianism', in Jules Coleman, *Markets, Morals, and the Law* (Cambridge, Cambridge University Press: 1988), chap. 10.

were choosing the terms on which they would interact with each other. And this agreement is the basis of morality.

Consider a simple example of a moral practice that would command rational agreement. Suppose each of us were to assist her fellows only when either she could expect to benefit herself from giving assistance, or she took a direct interest in their well-being. Then, in many situations, persons would not give assistance to others, even though the benefit to the recipient would greatly exceed the cost to the giver, because there would be no provision for the giver to share in the benefit. Everyone would then expect to do better were each to give assistance to her fellows, regardless of her own benefit or interest, whenever the cost of assisting was low and the benefit of receiving assistance considerable. Each would thereby accept a constraint on the direct pursuit of her own concerns, not unilaterally, but given a like acceptance by others. Reflection leads us to recognize that those who belong to groups whose members adhere to such a practice of mutual assistance enjoy benefits in interaction that are denied to others. We may then represent such a practice as rationally acceptable to everyone.

This rationale for agreed constraint makes no reference to the content of anyone's preferences. The argument depends simply on the *structure* of interaction, on the way in which each person's endeavor to fulfill her own preferences affects the fulfillment of everyone else. Thus, each person's reason to accept a mutually constraining practice is independent of her particular desires, aims and interests, although not, of course, of the fact that she has such concerns. The idea of a purely rational agent, moved to act by reason alone, is not, I think, an intelligible one. Morality is not to be understood as a constraint arising from reason alone on the fulfillment of nonrational preferences. Rather, a rational agent is one who acts to achieve the maximal fulfillment of her preferences, and morality is a constraint on the manner in which she acts, arising from the effects of interaction with other agents.

Hobbes's Foole now makes his familiar entry onto the scene, to insist that however rational it may be for a person to agree with her fellows to practices that hold out the promise of mutual advantage, yet it is rational to follow such practices only when so doing directly conduces to her maximal preference fulfillment.[1] But then such practices impose no real constraint. The effect of agreeing to or accepting them can only be to change the expected payoffs of her possible choices, making it rational for her to choose what in the absence of the practice would not be utility maximizing. The practices would offer only true prudence, not true morality.

---

[1] See Thomas Hobbes, *Leviathan*, (London, 1651), chap. 15.

The Foole is guilty of a twofold error. First, he fails to understand that real acceptance of such moral practices as assisting one's fellows, or keeping one's promises, or telling the truth is possible only among those who are disposed to comply with them. If my disposition to comply extends only so far as my interests or concerns at the time of performance, then you will be the real fool if you interact with me in ways that demand a more rigorous compliance. If, for example, it is rational to keep promises only when so doing is directly utility maximizing, then among persons whose rationality is common knowledge, only promises that require such limited compliance will be made. And opportunities for mutual advantage will be thereby forgone.

Consider this example of the way in which promises facilitate mutual benefit. Jones and Smith have adjacent farms. Although neighbors, and not hostile, they are also not friends, so that neither gets satisfaction from assisting the other. Nevertheless, they recognize that, if they harvest their crops together, each does better than if each harvests alone. Next week, Jones's crop will be ready for harvesting; a fortnight hence, Smith's crop will be ready. The harvest in, Jones is retiring, selling his farm, and moving to Florida, where he is unlikely to encounter Smith or other members of their community. Jones would like to promise Smith that, if Smith helps him harvest next week, he will help Smith harvest in a fortnight. But Jones and Smith both know that in a fortnight, helping Smith would be a pure cost to Jones. Even if Smith helps him, he has nothing to gain by returning the assistance, since neither care for Smith nor, in the circumstances, concern for his own reputation, moves him. Hence, if Jones and Smith know that Jones acts straightforwardly to maximize the fulfillment of his preferences, they know that he will not help Smith. Smith, therefore, will not help Jones even if Jones pretends to promise assistance in return. Nevertheless, Jones would do better could he make and keep such a promise—and so would Smith.

The Foole's second error, following on his first, should be clear; he fails to recognize that in plausible circumstances, persons who are genuinely disposed to a more rigorous compliance with moral practices than would follow from their interests at the time of performance can expect to do better than those who are not so disposed. For the former, constrained maximizers as I call them, will be welcome partners in mutually advantageous cooperation, in which each relies on the voluntary adherence of the others, from which the latter, straightforward maximizers, will be excluded. Constrained maximizers may thus expect more favorable opportunities than their fellows. Although in assisting their fellows, keeping their promises, and complying with other moral practices, they forgo preference fulfillment that they might obtain, yet they do better overall than those who always maximize expected utility, because of their superior opportunities.

In identifying morality with those constraints that would obtain agreement among rational persons who were choosing their terms of interaction, I am engaged in rational reconstruction. I do not suppose that we have actually agreed to existent moral practices and principles. Nor do I suppose that all existent moral practices would secure our agreement, were the question to be raised. Not all existent moral practices need be justifiable— need be ones with which we ought willingly to comply. Indeed, I do not even suppose that the practices with which we ought willingly to comply need be those that would secure our present agreement. I suppose that justifiable moral practices are those that would secure our agreement ex ante, in an appropriate premoral situation. They are those to which we should have agreed as constituting the terms of our future interaction, had we been, per impossible, in a position to decide those terms. Hypothetical agreement thus provides a test of the justifiability of our existent moral practices.

Many questions could be raised about this account, but here I want to consider only one. I have claimed that moral practices are rational, even though they constrain each person's attempt to maximize her own utility, insofar as they would be the objects of unanimous ex ante agreement. But to refute the Foole, I must defend not only the rationality of agreement, but also that of compliance, and the defense of compliance threatens to preempt the case for agreement, so that my title should be 'Why Constraint?' and not 'Why Contractarianism?' It is rational to dispose oneself to accept certain constraints on direct maximization in choosing and acting, if and only if so disposing oneself maximizes one's expected utility. What then is the relevance of agreement, and especially of hypothetical agreement? Why should it be rational to dispose oneself to accept only those constraints that would be the object of mutual agreement in an appropriate premoral situation, rather than those constraints that are found in our existent moral practices? Surely it is acceptance of the latter that makes a person welcome in interaction with his fellows. For compliance with existing morality will be what they expect, and take into account in choosing partners with whom to cooperate. [. . .]

To show the relevance of agreement to the justification of constraints, let us assume an ongoing society in which individuals more or less acknowledge and comply with a given set of practices that constrain their choices in relation to what they would be did they take only their desires, aims, and interests directly into account. Suppose that a disposition to conform to these existing practices is prima facie advantageous, since persons who are not so disposed may expect to be excluded from desirable opportunities by their fellows. However, the practices themselves have, or at least need have, no basis in agreement. And they need satisfy no intuitive standard of fairness or impartiality, characteristics that we may suppose relevant to the identification of the practices with those of a genuine morality. Although we may speak of the practices as constituting the morality of the society in question, we need not consider them morally justified or acceptable. They are simply practices constraining individual behavior in a way that each finds rational to accept.

Suppose now that our persons, as rational maximizers of individual utility, come to reflect on the practices constituting their morality. They will, of course, assess the practices in relation to their own utility, but with the awareness that their fellows will be doing the same. And one question that must arise is: Why these practices? For they will recognize that the set of actual moral practices is not the only possible set of constraining practices that would yield mutually advantageous, optimal outcomes. They will recognize the possibility of alternative moral orders. At this point it will not be enough to say that, as a matter of fact, each person can expect to benefit from a disposition to comply with existing practices. For persons will also ask themselves: Can I benefit more, not from simply abandoning any morality, and recognizing no constraint, but from a partial rejection of existing constraints in favor of an alternative set? Once this question is asked, the situation is transformed; the existing moral order must be assessed, not only against simple noncompliance, but also against what we may call alternative compliance.

To make this assessment, each will compare her prospects under the existing practices with those she would anticipate from a set that, in the existing circumstances, she would expect to result from bargaining with her fellows. If her prospects would be improved by such negotiation, then she will have a real, although not necessarily sufficient, incentive to demand a change in the established moral order. More generally, if there are persons whose prospects would be improved by renegotiation, then the existing order will be recognizably unstable. No doubt those whose prospects would be worsened by renegotiation will have a clear incentive to resist, to appeal to the status quo. But their appeal will be a weak one, especially among persons who are not taken in by spurious ideological considerations, but focus on individual utility maximization. Thus, although in the real world, we begin with an existing set of moral practices as constraints on our maximizing behavior, yet we are led by reflection to the idea of an amended set that would obtain the agreement of everyone, and this amended set has, and will be recognized to have, a stability lacking in existing morality.

The reflective capacity of rational agents leads them from the given to the agreed, from existing practices and principles requiring constraint to those that would receive each person's assent. The same reflective capacity, I claim, leads from those practices that would be agreed to, in existing social circumstances, to those that would receive ex ante agreement, premoral and presocial. As the status quo proves unstable when it comes into conflict with what would be agreed to, so what would be agreed to proves unstable when it comes into conflict with what would have been agreed to in an appropriate presocial context. For as existing practices must seem arbitrary insofar as they do not correspond to what a rational person would agree to, so what such a person would agree to in existing circumstances must seem arbitrary in relation to what she would accept in a presocial condition.

What a rational person would agree to in existing circumstances depends in large part on her negotiating position vis-à-vis her fellows. But her negotiating position is significantly affected by the existing social institutions, and so by the currently accepted moral practices embodied in those institutions. Thus, although agreement may well yield practices differing from those embodied in existing social institutions, yet it will be influenced by those practices, which are not themselves the product of rational agreement. And this must call the rationality of the agreed practices into question. The arbitrariness of existing practices must infect any agreement whose terms are significantly affected by them. Although rational agreement is in itself a source of stability, yet this stability is undermined by the arbitrariness of the circumstances in which it takes place. To escape this arbitrariness, rational persons will revert from actual to hypothetical agreement, considering what practices they would have agreed to from an initial position not structured by existing institutions and the practices they embody.

The content of a hypothetical agreement is determined by an appeal to the equal rationality of persons. Rational persons will voluntarily accept an agreement only insofar as they perceive it to be equally advantageous to each. To be sure, each would be happy to accept an agreement more advantageous to herself than to her fellows, but since no one will accept an agreement perceived to be less advantageous, agents whose rationality is a matter of common knowledge will recognize the futility of aiming at or holding out for more, and minimize their bargaining costs by coordinating at the point of equal advantage. Now the extent of advantage is determined in a twofold way. First, there is advantage internal to an agreement. In this respect, the expectation of equal advantage is assured by procedural fairness. The step from existing moral practices to those resulting from actual agreement takes rational persons to a procedurally fair situation, in which each perceives the agreed practices to be ones that it is equally rational for all to accept, given the circumstances in which agreement is reached. But those circumstances themselves may be called into question insofar as they are perceived to be arbitrary—the result, in part, of compliance with constraining practices that do not themselves ensure the expectation of equal advantage, and so do not reflect the equal rationality of the complying parties. To neutralize this arbitrary element, moral practices to be fully acceptable must be conceived as constituting a possible outcome of a hypothetical agreement under circumstances that are unaffected by social institutions that themselves lack full acceptability. Equal rationality demands consideration of external circumstances as well as internal procedures.

But what is the practical import of this argument? It would be absurd to claim that mere acquaintance with it, or even acceptance of it, will lead to the replacement of existing moral practices by those that would secure presocial agreement. It would be irrational for anyone to give up the benefits of the existing moral order simply because he comes to realize that it affords him more than he could expect from pure rational agreement with his fellows. And it would be irrational for anyone to accept a long-term utility loss by refusing to comply with the existing moral order, simply because she comes to realize that such compliance affords her less than she could expect from pure rational agreement. Nevertheless, these realizations do transform, or perhaps bring to the surface, the character of the relationships between persons that are maintained by the existing constraints, so that some of these relationships come to be recognized as coercive. These realizations constitute the elimination of false consciousness, and they result from a process of rational reflection that brings persons into what, in my theory, is the parallel of Jürgen Habermas's ideal speech situation.[1] Without an argument to defend themselves in open dialogue with their fellows, those who are more than equally advantaged can hope to maintain their privileged position only if they can coerce their fellows into accepting it. And this, of course, may be possible. But coercion is not agreement, and it lacks any inherent stability.

Stability plays a key role in linking compliance to agreement. Aware of the benefits to be gained from constraining practices, rational persons will seek those that invite stable compliance. Now compliance is stable if it arises from agreement among persons each of whom considers both that the terms of agreement are sufficiently favorable to herself that it is rational for her to accept them, and that they are not so favorable to others that it would be rational for them to accept terms less favorable to them and more favorable to herself. An agreement affording equally favorable terms to all thus invites, as no other can, stable compliance.

['Why Contractarianism', in Peter Vallentyne (ed.), *Contractarianism and Rational Choice* (Cambridge University Press: Cambridge, 1991), 22–9.]

---

[1] See Raymond Geuss, *The Idea of a Critical Theory: Habermas and the Frankfurt School* (Cambridge University Press: Cambridge, 1981), 65 ff.

b. Criticism

MARY MIDGLEY

 89 Duties concerning Islands

Had Robinson Crusoe any duties?

When I was a philosophy student, this used to be a familiar conundrum, which was supposed to pose a very simple question; namely, can you have duties to yourself? Mill, they correctly told us, said no. 'The term duty to oneself, when it means anything more than prudence, means self-respect or self-development, and for none of these is anyone accountable to his fellow-creatures.'[1] Kant, on the other hand, said yes. 'Duties to ourselves are of primary importance and should have pride of place . . . nothing can be expected of a man who dishonours his own person.'[2] There is a serious disagreement here, not to be sneezed away just by saying, 'It depends on what you mean by duty.' Much bigger issues are involved—quite how big has, I think, not yet been fully realized. To grasp this, I suggest that we rewrite a part of Crusoe's story, in order to bring in sight a different range of concerns.

19 Sept. 1685. This day I set aside to devastate my island. My pinnance being now ready on the shore, and all things prepared for my departure, Friday's people also expecting me, and the wind blowing fresh away from my little harbour, I had a mind to see how all would burn. So then, setting sparks and powder craftily among certain dry spinneys which I had chosen, I soon had it ablaze, nor was there left, by the next down, any green stick among the ruins. . . .

Now, work on the style how you will, you cannot make that into a convincing paragraph. Crusoe was not the most scrupulous of men, but he would have felt an invincible objection to this senseless destruction. So would the rest of us. Yet the language of our moral tradition has tended strongly, ever since the Enlightenment, to make that objection unstateable. All the terms which express that an obligation is serious or binding—duty, right, law, morality, obligation, justice—have been deliberately narrowed in their use so as to apply only in the framework of contract, to describe only relations holding between free and rational agents. Since it has been decided *a priori* that rationality admits of no degrees and that cetaceans are not rational, it follows that, unless you take either religion or science fiction

---

[1] John Stuart Mill, *Essay on Liberty* (Dent, Everyman's Library: London, 1910), 135.
[2] Immanuel Kant, 'Duties to Oneself', in *Lectures on Ethics*, trans. Louis Infield (Methuen: London, 1930), 118.

seriously, we can only have duties to humans, and sane, adult, responsible humans at that. Now the morality we live by certainly does not accept this restriction. In common life we recognize many other duties as serious and binding, though of course not necessarily overriding. If philosophers want to call these something else instead of duties, they must justify their move.

We have here one of those clashes between the language of common morality (which is of course always to some extent confused and inarticulate) and an intellectual scheme which arose in the first place from a part of that morality, but has now taken off on its own claims of authority to correct other parts of its source. There are always real difficulties here. As ordinary citizens, we have to guard against dismissing such intellectual schemes too casually; we have to do justice to the point of them. But, as philosophers, we have to resist the opposite temptation of taking the intellectual scheme as decisive, just because it is elegant and satisfying, or because the moral insight which is its starting point is specially familiar to us. Today, this intellectualist bias is often expressed by calling the insights of common morality mere 'intuitions.' This is quite misleading, since it gives the impression that they have been reached without thought, and that there is, by contrast, a scientific solution somewhere else to which they ought to bow—as there might be if we were contrasting common sense 'intuitions' about the physical world with physics or astronomy. Even without that word, philosophers often manage to give the impression that whenever our moral views clash with any simple, convenient scheme, it is our *duty* to abandon them. Thus, Grice states:

It is an inescapable consequence of the thesis presented in these pages that certain classes cannot have natural rights: animals, the human embryo, future generations, lunatics and children under the age of, say, ten. In the case of young children at least, my experience is that this consequence is found hard to accept. But it is a consequence of the theory; it is, I believe, true; and I think we should be willing to accept it. At first sight it seems a harsh conclusion, but it is not nearly so harsh as it appears.[1]

But it is in fact extremely harsh, since what he is saying is that the treatment of children ought not to be determined by their interests but by the interests of the surrounding adults capable of contract, which, of course, can easily conflict with them. In our society, he explains, this does not actually make much difference, because parents here are so benevolent that they positively want to benefit their children, and accordingly here 'the interests of children are reflected in the interests of their parents.' But this, he adds, is just a contingent fact about us. 'It is easy to imagine a society where this is not so,' where, that is, parents are entirely exploitative. 'In

[1] G.R. Grice, *The Grounds of Moral Judgment* (Cambridge University Press: Cambridge, 1967), 147–9.

this circumstance, the morally correct treatment of children would no doubt be harsher than it is in our society. But the conclusion has to be accepted.' Grice demands that we withdraw our objections to harshness, in deference to theoretical consistency. But 'harsh' here does not mean just 'brisk and bracing,' like cold baths and a plain diet. (There might well be more of those where parents do feel bound to consider their children's interests.) It means 'unjust.' Our objection to unbridled parental selfishness is not a mere matter of tone or taste; it is a moral one. It therefore requires a moral answer, an explanation of the contrary *value* which the contrary theory expresses. Grice, and those who argue like him, take the ascetic, disapproving tone of those who have already displayed such a value, and who are met by a slovenly reluctance to rise to it. But they have not displayed that value. The ascetic tone cannot be justified merely by an appeal to consistency. An ethical theory, which, when consistently followed through, has iniquitous consequences, is a bad theory and must be changed. Certainly we can ask whether these consequences really are iniquitous, but this question must be handled seriously. We cannot directly conclude that the consequences cease to stink the moment they are seen to follow from our theory.

The theoretical model which has spread blight in this area is, of course, that of social contract, and, to suit it, that whole cluster of essential moral terms—right, duty, justice and the rest—has been progressively narrowed. This model shows human society as a spread of standard social atoms, originally distinct and independent, each of which combines with others only at its own choice and in its own private interest. This model is drawn from physics, and from seventeenth-century physics, at that, where the ultimate particles of matter were conceived as hard, impenetrable, homogeneous little billiard balls, with no hooks or internal structure. To see how such atoms could combine at all was very hard. Physics, accordingly, moved on from this notion to one which treats atoms and other particles as complex items, describable mainly in terms of forces, and those the same kind of forces which operate outside them. It has abandoned the notion of ultimate, solitary, independent individuals. Social-contract theory, however, retains it.

On this physical—or archaeo-physical—model, all significant moral relations between individuals are the symmetrical ones expressed by contract. If, on the other hand, we use a biological or 'organic' model, we can talk also of a variety of asymmetrical relations found within a whole. Leaves relate not only to other leaves, but to fruit, twigs, branches and the whole tree. People appear not only as individuals, but as members of their groups, families, tribes, species, ecosystems and biosphere, and have moral relations as part to these wholes. The choice between these two ways of thinking is not, of course, a simple once-and-for-all affair. Different models are useful for different purposes. We can, however, reasonably point out, firstly, that the old physical pattern does make all attempts to explain combination extremely difficult; and, secondly, that since human beings actually are living creatures, not crystals or galaxies, it is reasonable to expect that biological ways of thinking will be useful in understanding them.

In its own sphere, the social contract model has of course been of enormous value. Where we deal with clashes of interest between free and rational agents already in existence, and particularly where we want to disentangle some of them from some larger group that really does not suit them, it is indispensable. And for certain political purposes during the last three centuries these clashes have been vitally important. An obsession with contractual thinking, and a conviction that it is a cure-all, are therefore understandable. But the trouble with such obsessions is that they distort the whole shape of thought and language in a way which makes them self-perpetuating, and constantly extends their empire. Terms come to be defined in a way which leaves only certain moral views expressible. This can happen without any clear intention on the part of those propagating them, and even contrary to their occasional declarations, simply from mental inertia. Thus, John Rawls, having devoted most of his long book to his very subtle and exhaustive contractual view of justice, remarks without any special emphasis near the end that 'we should recall here the limits of a theory of justice. Not only are many aspects of morality left aside, but no account can be given of right conduct in regard to animals and the rest of nature.'[1] He concedes that these are serious matters. 'Certainly it is wrong to be cruel to animals and the destruction of a whole species can be a great evil. The capacity for feelings of pleasure and pain and for the forms of life of which animals are capable clearly impose duties of compassion and humanity in their case.' All this is important, he says, and it calls for a wider metaphysical enquiry, but it is not his subject. Earlier in the same passage he touches on the question of permanently irrational human beings, and remarks that it 'may present a difficulty. I cannot examine this problem here, but I assume that the account of equality would not be materially affected.'[2] Won't it though? It is a strange project to examine a single virtue— justice—without at least sketching in one's view of the vast background of general morality which determines its shape and meaning, including, of course, such awkward and noncontractual virtues as 'compassion and humanity.' It isolates the duties which people owe each other *merely as thinkers* from those deeper and more general ones which they owe each other

---

[1] John Rawls, *A Theory of Justice* (Oxford University Press: Oxford, 1972), 512.
[2] Ibid. 510.

as beings who feel. It cannot, therefore, fail both to split a man's nature and to isolate him from the rest of the creation to which he belongs.

Such an account may not be *Hamlet* without the prince, but it is *Hamlet* with half the cast missing, and without the state of Denmark. More exactly, it is like a history of Poland which regards Russia, Germany, Europe and the Roman Church as not part of its subject. I am not attacking Rawls' account on its own ground. I am simply pointing out what the history of ethics shows all too clearly—how much our thinking is shaped by what our sages *omit* to mention. The Greek philosophers never really raised the problem of slavery till towards the end of their speech, and then few of them did so with conviction. This happened even though it lay right in the path of their enquiries into political justice and the value of the individual soul. Christianity did raise that problem, because its class background was different and because the world in the Christian era was already in turmoil, so that men were not presented with the narcotic of a happy stability. But Christianity itself did not, until quite recently, raise the problem of the morality of punishment, and particularly of eternal punishment. This failure to raise central questions was not, in either case, complete. One can find very intelligent and penetrating criticisms of slavery occurring from time to time in Greek writings—even in Aristotle's defence of that institution.[1] But they are mostly like Rawls' remark here. They conclude that 'this should be investigated some day.' The same thing happens with Christian writings concerning punishment, except that the consideration, 'this is a great mystery,' acts as an even more powerful paralytic to thought. Not much more powerful, however. Natural intertia, when it coincides with vested interest or the illusion of vested interest, is as strong as gravitation.

It is important that Rawls does not, like Grice, demand that we toe the line which would make certain important moral views impossible. Like Hume, who similarly excluded animals from justice, he simply leaves them out of his discussion. This move ought in principle to be harmless. But when it is combined with an intense concentration of discussion on contractual justice, and a corresponding neglect of compassion and humanity, it inevitably suggests that the excluded problems are relatively unimportant. This suggestion is still more strongly conveyed by rulings which exclude the nonhuman world from rights, duties and morality. Words like 'rights' and 'duties' are awkward because they do indeed have narrow senses approximating to the legal, but they also have much wider ones in which they cover the whole moral sphere. To say 'they do not have rights,' or 'you do not have duties to them' conveys to any ordinary hearer a very simple message; namely, 'they do not matter.' This is an absolute, a removal of blame for ill-treatment of 'them,' whoever they may be.

---

[1] Aristotle, *Politics*, 1, 3–8; cf. *Nichomachean Ethics*, 7.2.

To see how strong this informal, moral usage of 'rights' is, we need only look at the history of that powerful notion, the 'rights of man.' These rights were not supposed to be ones conferred by law, since the whole point of appealing to them was to change laws so as to embody them. They were vague, but vast. They did not arise, as rights are often said to do, only within a community, since they were taken to apply in principle every-where. The immense, and on the whole coherent, use which has been made of this idea by reform movements shows plainly that the tension between the formal and the informal idea of 'right' is part of the word's meaning, a fruitful connection of thought, not just a mistake. It is therefore hard to adopt effectively the compromise which some philosophers now favour, of saying that it is indeed wrong to treat animals in certain ways, but that we have no duties to them or that they have no rights.[2] 'Animal rights' may be hard to formulate, as indeed are the rights of humans. But 'no rights' will not do. The word may need to be dropped entirely. The compromise is still harder with the word 'duty,' which is rather more informal, and is more closely wedded to a private rather than political use.

Where the realm of right and duty stops, there, to ordinary thinking, begins the realm of the optional. What is not a duty may be a matter of taste, style or feeling, of aesthetic sensibility, of habit and nostalgia, of etiquette and local custom, but it cannot be something which demands our attention whether we like it or not. When claims get into this area, they can scarcely be taken seriously. This becomes clear when Kant tries to straddle the border. He says that we have no direct duties to animals, because they are not rational, but that we should treat them properly all the same because of 'indirect' duties which are really duties to our own humanity.[3] This means that ill-treating them (a) might lead us to ill-treat humans, and (b) is a sign of a bad or inhumane disposition. The whole issue thus becomes a contingent one of spiritual style or training, like contemplat-ive exercises, intellectual practice or, indeed, refined manners.[4] Some might need practice of this kind to make them kind to people, others might not, and, indeed, might get on better without it. (Working off one's ill-temper on animals might make one treat people *better*.) But the question of cruelty to animals cannot be like this, because it is of the essence to such training exercises that they are internal. Anything that affects some other being is not just practice, it is real action. Anyone who refrained from cruelty *merely* from a wish not to sully his own character, without any direct considera-tion for the possible victims, would be frivolous and narcissistic.

---

[2] For example, John Passmore, *Man's Responsibility for Nature* (Duckworth: London, 1974), 116–17; H. J. McCloskey, 'Rights', *Philosophical Quarterly*, 15 (1965).

[3] Nor will it help for philosophers to say 'it is not the case that they have rights.' Such pompous locutions have either no meaning at all, or the obvious one.

[4] Immanuel Kant, 'Duties towards Animals and Spirits', in *Lectures on Ethics*, 240.

A similar trivialization follows where theorists admit duties of compassion and humanity to noncontractors, but deny duties of justice. Hume and Rawls, in making this move, do not explicitly subordinate these other duties, or say that they are less binding. But because they make the contract element so central to morality, this effect appears to follow. The priority of justice is expressed in such everyday proverbs as 'be just before you're generous.' We are therefore rather easily persuaded to think that compassion, humanity and so forth are perhaps emotional luxuries, to be indulged only after all debts are paid. A moment's thought will show that this is wrong. Someone who receives simultaneously a request to pay a debt and another to comfort somebody bereaved or on their death bed is not as a matter of course under obligation to treat the debt as the more urgent. He has to look at circumstances on both sides, but in general we should probably expect the other duties to have priority. This is still more true if, on his way to pay the debt, he encounters a stranger in real straits, drowning or lying on the road. To give the debt priority, we probably need to think of his creditor as also being in serious trouble—which brings compassion and humanity in on both sides of the case.

What makes it so hard to give justice a different clientele from the other virtues, as Hume and Rawls do, is simply the fact that justice is such a pervading virtue. In general, all serious cases of cruelty, meanness, inhumanity and the like are also cases of injustice. If we are told that a certain set of these cases does not involve injustice, our natural thought is that these cases must be *trivial*. Officially, Hume's and Rawls' restriction is not supposed to mean this. What, however, is it supposed to mean? It is forty years since I first read Hume's text, and I find his thought as obscure now as I did then. I well remember double-taking then, going back over the paragraph for a point which, I took it, I must have missed. Can anyone see it?

Were there a species of creatures intermingled with men, which, though rational, were possessed of such inferior strength, both of body and mind, that they were incapable of all resistance, and could never, upon the highest provocation, make us feel the effects of their resentment; the necessary consequence, I think, is that we should be bound by the laws of humanity to give gentle usage to these creatures, but should not, properly speaking, lie under any restraint of justice with regard to them, nor could they possess any right or property, exclusive of such arbitrary lords. Our intercourse with them could not be called society, which supposes a degree of equality, but absolute command on one side and servile obedience on the other. . . . This is plainly the situation of men with regard to animals.[1]

I still think that the word 'justice,' so defined, has lost its normal meaning. In ordinary life we think that duties of justice become *more* pressing, not less

---

[1] David Hume, 'An Enquiry concerning the Principles of Morals', in *Hume's Moral and Political Philosophy*, ed. H. E. Aiben (Hafner: New York, 1949), app. 3, pp. 190–1.

so, when we are dealing with the weak and inarticulate, who cannot argue back. It is the boundaries of prudence which depend on power, not those of justice. Historically, Hume's position becomes more understandable when one sees its place in the development of social-contract thinking. The doubtful credit for confining justice to the human species seems to belong to Grotius, who finally managed to ditch the Roman notion of *jus naturale*, natural right or law, common to all species. I cannot here discuss his remarkably unimpressive arguments for this.[1] The point I want to make here is simply in reference to the effect of these restrictive definitions of terms like 'justice' on people's view of the sheer size of the problems raised by what falls outside them.

Writers who treat morality as primarily contractual tend to discuss noncontractual cases briefly, casually and parenthetically, as though they were rather rare. Rawls' comments on the problem of mental defectives are entirely typical here. We have succeeded, they say, in laying most of the carpet; why are you making this fuss about those little wrinkles behind the sofa? This treatment confirms a view, already suggested by certain aspects of current politics in the United States, that those who fail to clock in as normal rational agents and make their contracts are just occasional exceptions, constituting one more 'minority' group—worrying, no doubt, to the scrupulous, but not a central concern of any society. Let us, then, glance briefly at their scope, by roughly listing some cases which seem to involve us in noncontractual duties. (The order is purely provisional and the numbers are added just for convenience.)

Human Sector	1. The dead
	2. Posterity
	3. Children
	4. The senile
	5. The temporarily insane
	6. The permanently insane
	7. Defectives, ranging down to 'human vegetables'
	8. Embryos, human and otherwise
Animal Sector	9. Sentient animals
	10. Nonsentient animals
Inanimate Sector	11. Plants of all kinds
	12. Artefacts, including works of art
	13. Inanimate but structured objects—crystals, rivers, rocks, etc.
Comprehensive	14. Unchosen groups of all kinds, including families and species
	15. Ecosystems, landscapes, villages, warrens, cities, etc.

---

[1] A point well discussed by Stephen R. L. Clark, *The Moral Status of Animals* (Clarendon Press: Oxford, 1977), 12–13.

	16. Countries
	17. The Biosphere
Miscellaneous	18. Oneself
	19. God

No doubt I have missed a few, but that will do to go on with. The point is this; if we look only at a few of these groupings, and without giving them full attention, it is easy to think that we can include one or two as honorary contracting members by a slight stretch of our conceptual scheme, and find arguments for excluding the others from serious concern entirely. But if we keep our eye on the size of the range, this stops being plausible. As far as sheer numbers go, this is no minority of the beings with whom we have to deal. We are a small minority of them. As far as importance goes, it is certainly possible to argue that some of these sorts of beings should concern us more and others less: we need a priority system. But, to build it, *moral* arguments are required. The various kinds of claims have to be understood and compared, not written off in advance. We cannot rule that those who, in our own and other cultures, suppose that there is a direct objection to injuring or destroying some of them, are always just confused, and mean only, in fact, that this item will be needed for rational human consumption.[1]

The blank antithesis which Kant made between rational persons (having value) and mere things (having none) will not serve us to map out this vast continuum. And the idea that, starting at some given point on this list, we have a general licence for destruction, is itself a moral view which would have to be justified. Western culture differs from most others in the breadth of destructive licence which it allows itself, and, since the seventeenth century, that licence has been greatly extended. Scruples about rapine have been continually dismissed as irrational, but it is not always clear with what rational principles they are supposed to conflict. Western destructiveness has not in fact developed in response to a new set of disinterested intellectual principles demonstrating the need for more people and less redwoods, but mainly as a by-product of greed and increasing commercial confidence. Humanistic hostility to superstition has played some part in the process, because respect for the nonhuman items on our list is often taken to be religious. It does not have to be. Many scientists who are card-carrying atheists can still see the point of preserving the biosphere. So can the rest of us, religious or otherwise. It is the whole of which we are parts, and its other parts concern us for that reason.

But the language of rights is rather ill-suited to expressing this, because it has been developed mainly for the protection of people who, though

---

[1.] For details, see John Rodman, 'Animal Justice: The Counter-Revolution in Natural Right and Law', *Inquiry*, 22 1–2 (Summer 1979).

perhaps oppressed, are in principle articulate. This makes it quite reasonable for theorists to say that rights belong only to those who understand
them and can claim them. When confronted with the 'human sector' of our
list, these theorists can either dig themselves in, like Grice, and exclude the
lot, or stretch the scheme, like Rawls, by including the hypothetical rational choices which these honorary members *would* make if they were not
unfortunately prevented. Since many of these people seem less rational
than many animals, zoophiles have, then, a good case for calling this
second device arbitrary or specious, and extending rights to the border of
sentience. Here, however, the meaning of the term 'rights' does become
thin, and when we reach the inanimate area, usage will scarcely cover it. (It
is worth noticing that long before this, when dealing merely with the
'rights of man,' the term often seems obscure, because to list and specify
these rights is so much harder than to shout for them. The word is probably
of more use as a slogan, indicating a general direction, than as a detailed
conceptual tool.) There may be a point in campaigning to extend usage.
But to me it seems wiser on the whole not to waste energy on this verbal
point, but instead to insist on the immense variety of kinds of beings with
which we have to deal. Once we grasp this, we ought not to be surprised
that we are involved in many different kinds of claim or duty. The dictum
that 'rights and duties are correlative' is misleading, because the two words
keep rather different company, and one may be narrowed without affecting
the other.

What, then, about duties? I believe that this term can properly be used
over the whole range. We have quite simply got many kinds of duties to
animals,[1] to plants and to the biosphere. But to speak in this way we must
free the term once and for all from its restrictive contractual use, or
irrelevant doubts will still haunt us. If we cannot do this, we shall have to
exclude the word 'duty,' along with 'rights' from all detailed discussion,
using wider words like 'wrong,' 'right' and 'ought' instead. This gymnastic
would be possible but inconvenient. The issue about duty becomes clear as
soon as we look at the controversy from which I started, between Kant's
and Mill's views on duties to oneself. What do we think about this? Are
there duties of integrity, autonomy, self-knowledge, self-respect? It seems
that there are. Mill is right, of course, to point out that they are not duties
to someone in the ordinary sense. The divided self is a metaphor. It is as
natural and necessary a metaphor here as it is over, say, self-deception or
self-control, but it certainly is not literal truth. The form of the requirement
is different. Rights, for instance, certainly do not seem to come in here as

---

[1] A case first made by Jeremy Bentham, *An Introduction of the Principles of Moral and Legislation*, chap. 17, and well worked out by Peter Singer, *Animal Liberation* (Avon: New York, 1977),
chaps. 1, 5 and 6.

they often would with duties to other persons; we would scarcely say, 'I have a right to my own respect.' And the *kind* of things which we can owe ourselves are distinctive. It is not just chance who they are owed to. You cannot owe it to somebody else, as you can to yourself, to force him to act freely or with integrity. He owes that to himself; the rest of us can only remove outside difficulties. As Kant justly said, our business is to promote our own perfection and the happiness of others; the perfection of others is an aim which belongs to them.[1] Respect, indeed, we owe both to ourselves and to others, but Kant may well be right to say that self-respect is really a different and deeper requirement, something without which all outward duties would become meaningless. (This may explain the paralyzing effect of depression.)

Duties to oneself, in fact, are duties with a different *form*. They are far less close than outward duties to the literal model of debt, especially monetary debt. Money is a thing which can be owed in principle to anybody, it is the same whoever you owe it to, and if by chance you come to owe it to yourself, the debt vanishes. Not many of our duties are really of this impersonal kind; the attempt to commute other sorts of duties into money is a notorious form of evasion. Utilitarianism however wants to make all duties as homogeneous as possible. And that is the point of Mill's position. He views all our self-concerning motives as parts of the desire for happiness. Therefore he places all duty, indeed all morality, on the outside world, as socially required restrictions of that desire—an expression, that is, of other people's desire for happiness.

We do not call anything wrong, unless we mean that a person ought to be punished in some way or another for doing it; if not by law, by the opinion of his fellow-creatures; if not by opinion, by the reproaches of his own conscience. This seems the real turning point of the distinction between morality and simple expedience. It is a part of the notion of Duty in every one of its forms, that a person may rightly be compelled to fulfil it. Duty is a thing which may be *exacted* from a person, as one exacts a debt.[2]

To make the notion of wrongness depend on punishment and public opinion in this way instead of the other way round is a bold step. Mill did not mind falling flat on his face from time to time in trying out a new notion for the public good. He did it for us, and we should, I think, take proper advantage of his generosity, and accept the impossibility which he demonstrates. The concepts cannot be connected this way round. Unless you think of certain acts as wrong, it makes no sense to talk of punishment. 'Punishing' alcoholics with aversion therapy or experimental rats with

---

[1] Immanuel Kant, *Preface to the Metaphysical Elements of Ethics*, 'Introduction to Ethics', 4 and 5.

[2] John Stuart Mill, *Utilitarianism* (Dent, Everyman's Library: London, 1910), 45.

electric shocks is not really punishing at all; it is just deterrence. This 'punishment' will not make their previous actions wrong, nor has it any-thing to do with morality. The real point of morality returns to Mill's scheme in the Trojan horse of 'reproaches of his own conscience.' Why do *they* matter? Unless the conscience is talking sense—that is, on Utilitarian principles, unless it is delivering the judgment of society—it should surely be silenced. Mill, himself a man of enormous integrity, deeply concerned about autonomy, would never have agreed to silence it. But, unless we do so, we shall have to complicate his scheme. It may well be true that, in the last resort and at the deepest level, conscience and the desire for happiness converge. But in ordinary life and at the everyday level they can diverge amazingly. We do want to be honest but we do not want to be put out. What we know we ought to do is often most unwelcome to us, which is why we call it duty. And whole sections of that duty do not concern other people directly at all. A good example is the situation in Huxley's *Brave New World*, where a few dissident citizens have grasped the possibility of a fuller and freer life. Nobody else wants this. Happiness is already assured. The primary duty of change here seems to be that of each to himself. True, they may feel bound also to help others to change, but hardly in a way which those others would *exact*. In fact, we may do better here by dropping the awkward second party altogether and saying that they have a duty *of* living differently—one which will affect both themselves and others, but which does not require, as a debt does, a named person or people *to* whom it must be paid. Wider models like 'the whole duty of man' may be more relevant.

This one example from my list will, I hope, be enough to explain the point. I cannot go through all of them, nor ought it to be necessary. Duties need *not* be quasi-contractual relations between symmetrical pairs of ra-tional human agents. There are all kinds of other obligations holding between asymmetrical pairs, or involving, as in this case, no outside beings at all. To speak of duties *to* things in the inanimate and comprehensive sectors of my list is not necessarily to personify them superstitiously, or to indulge in chatter about the 'secret life of plants.'[1] It expresses merely that there are suitable and unsuitable ways of behaving in given situations. People have duties *as* farmers, parents, consumers, forest dwellers, colon-ists, species members, shipwrecked mariners, tourists, potential ancestors

---

[1] P. Tompkins and C. Bird, *The Secret Life of Plants* (Harper and Row: New York, 1973), claimed to show, by various experiments involving electrical apparatus, that plants can feel. Attempts to duplicate their experiments have, however, totally failed to produce any similar results. (See A. W. Galston and C. L. Slayman, 'The Secret Life of Plants', *American Scientist*, 67 (1973, 337). It seems possible that the original results were due to a fault in the electrical apparatus. The attempt shows, I think, one of the confusions which continually arise from insisting that all duties must be of the same form. We do not need to prove that plants are animals in order to have reason to spare them. The point is well discussed by Marian Dawkins in her book *Animal Suffering* (Chapman and Hall: London, 1981), 117–19.

and actual descendants, etc. As such, it is the business of each not to forget his transitory and dependent position, the rich gifts which he has received, and the tiny part he plays in a vast, irreplaceable and fragile whole.

It is remarkable that we now have to state this obvious truth as if it were new, and invent the word 'ecological' to describe a whole vast class of duties. Most peoples are used to the idea. In stating it, and getting back into the centre of our moral stage, we meet various difficulties, of which the most insidious is possibly the temptation to feed this issue as fuel to long-standing controversies about religion. Is concern for the nonhuman aspects of our biosphere necessarily superstitious and therefore to be resisted tooth and nail? I have pointed out that it need not be religious. Certified rejectors of all known religions can share it. No doubt, however, there is a wider sense in which any deep and impersonal concern can be called religious—one in which Marxism is a religion. No doubt, too, all such deep concerns have their dangers, but certainly the complete absence of them has worse dangers. Moreover, anyone wishing above all to avoid the religious dimension should consider that the intense individualism which has focused our attention exclusively on the social contract model is itself thoroughly mystical. It has glorified the individual human soul as an object having infinite and transcendent value; has hailed it as the only real creator; and bestowed on it much of the panoply of God. Nietzsche, who was responsible for much of this new theology,[1] took over from the old theology (which he plundered extensively) the assumption that all the rest of creation mattered only as a frame for humankind. This is not an impression which any disinterested observer would get from looking around at it, nor do we need it in order to take our destiny sufficiently seriously.

Crusoe then, I conclude, did have duties concerning this island, and with the caution just given we can reasonably call them duties *to* it. They were not very exacting, and were mostly negative. They differed, of course, from those which a long-standing inhabitant of a country has. Here the language of *fatherland* and *motherland*, which is so widely employed, indicates rightly a duty of care and responsibility which can go very deep, and which long-settled people commonly feel strongly. To insist that it is really only a duty to the exploiting human beings is not consistent with the emphasis often given to reverence for the actual trees, mountains, lakes, rivers and the like which are found there. A decision to inhibit all this rich area of human love is a special manoeuvre for which reasons would need to be given, not a dispassionate analysis of existing duties and feelings. What

---

[1] See particularly, Friedrich Nietzsche, *Thus Spake Zarathustra*, 3, section 'Of Old and New Tables'; and *The Joyful Wisdom* (otherwise called *The Gay Science*), 125 (the Madman's Speech). I have discussed this rather mysterious appointment of man to succeed God in a paper called 'Creation and Originality', *Heart & Mind: The Varieties of Moral Experience* (The Harvester Press: Brighton, 1981).

happens, however, when you are shipwrecked on an entirely strange island? As the history of colonization shows, there is a tendency for people so placed to drop any reverence and become more exploitative. But it is not irresistible. Raiders who settle down can quite soon begin to feel at home, as the Vikings did in East Anglia, and can, after a while, become as possessive, proud and protective towards their new land as the old inhabitants. Crusoe himself does, from time to time, show this pride rather touchingly, and it would, I think, certainly have inhibited any moderate temptation, such as that which I mentioned, to have a good bonfire. What keeps him sane through his stay is in fact his duty to God. If that had been absent, I should rather suppose that sanity would depend on a stronger and more positive attachment to the island itself and its creatures. It is interesting, however, that Crusoe's story played its part in developing that same icy individualism which has gone so far towards making both sorts of attachment seem corrupt or impossible. Rousseau delighted in *Robinson Crusoe*, and praised it as the only book fit to be given to a child, *not* because it showed a man in his true relation to animal and vegetable life, but because it was the bible of individualism. 'The surest way to raise him [the child] above prejudice and to base his judgments on the true relations of things, is to put him in the place of a solitary man, and to judge all things as they would be judged by such a man in relation to their own utility . . . So long as only bodily needs are recognized, man is self sufficing . . . the child knows no other happiness but food and freedom.'[1] That false atomic notion of human psychology—a prejudice above which nobody ever raised Rousseau—is the flaw in all social-contract thinking. If he were right, every member of the human race would need a separate island—and what, then, would our ecological problems be? Perhaps, after all, we had better count our blessings.

['Duties concerning Islands', *Encounter*, 60/2 (1983), 36–44.]

[1] Barbara Foxley (trans.), *Emile* (Dent, Everyman's Library: London, 1966), 147–8.

Epilogue

90 How Both Human History, and the History of Ethics, May be Just Beginning

Some people believe that there cannot be progress in Ethics, since everything has been already said. I believe the opposite. How many people have made Non-Religious Ethics their life's work? Before the recent past, very few. In most civilizations, most people have believed in the existence of a God, or of several gods. A large minority were in fact Atheists, whatever they pretended. But, before the recent past, very few Atheists made Ethics their life's work. Buddha may be among this few, as may be Confucius, and a few Ancient Greeks and Romans. After more than a thousand years, there were a few more between the Sixteenth and Twentieth Centuries. Hume was an Atheist who made Ethics part of his life's work. Sidgwick was another. After Sidgwick, there were several Atheists who were professional moral philosophers. But most of these did not do Ethics. They did Meta-Ethics. They did not ask which outcomes would be good or bad, or which acts would be right or wrong. They asked, and wrote about, only the meaning of moral language, and the question of objectivity. Non-Religious Ethics has been systematically studied, by many people, only since about 1960. Compared with the other sciences, Non-Religious Ethics is the youngest and the least advanced.

I believe that if we destroy mankind, as we now could, this outcome would be *much* worse than most people think. Compare three outcomes:

(1) Peace.
(2) A nuclear war that kills 99% of the world's existing population.
(3) A nuclear war that kills 100%.

(2) would be worse than (1), and (3) would be worse than (2). Which is the greater of these two differences? Most people believe that the greater difference is between (1) and (2). I believe that the difference between (2) and (3) is *very much* greater.

My view is the view of two very different groups of people. Both groups would appeal to the same fact. The Earth will remain inhabitable for at least another billion years. Civilization began only a few thousand years ago. If we do not destroy mankind, these few thousand years may be only a tiny fraction of the whole of civilized human history. The difference between (2) and (3) may thus be the difference between this tiny fraction and all of the rest of this history. If we compare this possible history to a day, what has occurred so far is only a fraction of a second.

One of the groups who would accept my view are Classical Utilitarians. They would claim, as Sidgwick did, that the destruction of mankind would be by far the greatest of all conceivable crimes. The badness of this crime would lie in the vast reduction of the possible sum of happiness.

Another group would agree, but for very different reasons. These people believe that there is little value in the mere sum of happiness. For these people, what matters are what Sidgwick called the 'ideal goods'—the Sciences, the Arts, and moral progress, or the continued advance towards a wholly just world-wide community. The destruction of mankind would prevent further achievements of these three kinds. This would be extremely bad because what matters most would be the *highest* achievements of these kinds, and these highest achievements would come in future centuries.

There could clearly be higher achievements in the struggle for a wholly just world-wide community. And there could be higher achievements in all of the Arts and Sciences. But the progress could be greatest in what is now the least advanced of these Arts or Sciences. This, I have claimed, is Non-Religious Ethics. Belief in God, or in many gods, prevented the free development of moral reasoning. Disbelief in God, openly admitted by a majority, is a very recent event, not yet completed. Because this event is so recent, Non-Religious Ethics is at a very early stage. We cannot yet predict whether, as in Mathematics, we will all reach agreement. Since we cannot know how Ethics will develop, it is not irrational to have high hopes.

[*Reasons and Persons* (Oxford University Press: Oxford, 1984), 453–4.]

Select Bibliography

I. GENERAL

BECKER, LAWRENCE and BECKER, CHARLOTTE (eds.), *Encyclopedia of Ethics*, (Garland: New York, 1992).
SINGER, PETER (ed.), *A Companion to Ethics* (Blackwell: Oxford, 1991).

II. THE CLASSIC TEXTS

AQUINAS, THOMAS *Summa Theologica*, ed. T. Gilby *et al.*, (Blackfriars and Eyre and Spottiswoode: London, 1963–75).
ARISTOTLE, *The Nicomachean Ethics*, trans. W. D. Ross (Oxford University Press: London, 1959).
BENTHAM, JEREMY, *Introduction to the Theory of Morals and Legislation*, ed. J. H. Burns and H. L. A. Hart (Athlone Press: London, 1970).
The Bhagavadgita in the Mahabharata, ed. and trans. J. A. B. van Buitenen, (University of Chicago Press: Chicago, 1985).
BUDDHA, THE *Some Sayings of the Buddha*, trans. F. L. Woodward, (Oxford University Press: New York, 1973).
EPICTETUS, *The Discourses*, trans. W. A. Oldfather, (Harvard University Press: Cambridge, Mass, 1925–8).
EPICURUS, *The Extant Remains*, trans. C. Bailey (Clarendon Press: Oxford, 1926).
GODWIN, WILLIAM, *An Enquiry Concerning Political Justice*, 3rd edn., ed. I. Kramnick (Penguin: Harmondsworth, 1976).
HEGEL, G. W. F. *The Philosophy of Right*, trans. T. M. Knox (Clarendon Press: Oxford, 1952).
HOBBES, THOMAS, *Leviathan* (Dent: London, 1914).
HUME, DAVID, *An Enquiry Concerning the Principles of Morals* (Open Court: La Salle, III., 1966).
—— *A Treatise of Human Nature*, ed. L. A. Selby-Bigge (Oxford University Press: Oxford, 1978).
KANT, IMMANUEL, *The Critique of Practical Reason and Other Writings in Moral Philosophy*, trans. L. W. Beck (University of Chicago Press: Chicago, 1949).
—— *Foundations of the Metaphysics of Morals*, trans. L. W. Beck (Bobbs-Merrill: Indianapolis, 1959).
MILL, JOHN STUART, Utilitarianism, ed. H. B. Acton (Dent: London, 1972).
MOORE, G. E., *Principia Ethica* (Cambridge University Press: Cambridge, 1903).
NIETZSCHE FRIEDRICH, *Beyond Good and Evil*, trans. Marianne Cowan (Henry Regnery Company: Chicago, 1955).
PLATO, *The Republic*, trans. Robin Waterfield (Oxford University Press: Oxford, 1993).
ROUSSEAU, JEAN-JACQUES, *A Discourse on the Origins of Inequality*, trans. Franklin Philip (Oxford University Press: Oxford, 1994).

SIDGWICK, HENRY, *The Methods of Ethics*, 7th edn. (Macmillan: London, 1907).

A Source Book in Chinese Philosophy, trans. and comp. Wing-Tsit Chan (Princeton University Press: Princeton, NJ, 1963).

III. MODERN PHILOSOPHICAL ETHICS

The Nature of Ethics

AYER, A. J., *Language, Truth and Logic* (Gollancz: London, 1936).

BRANDT, R. B., *A Theory of the Good and the Right* (Oxford University Press: Oxford, 1979).

HARE, R. M., *The Language of Morals* (Oxford University Press: Oxford, 1952).

—— *Freedom and Reason* (Oxford University Press: Oxford, 1963).

MACINTYRE, ALASDAIR, *After Virtue* (Duckworth: London, 1981).

MACKIE, J. L., *Ethics: Inventing Right and Wrong* (Penguin: Harmondsworth, 1977).

NAGEL, THOMAS, *The Possibility of Altruism* (Oxford University Press: Oxford, 1970).

—— *The View from Nowhere* (Oxford University Press: Oxford, 1986).

OUTKA, G. and REEDER J. P., (eds.), *Religion and Morality* (Anchor/Doubleday: New York, 1973).

PERRY, RALPH BARTON, *General Theory of Value* (Harvard University Press: Cambridge, Mass., 1954).

ROSS, W. D. *The Right and the Good* (Oxford University Press: Oxford, 1930).

SARTRE, JEAN-PAUL, *Existentialism is a Humanism*, trans. P. Mairet (Methuen: London, 1948).

SAYRE-MCCORD G. (ed.), *Essays on Moral Realism* (Cornell University Press: Ithaca, NY, 1988).

STEVENSON, C. L., *Ethics and Language* (Yale University Press: New Haven, Conn., 1944).

WILLIAMS, BERNARD, *Ethics and the Limits of Philosophy* (Harvard University Press: Cambridge, Mass., 1985).

WITTGENSTEIN, LUDWIG, 'A Lecture on Ethics', *The Philosophical Review*, 74/1 (1965).

WONG, D. B., *Moral Relativity* (University of California Press: Berkeley, Calif., 1984).

Normative Ethics

FINNIS, JOHN, *Natural Law and Natural Rights* (Oxford University Press: Oxford, 1980).

FOOT, PHILIPPA, *Virtues and Vices* (University of California Press: Berkeley, Calif., 1978).

FRIED, CHARLES, *Right and Wrong* (Harvard University Press: Cambridge, Mass., 1978).

GAUTHIER, DAVID, *Morals by Agreement* (Oxford University Press: Oxford, 1986).

GIBBARD, ALLAN, *Wise Choices, Apt Feelings: A Theory of Normative Judgment* (Harvard University Press: Cambridge, Mass., 1990).

HARE, R. M., *Moral Thinking: Its Levels, Methods and Point* (Oxford University Press: Oxford, 1981).

KAGAN, SHELLY, *The Limits of Morality* (Oxford University Press: Oxford, 1989).

NOZICK, ROBERT, *Anarchy, State and Utopia* (Basic Books: New York, 1974).

PARFIT, DEREK, *Reasons and Persons* (Clarendon Press: Oxford, 1984).

RAWLS, JOHN, *A Theory of Justice* (Oxford University Press: Oxford, 1972).

SCHEFFLER SAMUEL, (ed.), *Consequentialism and its Critics* (Oxford University Press: Oxford, 1988).

SMART, J. J. C. and WILLIAMS, BERNARD, *Utilitarianism for and against* (Cambridge University Press: Cambridge, 1973).

IV. EXPLAINING AND DESCRIBING ETHICS

Evolutionary Theory

AXELROD, ROBERT, *The Evolution of Cooperation* (Basic Books: New York, 1984).

BARASH, DAVID, *The Whisperings Within* (Harper and Row: New York, 1979).

DARWIN, CHARLES, *The Descent of Man*, 2nd edn. (John Murray: London, 1875).

DAWKINS, RICHARD, *The Selfish Gene* (Oxford University Press: Oxford, 1975).

MIDGLEY, MARY, *Beast and Man* (Harvester Press: Hassocks, 1979).

SINGER, PETER, *The Expanding Circle* (Oxford University Press: Oxford, 1981).

TRIVERS, ROBERT, *Social Evolution* (Benjamin Cummings Publishing Company: Menlo Park, Calif., 1985).

WILSON, E. O., *Sociobiology: The New Synthesis* (Harvard University Press: Cambridge, Mass., 1975).

Ethology and Anthropology

CHAGNON, NAPOLEON A., *The Yanomano: The Fierce People* (Holt, Rinehart and Winston: New York 1968).

GOODALL, JANE, *The Chimpanzees of Gombe* (Belknap Press/Harvard University Press: Cambridge, Mass., 1986).

MALINOWSKI, BRUNO, *Argonauts of the Western Pacific* (Routledge: London, 1922).

MARSHALL, LORNA, *The !Kung of Nyae Nyae* (Harvard University Press: Cambridge, Mass., 1976).

MAUSS, MARCEL, *The Gift: The Form and Reason for Exchange in Archaic Societies*, trans. W. D. Halls, (Routledge: London, 1990).

DE WAAL, FRANS, *Chimpanzee Politics* (Jonathan Cape: London, 1982).

—— *Peacemaking among Primates* (Harvard University Press: Cambridge, Mass., 1989).

History

ASHWORTH, TONY, *Trench Warfare, 1914–1918: The Live and Let Live System* (Macmillan: London, 1980).

LECKY, W. E. H., *History of European Morals*, 2 vols. (Longmans, Green and Co.: London, 1892).

PRITCHARD J. B., (ed.), *Ancient Near Eastern Texts Relating to the Old Testament* (Princeton University Press: Princeton, NJ, 1958).

WESTERMARCK, EDWARD, *The Origin and Development of the Moral Ideas*, 2 vols. (Macmillan: London, 1906).

—— *The History of Human Marriage*, 3 vols. (The Allerton Book Company: New York, 1922).

Psychology

GILLIGAN, CAROL, *In a Different Voice: Psychological Theory and Women's Development* (Harvard University Press: Cambridge, Mass., 1982).

KITTAY, EVA FEDER, and MEYERS, DIANA T. (eds.), *Women and Moral Theory* (Rowman and Littlefield: Savage, MD., 1987).

KOHLBERG, LAWRENCE, *The Philosophy of Moral Development* (Harper and Row: San Francisco, 1981).

LARRABEE, MARY JEANNE, (ed.), *An Ethic of Care: Feminist and Interdisciplinary Perspectives* (Routledge: London, 1993).

PIAGET, JEAN, *The Moral Judgment of the Child*, trans. L. W. Beck (University of Chicago Press: Chicago, 1949).

Biographical Notes

AQUINAS   Thomas Aquinas (c.1224–74) is generally considered to have been the greatest of the medieval Catholic theologians and philosophers. Born in Italy, he studied and taught at the University of Paris, as well as in Naples and near Rome. He produced an enormous volume of work, all in Latin and usually in a set style, in which a question is raised, an answer put forward, and objections dealt with. In all areas of philosophy, including ethics, his approach follows Aristotle, whom he refers to simply as 'the philosopher'. After his death, his philosophy was officially adopted by the Roman Catholic Church, where it remains highly influential.

ARISTOTLE   Aristotle (384–322 BC) was a student of Plato who later founded a separate school, the Lyceum. He wrote widely on philosophy and science, and tutored the boy who was to become Alexander the Great. The rediscovery of his works in medieval Europe exercised a decisive influence on medieval scholastic philosophy which still endures, particularly within Roman Catholic theology.

ASHWORTH, T.   Tony Ashworth is lecturer in sociology at the University of Wales, Cardiff College.

AXELROD, R.   Robert Axelrod is the Arthur W. Bromage Distinguished University Professor of political science and public policy at the University of Michigan. His main research interests are international security affairs and mathematical modelling. He is best known for his work on the conditions that promote co-operation in social and political settings. In 1986 he was elected to membership in the National Academy of Sciences.

AYER, A. J.   Alfred Jules Ayer (1910–89) published *Language, Truth and Logic*, a kind of manifesto for logical positivism, at the age of 26. All true statements, Ayer held, were either tautologies or open to verification; everything else is meaningless. Ayer subsequently held chairs of philosophy at the University of London and at Oxford. His later work qualified, but in essentials did not depart from, the views he had developed in his celebrated first book.

BARASH, D. P.   David P. Barash is professor of psychology at the University of Washington, Seattle, where his career spans work from animal behaviour (sociobiology) to peace studies and the prevention of nuclear war. He has written 165 technical articles and 12 books, and he is currently finishing a volume entitled *Beloved Enemies: Exploring our Need for Opponents*.

BENNETT, J.   Jonathan Bennett teaches philosophy at Syracuse University. He has written books on early modern philosophy, the philosophy of mind and language, and metaphysics. A work on ethics entitled *The Act Itself* appears in 1994.

BENTHAM, J.   Jeremy Bentham (1748–1832) was the founder of the English Utilitarian tradition in ethics, and the leader of a group of philosophical radicals who sought reforms based on Utilitarian principles. He wrote voluminously both on philosophical questions and on proposals for legal and social reform. In accordance with his will, his embalmed body can still be seen in University College, London.

BUDDHA   The Buddha (6th century BC), also known as Siddhartha (his personal name) and Gautama (his family name), grew up in the luxury befitting the son of a North Indian ruler. After becoming aware of the suffering that occurred outside the walls of his father's palace, he became a wandering monk, and for a time was a rigorous ascetic. But he renounced extremes of both luxury and asceticism, and also ceased to believe in gods. He founded a new order of monks, but did not intend it to be a religion. His teachings were maintained by oral tradition for about four hundred years before they were written down for the first time.

CAMUS, A.   Albert Camus (1913–60) wrote novels and essays. Born in what was then the French colony of Algeria, he was active in the French resistance to the Nazi occupation. The essay *The Myth of Sisyphus*, from which a passage is reprinted here, was written during this period, in 1942. After the war, Camus was associated with Jean-Paul Sartre and the existentialist movement. He denied that he was an existentialist, but Sisyphus, as presented in his essay, has often been taken as an existentialist hero, triumphing over the absurdity of a meaningless existence.

CONFUCIUS   Confucius (6th–5th century BC) was the most influential of all Chinese philosophers. Our knowledge of his views comes from the *Analects*, a collection of his sayings and of his conversations with disciples. This material is often brief and fragmentary, and because it was compiled some time after the death of Confucius, it may well represent the views of his later disciples, rather than those of Confucius himself.

DARWIN, C.   Charles Darwin (1809–82) proposed and defended the theory of evolution: in essence, that different species have evolved by the operation of natural selection on random variations in offspring. Hence he dared to suggest that human beings are descended from animals, more specifically, from apes. His two greatest books are *The Origin of Species* and *The Descent of Man*.

DOSTOEVSKY, F. M.   Fyodor Dostoevsky (1821–81), one of the great Russian nineteenth-century novelists, has been seen as a forerunner of modern existentialism because of his insistence on our ability to choose what we are. In his twenties Dostoevsky was arrested for being a member of a utopian socialist organization and spent eight years in Siberia; he returned a conservative in his political beliefs and a defender of the Russian Orthodox faith. He travelled to Western Europe, but detested the scientific and humanist outlook that he found there. In this brief but oft-cited passage from *The Karamazov Brothers*, Dostoevsky captures the essence of why many people find Utilitarianism—or, indeed, any form of consequentialism—unacceptable.

EPICTETUS   Epictetus (*c*.55–*c*.135 AD) grew up as a slave in Rome, but was given his freedom and became one of the ablest expounders of the Stoic school of philosophy. Some volumes of his *Discourses*, or conversations with pupils, have been preserved, as has his *Encheiridion*, a kind of manual or set of instructions on how to make moral progress. The Stoic philosophy emphasized the extent to which we can maintain our own dignity, equilibrium, and inner tranquillity in the face of any adverse circumstances—a doctrine that was suited to both slave and emperor in ancient Rome.

EPICURUS   Epicurus (341–270 BC) was a Greek philosopher who spent most of his mature years living in a community that he established just outside Athens. He appears to have been a prolific writer, but relatively few of his works have survived. The 'Letter to Menoeceus' is one of these. It contains a concise outline of his ideas on how we can find happiness. The Epicurean school, which taught that happiness and contentment is within the reach of everyone, survived for five hundred years after the death of its founder.

FINNIS, J.   John Finnis is an Australian and is professor of law and legal philosophy at the University of Oxford. He is also Fellow of University College, Oxford and a Fellow of the British Academy. His account of ethics is developed, refined, and applied in his *Fundamentals of Ethics* (1983), *Nuclear Deterrence, Morality, and Realism* (with Joseph Boyle and Germain Grisez, 1987), and *Moral Absolutes* (1991).

FREUD, S.   Sigmund Freud (1856–1939) was the founder of psychoanalysis. Most of his writings are an investigation of the subconsciousness of individual minds; in *Civilization and its Discontents*, however, he saw psychoanalytical problems writ large on the fabric of human civilization as a whole.

GANDHI   Mohandas Karamchand Gandhi (1869–1948) led the Indian opposition to British rule, and is considered the father of his country. He was brought up to believe in *ahimsa*, or harmlessness towards all living things. Before World War I, he worked in South Africa and challenged government policies of racial discrimination. He waged his struggle for change on strictly ethical grounds, and advocated non-violent resistance as the only ethical weapon in the struggle for reform. The passage included here is taken from the concluding pages of his autobiography, in which he reflects on the values that have governed his life.

GAUTHIER, D.   David Gauthier is distinguished service professor of philosophy at the University of Pittsburgh. His writings include *The Logic of Leviathan, Morals by Agreement*, and *Moral Dealing: Contract, Ethics, and Reason*. His primary current research interests are the place of intention in rational deliberation and the thought of Jean-Jacques Rousseau.

GILLIGAN, C.   Carol Gilligan is professor of education at Harvard University, where she works on psychology and women's development. Her *In a Different Voice*, stimulated many other explorations of possible differences in the way in which men and women think about ethical questions.

GODWIN, W.   William Godwin (1756–1836) became famous with the publication of his *An Enquiry concerning Political Justice*. Appearing at the height of the French Revolution, the book argues so strongly against political authority that its conclusion is a form of anarchism, defended on the basis of impartial reason. The book would probably have been suppressed, had not the British government reasoned that it was too dense and expensive to be accessible to the working class. Godwin was married to the pioneering feminist writer Mary Wollstonecraft, and was the father of Mary Wollstonecraft Shelley, author of *Frankenstein*.

GOODALL, J.   Jane Goodall has probably done more than anyone else to help us understand the individuality of free-living chimpanzees. When everyone else thought it impossible to observe chimpanzees in their own habitat for long periods, she persisted until they became used to her. Her book *In the Shadow of Man*, based on her long observation of chimpanzees in the Gombe region of Tanzania, was an international best seller. *The Chimpanzees of Gombe* is a more detailed academic study. The Jane Goodall Institute is based at Lymington, Hampshire.

HAMMURABI   The Law of Hammurabi is the most complete surviving summary of the laws of ancient Babylon. Compiled during the reign of Hammurabi (1792–1750 BC) it probably included laws from both the Semitic and the Sumerian peoples. The Law was inscribed on a stone which is now preserved in the Louvre, in Paris.

HARE, R. M.   R. M. Hare has been fellow of Balliol College and White's Professor of moral philosophy at Corpus Christi College, Oxford, and then research professor at the University of Florida. His main theoretical works are *The Language of Morals* (1952), *Freedom and Reason* (1963), and *Moral Thinking* (1981); he has also written extensively on applied ethics.

HEGEL, G. W. F.   Georg Wilhelm Friedrich Hegel (1770–1831) spent his entire adult life as a teacher, in a high school and then later as professor of philosophy at Heidelberg and Berlin. He regarded his predecessors, including Kant, as having made progress towards greater philosophical understanding, but in one-sided ways. He thought that Kant's rationalism was too abstract, and needed to be supplemented by the more concrete ethical traditions that exist in any real community. His major work on ethics is the *Philosophy of Right*.

HELD, V.   Virginia Held is professor of philosophy at the City University of New York (Graduate School and Hunter College). She has been Visiting Professor at UCLA and Dartmouth, has also taught at Yale and Barnard, and was recently Truax Visiting Professor at Hamilton College. Her most recent books are *Rights and Goods: Justifying Social Action* (1989) and *Feminist Morality: Transforming Culture, Society, and Politics* (1993).

HILLEL   Hillel (1st century BC–1st century AD) was a Jewish sage, a master of biblical commentary and the leading interpreter of Jewish tradition in his time. He was born in Babylon, but lived mostly in Palestine. Many legends and popular tales describe his devotion to learning, his personal virtues, and his skill at teaching.

HOBBES, T.   Thomas Hobbes (1588–1679) wrote his greatest work, *Leviathan*, in the shadow of the English Civil War. His argument for the obligation to obey a sovereign did not make him popular with the currently successful revolutionaries, and he lived for some time in exile in France. After the Restoration, he was briefly in favour at Court, but his naturalistic approach to philosophy led to accusations of atheism, which soon made him unpopular there, too.

HUME, D.   David Hume (1711–76) is widely regarded as the greatest of all British philosophers. His major work, *A Treatise of Human Nature*, was finished before he was 25, but neglected when published. He later published *An Enquiry concerning the*

Human Understanding and *An Enquiry concerning the Principles of Morals*, and asked that these two works should be regarded as containing 'his philosophical senti-ments and principles'. A friend of Adam Smith, Hume also wrote an acclaimed *History of Great Britain*, and many essays on economics and politics. He never held an academic post, although he applied unsuccessfully for chairs of philosophy at Edinburgh and Glasgow.

HUXLEY, A.   Aldous Huxley (1894–1963) was an English novelist, best known for writing *Brave New World*. In this futuristic novel the population is programmed to be happy; but there is at least one person who rejects the principle on which this utopia is designed.

JAMES, W.   William James (1842–1910) was one of the most important nine-teenth-century American philosophers. Together with Charles Peirce, he was a founder of pragmatism, the view that the truth of a belief depends on its usefulness. James spent most of his adult life at Harvard, where he taught not only philosophy, but also psychology and physiology.

JESUS   Jesus of Nazareth (*c.*4 BC–27 AD) was a Jewish teacher and prophet, now revered by Christians as the son of God. Like Confucius, he left no written works, and what we know about him comes from accounts written at least a generation after his death.

KANT, I.   Immanuel Kant (1724–1804) acknowledged that reading David Hume had awoken him from his 'dogmatic slumber'. It was quite an awakening. Since the publication of his *Critique of Pure Reason*, Kant's work has been the pivot around which German—and, indeed, European—philosophy has turned. His chief philos-ophical aim is to show how it is possible for us to understand the world. In ethics he tried to show how it was possible for human beings to be subject to a morality that is based on reason alone.

KELLY, G.   Gerald Kelly (1901–64) was professor of theology at St Mary's Col-lege, Kansas. He wrote numerous books and articles, all published by the Catholic Health Association of the United States.

LANGTON, R.   Rae Langton is lecturer in philosophy at Monash University. She is writing her doctoral thesis on Kant for Princeton University, and works in the fields of political philosophy, epistemology, and the history of philosophy.

LECKY, W. E. H.   William Edward Hartpole Lecky (1838–1903) was a historian and essayist. Of Scottish descent, he was born near Dublin, in Ireland. Liberal in politics and free-thinking in religion, he served as Member of Parliament for Dublin University. He declined an offer of the regius professorship of modern history at Oxford. Today he is best known for his *History of European Morals from Augustus to Charlemagne*, and his *History of the Rise and Influence of the Spirit of Rationalism in Europe*, each displaying a remarkably wide knowledge of historical sources. He also wrote a *History of England in the Eighteenth Century*, in twelve volumes.

LEVITICUS   Leviticus is a book of Hebrew scripture, largely concerned with the duties of the priestly caste. Essentially a book of laws, scholars believe that much of it was written during the period after 586 BC when the Hebrews returned from exile in Babylon, but that chapters 17–26—including the passage quoted here—are much more ancient.

LOCKE, J.   John Locke (1632–1704) is a major figure in the history of British philosophy. His *Essay concerning Human Understanding* is an attempt to show what we can know and how; according to Locke, we learn from experience; rather than by the exercise of reason alone. It is through his political philosophy, however, that Locke influenced the constitutional development of Britain after the Glorious Revolution of 1688 and, long after his death, the form taken by the constitution of the United States of America.

LUTHER, M.   Martin Luther (1483–1546) began the Protestant Reformation by pinning his famous ninety-six theses to the door of the church in Wittenberg. He wrote widely on ethical matters.

McGINN, C.   Colin McGinn has taught philosophy at University College, London, and the University of Oxford, as well as at Rutgers University in New Jersey, where he now holds the distinguished chair of philosophy. His books include *The Subjective View* and *The Problem of Consciousness*.

MACKIE, J.   John Mackie (1917–82) was born in Sydney and held chairs of philosophy in New Zealand, Australia, and England, before becoming a fellow of University College, Oxford. In ethics he described himself as a 'moral sceptic', holding that although our ethical judgements seem to make claims to truth or falsehood, there is nothing about which they could be true or false.

MALINOWSKI, B.   Bruno Malinowski (1884–1942), a pioneer of modern anthropology, was born and educated in Poland. In 1910 he went to London to study in what was then a newly established discipline. He lived for two years in the Trobriand Islands, near New Guinea, where he observed the remarkable 'Kula ring' of exchange between men of different island communities.

MARSHALL, L.   Lorna Marshall worked with the !Kung speaking Bushmen in the Nyae Nyae Area of Namibia in the 1950s, making an ethnographic study of their culture when they were living in complete independence, wholly by hunting and gathering.

MARX, K.   Karl Marx (1818–83) developed an interest in politics and philosophy under the influence of the Young Hegelians, a group of German thinkers who believed that Hegel had not been true to the radical vision of his own philosophy. Together with his lifelong friend, Friedrich Engels (1820–95), Marx 'stood Hegel on his head', and developed an approach to understanding human history in which our economic circumstances—basically, the way we meet our needs—determine our consciousness, rather than the other way around. *The German Ideology* is a lengthy and often tedious 'settling of accounts' with some other Young Hegelians with whom Marx and Engels came to disagree; on the other hand, the fervent *Communist Manifesto* was dashed off at the request of a German workers' club.

MIDGLEY, M.   Mary Midgley, formerly senior lecturer in philosophy at the University of Newcastle on Tyne, is a moral philosopher with a particular interest in the relations between humans and other species. Among her books are *Beast and Man, Heart and Mind, Wickedness,* and *Can't We Make Moral Judgments?*

MILL, J. S.   John Stuart Mill (1806–73) was educated by his father, James Mill, a friend and admirer of Jeremy Bentham. As a boy, he accepted the mission of promoting social reform along Utilitarian lines. When he was 20, however, he went through a mental crisis, as a result of which he came to believe that Bentham's version of Utilitarianism was narrow and crude. Hence, as illustrated in the extract included here, he sought ways of including a wider range of goods within the hedonistic framework.

MENCIUS   Mencius (4th century BC) was a defender of the philosophy of Confucius. The *Book of Mencius,* one of the classics of Chinese philosophy, is a book of his teachings and conversations, probably compiled by his pupils after his death.

MOORE, G. E.   G. E. Moore (1873–1958) was an English philosopher who became professor of philosophy at Cambridge University. A member of the Bloomsbury Group, he was revered by friends and acquaintances for the purity of his commitment to philosophy, coupled with an almost childlike simplicity about all other matters. In ethics he is best known for his attack on the 'naturalistic fallacy', in his book *Principia Ethica.*

NAGEL, T.   Thomas Nagel is professor of philosophy and law at New York University, and author of *The Possibility of Altruism, Mortal Questions, The View from Nowhere, What Does It All Mean?,* and *Equality and Partiality.*

NIETZSCHE, F.   Friedrich Nietzsche (1844–1900) was a brilliant student who became a professor in Basle when only 25. Many of his works, including *Beyond Good and Evil,* from which this extract is taken, are collections of aphorisms, only a few lines or a page or two long.

NOZICK, R.   Robert Nozick is professor of philosophy at Harvard University. His major works are *Anarchy, State, and Utopia* (1974), *Philosophical Explanations* (1981), and *The Examined Life* (1989).

PARFIT, D.   Derek Parfit is Senior Research Fellow at All Souls College, Oxford, and author of *Reasons and Persons* (1984).

PASCAL, B.   Blaise Pascal (1623–62) possessed a remarkable array of talents. As both mathematician and physicist, he made significant discoveries; and at the age of 18 he invented the calculating machine in order to help his father, a commissioner of taxes in Rouen. In 1654 Pascal had a religious experience that changed the direction of his life and led him towards theology. The *Provincial Letters,* written two years after this experience, ridicule the prevailing Jesuit mode of thinking about ethical questions. For this, the Catholic Church forbade its members to read them.

PLATO   Plato (*c.*430–347 BC) was the Greek philosopher who, more than anyone else, set the main lines of Western philosophical debate. So firmly did he do this, that the history of Western philosophy has been described as a series of footnotes to his work. He founded the philosophical school known as the Academy, in

Athens. His writings are in the form of dialogues, in which Socrates (who was condemned to death when Plato was about 30) plays a leading role. Scholars believe that in the dialogues from Plato's middle and later periods (like the *Republic*, from which the extract included is taken) the character 'Socrates' puts forward Plato's own views, rather than those of the historical Socrates.

RAWLS, J.   John Rawls, whose studies have centred on the problems of justice and moral philosophy, was the first John Cowles Professor of philosophy at Harvard University. He is now emeritus professor at Harvard, and his publications include *A Theory of Justice* (1971) and *Political Liberalism* (1993).

ROSS, W. D.   W. D. Ross (1877–1971), provost of Oriel College, was the foremost twentieth-century advocate of an intuitionist approach to ethics, and also a strong critic of Utilitarianism. In *The Right and the Good*, from which this extract is taken, he sets out to show the inadequacies of Utilitarianism, as a preliminary to proposing his own ethic, based on prima facie duties.

ROUSSEAU, J.-J.   Jean-Jacques Rousseau (1712–78) was born in Geneva and lived in various places in France, Switzerland, and Italy. His *Discourse on the Science and the Arts* and his *Discourse on the Origin of Inequality* brought him notoriety, challenged eighteenth-century classical rationalism, and signalled the birth of the Romantic movement. His vision of the 'noble savage' has had an influence on all subsequent thinking about human nature. His greatest philosophical work, *Social Contract*, was used, or misused, by French revolutionaries like Robespierre to justify their claim to represent the 'general will' of the people.

SARTRE, J.-P.   Jean-Paul Sartre (1905–80) was a French philosopher and writer, best known as an existentialist, although in later periods of his life he held other philosophical views. His major work of existentialist philosophy is *Being and Nothingness*, first published in 1943. The extract included here is taken from his most popular essay, 'Existentialism is a Humanism'.

SIDGWICK, H.   Henry Sidgwick (1828–1900) lived his entire life in Cambridge, where he was professor of moral philosophy for seventeen years. The last of the great nineteenth-century English Utilitarians, his masterpiece, *The Methods of Ethics*, is regarded by some as the finest book on ethics ever written.

SMART, J. J. C.   J. J. C. Smart is emeritus professor at the Australian National University, where he was professor of philosophy in the Research School of Social Sciences from 1976 to 1985. He is an honorary fellow of Corpus Christi College, Oxford, and was also professor of philosophy at the University of Adelaide and reader in philosophy at La Trobe University.

SMITH, M.   Michael Smith is reader in philosophy at Monash University. He is the author of *The Moral Problem* as well as several articles on moral philosophy and philosophy of mind.

SYMONS, D.   Donald Symons is professor in the anthropology department at the University of California, Santa Barbara, and author of *Play and Aggression: A Study of*

Rhesus Monkeys (1978) and *The Evolution of Human Sexuality* (1979). His primary research area is 'evolutionary psychology', which entails the use of evolutionary fact and theory to inspire and guide investigations of the human mind.

TRIVERS, R.   Robert Trivers is professor of anthropology and biology at Rutgers University and the author of *Social Evolution* (1985).

VOLTAIRE   pseudonym of François-Marie Arouet (1694–1778), the foremost literary genius of his age, was also a champion of liberty, tolerance, and humanitarianism. Born in Paris, he was frequently in trouble with the French authorities, spent several months in the Bastille, and lived for a time in exile in Holland and England. His masterpiece, *Candide*, is a satire on attempts to reconcile the existence of evil with the standard Christian belief in a god who is both good and omnipotent.

de WAAL, F. B. M.   Frans B. M. de Waal is professor of psychology at Emory University and research professor at the Yerkes Regional Primate Research Centre, both in Atlanta. He conducted a six-year project on the unique chimpanzee colony of Arnhem Zoo, which led to the writing of *Chimpanzee Politics* (1982). In 1989 he received the Los Angeles Times Book Award for *Peacemaking among Primates*. His current interests include food-sharing and social reciprocity in primates.

WESTERMARCK, E.   Edward Westermarck (1862–1939) was born and educated in Finland, but became a professor of sociology at the University of London. He travelled to North Africa, intending to move gradually eastward, studying the diverse customs and ideas of various peoples as he went. He soon realized, however, that it was not so easy to grasp a culture quickly, and he got no further than Morocco, where he spent a total of nine years. His encyclopaedic work, *The Origin and Development of the Moral Ideas*, is still unrivalled in the breadth of information that it contains on the moral views of different cultures.

WILLIAMS, B.   Bernard Williams is White's Professor of moral philosophy and Fellow of Corpus Christi College, Oxford, and Monroe Deutsch Professor of philosophy at the University of California, Berkeley. His most recent publications include *Moral Luck* (1981), *Ethics and the Limits of Philosophy* (1985), and *Shame and Necessity* (1993).

WITTGENSTEIN, L.   Ludwig Wittgenstein (1889–1951) was born in Austria, studied engineering in Berlin and Manchester, and then became interested in philosophy. During World War I, while serving in the Austrian army, he wrote his highly original *Tractatus Logico-Philosophicus*, which he believed had solved all the problems of philosophy. After the war, he worked for a time as an elementary schoolteacher in an Austrian village, but then he changed his mind about the success of the *Tractatus* and went to Cambridge, where he eventually became professor of philosophy. Wittgenstein wrote very little about ethics, for reasons which are apparent from this 'Lecture on Ethics', delivered in Cambridge in 1929.

WOLF, S.   Susan Wolf is a professor of philosophy at the Johns Hopkins University, Baltimore. She is author of *Freedom Within Reason* (1990) and numerous articles on ethics and the philosophy of mind.

Acknowledgements

ASHWORTH, TONY, 'Live and Let Live', from *Trench Warfare 1914–1918: The Live and Let Live System*, © Tony Ashworth 1980. Reprinted by permission of Macmillan Ltd., and Holmes and Meier, New York.

AXELROD, ROBERT, 'Tit for Tat', from *The Evolution of Cooperation* (Basic Books, 1984). © Robert Axelrod 1984. Reprinted by permission of Harper Collins Publishers, Inc.

AYER, A. J., 'Ethics for Logical Positivists', from *Language, Truth and Logic*, in *Philosophical Studies* (Routledge, 1951), 310–39. © The Estate of A. J. Ayer.

BARASH, DAVID, 'The Genetic Basis of Kinship', from *The Whisperings Within* (Harper & Row, 1979). © David Barash 1979. Reprinted by permission of Harper Collins Publishers Inc., and Souvenir Press, Ltd.

BENNETT, JONATHAN, 'The Conscience of Huck Finn', from *Philosophy*, 49 (1974). Reprinted by permission of Cambridge University Press.

BUDDHA THE, 'The Ceasing of Woe', from *Some Sayings of the Buddha*, trans. F. L. Woodward (Oxford University Press, New York, 1973).

CAMUS, ALBERT, 'The Myth of Sisyphus', from *The Myth of Sisyphus and Other Essays*, trans. Justin O'Brien. Copyright © 1955 by Alfred A. Knopf, Inc. Reprinted by permission of Alfred A. Knopf and Hamish Hamilton Ltd.

EPICTETUS, 'A Stoic View of Life', from *The Encheiridion*, from *The Discourses*, Vol. II, trans. W. A. Oldfather. Reprinted by permission of the publishers and the Loeb Classical Library, Cambridge, Mass.: Harvard University Press.

FREUD, SIGMUND, 'The Cultural Super-Ego', from *Civilization and its Discontents*, trans. James Strachey (1962).

GANDHI, M. K., from *The Story of My Experiments with Truth*, trans. M. Desai, first published 1927. Translation copyright M. Desai.

GAUTHIER, DAVID, 'Why Contractarianism', from Peter Ballantyne (ed.), *Contractarianism and Rational Choice* (1991). Reprinted by permission of Cambridge University Press.

GILLIGAN, CAROL, 'In a Different Voice'. Reprinted by permission of the publishers from *In a Different Voice: Psychological Theory and Women's Development*, by Carol Gilligan, Cambridge, Mass.: Harvard University Press, © 1982 by Carol Gilligan.

GOODALL, JANE, 'Helping Kin in Chimpanzees' and 'Incest Avoidance among Chimpanzees'. Reprinted by permission of the publishers from *The Chimpanzees of Gombe*, by Jane Goodall, Cambridge, Mass.: Harvard University Press, © 1986 by The President and Fellows of Harvard College.

HELD, VIRGINIA, 'Reason, Gender and Moral Theory', from *Feminist Transformations of Moral Theory, Philosophy and Phenomenological Research*, 50 (1990), 321–44. Used by permission.

HUXLEY, ALDOUS, 'The Right to be Unhappy', from *Brave New World*. Reprinted by permission of Mrs Laura Huxley and the publishers Chatto & Windus, and Harper Collins, New York.

ACKNOWLEDGEMENTS   407

KANT, IMMANUEL, 'The Noble Descent of Duty', from I. Kant, *The Critique of Practical Reason and Other Writings in Moral Philosophy*; and 'Pure Practical Reason and the Moral Law', from *The Foundations of the Metaphysics of Morals*, both trans. L. W. Beck (University of Chicago Press, 1949). Translation copyright L. W. Beck 1949.

KELLY, GERALD, SJ, 'Moral Aspects of Sterility Tests', from *Medico-Moral Problems* (1985). Reprinted by permission of The Catholic Health Association of the United States.

LANGTON, RAE, 'Maria von Herbert's Challenge to Kant', adapted from 'Duty and Desolation', *Philosophy*, 67 (1992), 481–505. Reprinted by permission of Cambridge University Press.

MCGINN, COLIN, from 'Evolution, Animals and the Basis of Morality', *Inquiry*, 22/1 (1979), 92–3, 98, by permission of Scandinavian University Press, Oslo, Norway.

MACKIE, J. L., 'The Arguments for Queerness', from *Ethics: Inventing Right and Wrong* (Penguin Books, 1977), © J. L. Mackie, 1977. Reprinted by permission of the publisher.

MARSHALL, LORNA, 'Reciprocal Gift-Giving among the !Kung' and 'Adultery among the !Kung', from *The !Kung of Nyae Nyae* (1976). Reprinted by permission of Harvard University Press.

MARX, KARL and ENGELS, FRIEDRICH, 'The Material Basis of Morality', from *The German Ideology*, in *Karl Marx: Selected Writings*, ed. D. McLellan. Reprinted by permission of Lawrence & Wishart Ltd.

MENCIUS, 'Are Humans Good by Nature? A Debate between Chinese Sages', from *The Book of Mencius*, in *A Source Book in Chinese Philosophy*, trans. and compiled by Wing-Tsit Chan (Princeton University Press).

MIDGLEY, MARY, 'Duties Concerning Islands', from Robert Elliot and Arran Gare (eds.), *Environmental Philosophy* (1983). Reprinted by permission of the University of Queensland Press.

MOORE, G. E., 'Beauty and Friendship', from *Principia Ethica* (1903). Reprinted by permission of Cambridge University Press.

NAGEL, THOMAS, 'The Objective Basis of Morality', from *What Does It All Mean?* (Oxford University Press, New York, 1987).

NIETZSCHE, FRIEDRICH, 'The Origins of Herd-Morality', from *Beyond Good and Evil*, trans. Marianne Cowan (Regnery Gateway Inc., 1955). Translation © Marianne Cowan 1955.

NOZICK, ROBERT, 'The Experience Machine' and 'The Rationality of Side-Constraints', from *Anarchy, State & Utopia* (Basic Books, 1974). Reprinted by permission of Basic Books, a division of Harper Collins Publishers Inc.

RAWLS, JOHN, 'The Separateness of Persons' and 'The Main Idea of the Theory of Justice'. Reprinted by permission of the publishers from *A Theory of Justice* by John Rawls, Cambridge, Mass.: The Belknap Press of Harvard University Press, © 1971 by The President and Fellows of Harvard College.

SMART, J. J. C., 'Desert Island Promises', from J. J. C. Smart and Bernard Williams, *Utilitarianism For and Against* (1973). Reprinted by permission of Cambridge University Press.

SMITH, MICHAEL, 'Realism', adapted from P. Singer (ed.), *A Companion to Ethics* (1991). Reprinted by permission of Blackwell Publishers.

SYMONS, DONALD, 'The Double Standard', from *The Evolution of Human Sexuality* (Oxford University Press, New York, 1979).

TRIVERS, ROBERT, 'The Evolution of Reciprocal Altruism', from *Quarterly Review of Biology*, 46 (1971), 33–57. Reprinted by permission of The University of Chicago Press.

VOLTAIRE, 'Story of a Good Brahmin', from *The Portable Voltaire*, ed. Ben Ray Redman, trans. H. I. Woolf (Viking Press, 1963). Translation copyright © 1963.

DE WAAL, FRANS B. M., 'Chimpanzee Justice' and 'The Social Rules of Chimpanzee Sex', from *Chimpanzee Politics*. Copyright © 1982 Frans de Waal. Reprinted by permission.

WILLIAMS, BERNARD, 'Jim and the Indians', from J. J. C. Smart and Bernard Williams, *Utilitarianism For and Against*. Reprinted by permission of Cambridge University Press.

WOLF, SUSAN, 'Moral Saints', from *Journal of Philosophy*, LXXIX/8 (August 1982), 419–39. Used with permission.

The publisher and editor apologize for any errors or omissions in the above list. If contacted they will be pleased to rectify these at the earliest opportunity.

Index